Infectious Diseases of Livestock

Infectious Diseases of Livestock

Dr. S.V. Pandit
B.V.Sc. (Hons.) M.V.Sc. (Bacteriology)
(Bombay University)
P.G. (Denmark)

Dr. V.V. Deshmukh
B.V.Sc.& A.H.,. M.V.Sc.,Ph.D.
Prof. of Veterinary Public Health & Epidemiology,
College of Veterinary & Animal Sciences,
MAFSU, Parbhani- 431402

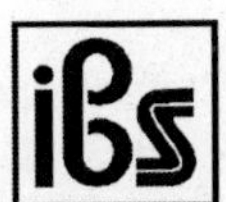

International Books & Periodical Supply Service
(Publisher of Scientific Books)
38, NISHANT KUNJ, PITAM PURA MAIN ROAD
DELHI-110034 (India)
Phone : 011-27352078, Mobile : 09810146811, E-mail : hkjain1975@yahoo.com

Published by :

International Books & Periodical Supply Service

(Publisher of Scientific Books)
38, NISHANT KUNJ, PITAM PURA MAIN ROAD
DELHI-110034 (India)
Phone : 011-27352078, Mobile : 09810146811, E-mail : hkjain1975@yahoo.com

ISBN 978-81-93906-53-8

Composed, Designed & Printed in India

About the Authors

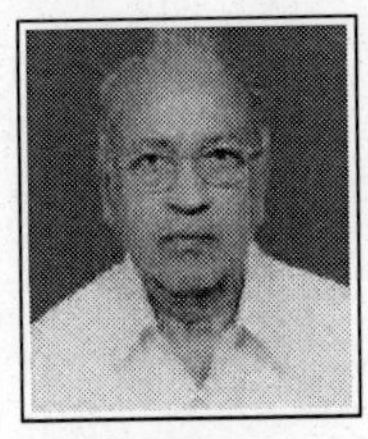

Dr. Sharadkumar Vishnu Pandit was born on 6th October, 1936. He obtained B.V.Sc. (Hons.) Degree from Bombay University and M.V.Sc. (Bacteriology, Pathology and Parasitology of Bombay University of 1st Batch in the year 1962. He received 2 years Training in Virology, Serology & Tissue Culture Techniques at various research centre, Pune (ICMR-Rockfellor Foundation's joint collaboration) between 1964-1966. He also participated in a Summer Institute in Immunology at I.V.R.I., Mukteshwar (UP) during 1971.

He had visited Denmark, Germany, U.K. Italy, France and Iran as DANIA Fellow for Advanced Post Graduate Training Programme in Foot & Mouth Disease Vaccine Production. He was also trained in Advanced Technology related to production and testing of Poultry Vaccines including Marek's Disease Vaccines during 1990 at Tri Bio Laboratories & Main Biologicals in U.S.A.

He worked in various capacities at Disease Investigation Section, Maharashtra State, Pune for a period of 14 years (1960-1974), which also includes his technical services as Assistant Professor at Agriculture University of Kolhapur & at Poultry Training Centre, Kolhapur, ICAR's Mucosal Disease and Blue Tongue Disease Research Schemes, Mastitis Research Schemes and All India co-ordinated project on F.M.D. typing (ICAR).

He has a deep insight in production, testing and development of various viral and bacterial vaccines against important disease of Cattle, Sheep and Goats like H.S., B.Q. Foot and Mouth Disease, Rinderpest, Brucellosis, Multi-factorial clostridial infections, etc., while working as Manager, Research & Development at Bheratiya Agro Industries) Foundation's Vaccines Production Centre at Wagholi, Pune for a long period of 14 years (1974-1988).

He worked extensively for a very long period of 18 years (1988-2006) in Development, Production, Testing and field application of poultry vaccines including those against ND, IB, IBD, Marek's Disease (Freeze Dried & Cell Associated Vaccines), Fowl Cholera, Fowl Spirochetosis, Fowl Coryza, Salmonellosis and lastly most important newly emerged Inclusion Body Hepatitis/Hydropericardium Syndrome (IBH/HPS) at Ventri Biologicals Division of Venkateshwara Hatcheries Group, Pune.

He was nominated as a member of committee for suggesting measures for control of emerging diseases of poultry under the Taks force established by Govt. of India (ICAR, New Delhi) during 1998. They suggested (recommended) various measurs for controlling newly emerging diseases like Avian Influenza, Gumboro disease CAA and Reo virus infections of poultry in India. Establishment of projects of reference laboratories for Surveillence of these Disease Agents at some Regional places was the outcome of this committee recommendations for strengthening HSDL, Bhopal (1998).

He worked as a member of scientific programme committee for 20th World Poultry Congress held at New Delhi, India during 2nd-5th September, 1996 He also acted as Chief Organiser of the technical sessions of this Poultry congress on the subject "Poultry health - Epidemidoge, Immunisation and control measures "at" Shahjahan Hall at Hotel Taj Palace.

He was a Technical Director of 2 Science films produced by Ventri Biological Division of Venkateshwara Hatchery, Pune namely by i) Bio security programme for control of poultry diseases and ii) Production of poulry vaccines and their diluents, their reconstitution and vaccination techniques used in the field and vaccination schedules for Control of Poultry Diseases (1996). Similar film on production of live-stock diseases and their field use for control of livestock diseases was produced (Technical Direction) by the author (Dr. S.V. Pandit) and Dr. Devare when both of them were working at BAIF, Wagholi (1982).

He established fairly well-equipped laboratory facility at "Biospace" laboratories at Devachi Uruli, Pune with young enthusiastic Veterinarian Entrepreneur Dr. S.B. Salutgi (M.V.Sc.in Medicine) of Avians Trades, Pvt. Ltd. By 2012 for research work isolation and production of Bacteriophages for therapeutic use in control treatment of bacterial diseases of poultry and livestock like Salmonelosis and E. Coli infections as well as strepto/staphylococcal infections of poultry and livestock. He also worked on use of B/Thuringensis for control of domestic fly problem in poultry houses. He and S.B. Salutgi also developed technology for production of Silver Nano particles for control of Bacteriological problems in poultry (Salmonall/*E. coli*/Pasturella).The said work was done from November, 2009 to March, 2017.

He published few papers in technical journals including paper on 'Development of Brucellalysate for allergic test in Pigs (Dr. G.P. Sen of IVRI, Mukteshwar as Co-author). He participated in very large number of technical seminars of National / International importance and presented papers on subjects like Foot & Mouth Disease Virus typing, IBH/HPS Vaccine Development, Diagnostic Tests for Rinderpest and Mucosal Disease, Nephrotropic IB Vaccine, Diagnosis of Infections

Laryngio-trachaeitis. Author presented valuable papers on IBD Vaccine Development, IBH/HPS Vaccine Development in Symposia at IVRI as well as at World Poultry Science Congress held at New Delhi in 1988. He also worked on newly emerging diseases like IBD, Chicken Anaemia Agent (CAA) & Reo virus infections in Poultry.

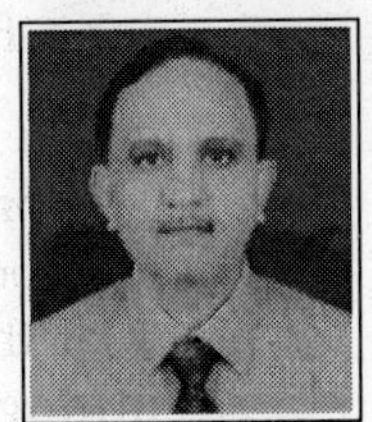

Dr. V.V. Deshmukh is working as Professor of Veterinary Public Health & Epidemiology in Maharashtra Animal & Fishery Sciences University at College of Veterinary & Animal Sciences, Parbhani. He started his career as Assistant Professor of Veterinary Microbiology at College of Veterinary & Animal Sciences, Udgir in the year 1987. He then worked as Junior Scientist at Animal Disease Research Centre, Parbhani from 1994 to 2000. He was Associate Professor of Veterinary Microbiology from 2000 to 2008. He became Professor of Veterinary Public Health & Epidemiology in the year 2008.

He is having vast experience in disease diagnosis, surveillance, epidemiology, vaccinology of livestock and poultry diseases. He worked on FMD virus at ICAR, AICRP on FMD at DIS, Pune. Then worked as Co-PI of ICAR Ad-hoc research project on 'Bluetongue in Ruminants' during 1994-1997. He was a PI of Parbhani Centre of ICAR, All India Network Programme on 'Bluetongue Disease' from 2001 to 2015. His major contribution was isolation of BTV-1, BTV-4 and BTV-18 from field outbreaks and a stakeholder in BT vaccine development under the programme.

He established Department of Veterinary Public health & Epidemiology at COVAS, Parbhani in the year 2008. A well-equiped Public Health Lab wa started with start of post graduate programme at the institute.

He has guided around 28 M.V.Sc students, published large number of research articles in national & international journals. He is a Ph.D. and M.V.Sc. paper setter, Thesis evaluator of number of State universities and IVRI. He travelled to U.S.A., U.K. and Malaysia for professional assignments.His work has been recognized by Dr. D. S. Gorhe State Level Best Veterinary Teacher and Researcher Award of Senior Veterinarian Foundation, Pune (2014). Shyama Singh and Balamati Devi Memorial Award for Excellence in Animal Health Care and Cover by Indian Association for the Advancement of Veterinary Research (2016).

Preface

Emerging and re-emerging viral diseases of livestock and human beings are in sharp rise in recent years. Importantly, many of these viruses are of zoonotic importance. Several viral diseases of livestock, such as bluetongue, peste des petits ruminants, camel pox, equine infectious anaemia and sheep-associated malignant catarrhal fever are crossing their traditional boundaries. Emergence of new serotypes and variant forms of viruses as in the case of bluetongue virus adds additional level of complexity. The increased incidence of emerging and re-emerging viral diseases could be attributed to several factors including deforestation and surge in direct contact of livestock and humans with wild animals and birds.

In recent times, Govt. of India has launched a massive Action Plan for Doubling Farmers Income by the year 2022. The Plan requires major emphasis on Health Sector. Infectious diseases of livestock play an important role in production. Prevention and control of infectious diseases require knowledge about various aspects of infectious diseases like aetiology, symptoms, postmortem signs, disease diagnosis, vaccination, etc. A lot of information about various infectious diseases of livestock is available now-a-days. However, information from experienced, senior professionals with their experiences may help in understanding poultry infectious diseases.

This book contains chapters on all major livestock diseases of viral, bacterial, parasitic and fungal origin which are prevalent in India. The uniqueness of this book is that in addition to the description, valuable practical tips evolved out of experience of authors have been given. This makes the book valuable from field point of view. This book is meant for field veterinarians, students and professionals for reference. An attempt has been made to keep reader updated on historical facts, recent advances and practical hints on various infectious diseases of poultry endemic in the country. Livestock sector professionals are facing lots of problems due to emerging and re-emerging infectious diseases. This book will give an insight to the reader for better understanding of the problem.

Authors

Acknowledgement

The authors are highly obliged and thankful to Dr. M.R. Deo, of IVBP, Pune and Prof. (Dr.) R.D. Sadekar, M.V.Sc. Ph.D. Ex. Head of the Deptt. of Pharmacology of Krishi Vidyapeeth, Akola for their behind the curtain continuous help to write and publish this book and also the invaluable technical help in bringing this book project in actual reality.

Dr. S.V. Pandit, one of the author also takes this opportunity to express his gratitude towards his mentors, namely Late Dr. S.N. Sapre, its Director, D.I.S. (M.S.), Pune,Late Dr. S.G. Dixit, Ex. Dy. Director, IVBP, Pune,Late Dr. D.S. Gorha, Ex. Chief Executive, B.A.I.F.S F.M.D. Vaccine Project Wagholi,Dr. N.S. Dutt, Ex. General Manager, BAIFS, F.M.D. Vaccine Project, Wagholi,Late Dr. B.D. Survashe, Chief Executive, Ventri Biological of Venkateshwar Hatchery Ltd., Pune,

Dr. S.B. Salutgi, Director "Bio-space" Labotatory (Avians Drades Pvt. Ltd.), Pune, Dr. K.M. Pawar Madam, Ex. Director, NIV, Pune, Dr. S.V. Pandit has no suitable words to Express how he should acknowledge Late Dr. Manibhai Desai, Founder of BAIF, Wrali Kanchan,Late Dr. B.V. Rao, Founder of Venkateshwara Hatcheries Group, Pune without whose support his technical ambitions would not have materialized.

The authors are thankful to Mr. Milind S. Pandit and Mr. Manwatkar for their assistance in typing of this book.

Contents

Chapter 1

Foot and Mouth Disease

Foot and Mouth Disease (FMD) is one of the ancient diseases, caused by Aptho virus belonging to family *Picornaviridae.* It is highly infectious disease of all cloven footed animals like cattle, sheep, goats and pigs as well as in about 70 species of wild animals. Man is occasionally infected. The disease is characterized by formation of vesicular lesions on mucosa of mouth, feet, sometimes udder and teats. In general, clinical signs are most severe in cattle and swine. Sheep and goats usually experience sub-clinical infections. Wild animals show responses ranging from inapperent infection to severe disease and even death.

The cause of FMD was first shown to be non-bacterial in 1897 by Friedrich Loeffler. He passed the blood of an infected animal through a Chamberland filter and found the collected fluid could still cause the disease in healthy animals. The discovery of "Virus Particle" existence was made for the first time in 1899, when Tobacco Mosaic Disease was established to be caused by "virus" but one year earlier i.e. in 1898, it was established that FMD is caused by one of the smallest virus particles (Seetharaman, C. and Sinha, K.C., 1968).

About the virus

FMD is caused by Aptho virus, which is a RNA virus belonging to the family *Picornaviridae.*There are seven major serotypes of virus, designated as O,A,C, Asia-I, SAT-1, SAT-2 and SAT-3 (Fig. 1). The first 3 serotypes are European, 4th one is Asiatic while last 3 serotypes are having African Origin. There are several sub-types under serotypes O, A, and C, which are immunologically and serologically distinct from each other. Few sub-types also exist under African types SAT-1, SAT-2 and SAT-3 and few varients under Asia-I type. There is no cross immunity *in- vivo* amongst above mentioned 7 serotypes.Hence, if disease is caused by one specific serotype, the animal still remains susceptible for the disease by other serotypes post infection.

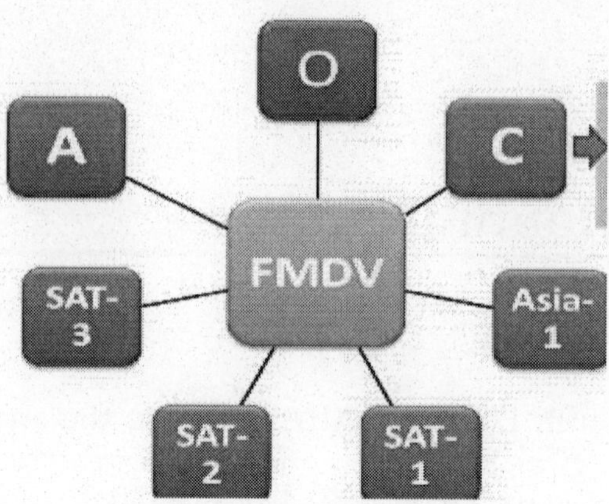

Fig. 1: Serotypes of FMD virus

Galloway *et.al.* (1948) developed complement fixation technique for serotyping of FMD virus strains. Similar technique was also evolved by Traub and Mohlman (1946) to demonstrate the antigenic differences between the variant strains of FMD virus. They demonstrated that the reaction between virus antigen and serum antibody prepared in guinea pigs can be measured as the amount of complement required for 50 per cent haemolysis fixed in the test. A range of strain specific antisera is prepared and the ratio of all the sera with all the virus antigens used to prepare the sera is compared as the cross fixation ratio of each serum with each virus. Two virus antigens are identical when the product of their cross fixation ratios is not significantly different from unity. Using this technique Davie (1962) examined a selection of virus strains, which have caused epizootics in the field and have been used for vaccine production in various parts of the world. These strains were compared with the established sub-type strains. The significance of such sub-type grouping lies in the fact that the vaccine prepared from established sub-type strain can protect the animals suffering from a limited range of field strains classified under homologous "sub-type group" (e.g. O, Lombardy strain vaccine will protect Europe 1943, M. 11/52 Mexico 1952, B.F.S. 1968 Britain 1961 field strains lying under same sub-type group). In India, vaccine prepared from O_5FMD virus strain from IVRI was being used to protect the animals against all type of virus isolates in the field.

The antigenicity of strains of FMD and virulence of these strains may change dramatically during the spread of the same in animal populations in the endemic areas as per the immunological pressures excerted by these populations. There are also biotypical strains which become adapted to particular animal species and then infect other species only with difficulty. Some porcinophilic strains are more virulent for pigs while some strains are virulent only for buffaloes. Some strains are virulent for exotic cattle but they show only mild reactions in tropical breeds.

Properties of virus

FMD virus is resistant to external influences including common disinfectants and usual storage practices of the meat trade, it may persist in infected premises over a year, upto one month on hair and 10 to 12 weeks on clothing and feed.

It is susceptible to pH changes away from "neutral" on both acidic and alkaline extremities (pH 5 and pH 12). Boiling can effectively destroy the virus, if it is free from tissues but may survive within tissue. It resists freezing at -79^{0}C for at least one month (frozen bull semen). Virus survives in uncooked meat scraps of sheep and goats, which are collected from slaughtered animals which are clinically normal but infected with FMD (carrier animals/animals under incubation period) and frozen by quick freezing technique while it may get destroyed, if carcass is frozen by slow freezing or is only chilled at refrigerated temperature.

If the FMD formaldehyde inactivated vaccine virus adsorbed on alhydrogel adjuvant is accidently frozen and then thawed, incompletely inactivated vaccine virus can escape and get freed to become a source of FMD outbreak (Bartling and Vreeswijk, 1991).

Occurrence of FMD

The disease is endemic in Africa, Asia, South America and parts of Europe while Japan, New Zealand and Australia are disease free. FMD is eradicated from USA after 1929, from Canada after 1951-52 and Mexico after 1954 by use "stamping out" policy and ring vaccination programme adjuncted with restriction of cattle and cattle product movements during and after the outbreaks.

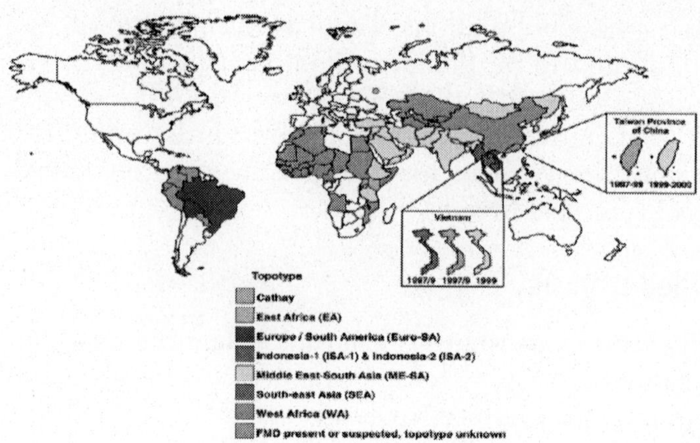

Fig. 2: Distribution of FMD

Western European countries were having fair control over FMD outbreak situation during early sixties of 20th century. This was due to stamping out policy in which slaughter of affected animals during FMD outbreak and use of Frankel type aluminium hydroxide gel adsorbed inactivated vaccine for ring vaccinations were used. Sporadic outbreaks were still being experienced for France (e.g. during 1962) and Denmark (e.g. during spring of 1966). Western Europe is essentially free of the disease since last decade of Twentieth century but cattle imported from Eastern Europe gave rise to an epidemic in Italy during 1993. There was a massive outbreak of the disease in Britain in 1967-68 which lasted for 8 months. A devastative outbreak occurred in China, in 1997 and over 4 million pigs died and/or slaughtered within 2 months.

About the disease

The severity of the disease in indigenous low productive cattle is very low with milder vesicular lesions on tongue, dental pad, lips and oral mucosa. Profuse salivation, vesicular lesions in interdigital space with mild to severe lamness and high febrile reaction is also characteristic. However, the exotic/crossbred highly productive milch cattle show the above mentioned symptoms more acutely with severe drop in milk production.

The morbidity in susceptible herds can approach almost 100 per cent but the mortality varies from Nil to 20 per cent or more depending upon the productivity of the animals. Milk production loss is severe in exotic cattle which can never recover back to normalcy in highly productive animals. The disease is characterized by vescicular lesions in feet, coronet region and mouth (including dorsum of tongue) after initial high temperature due to transient viremia.

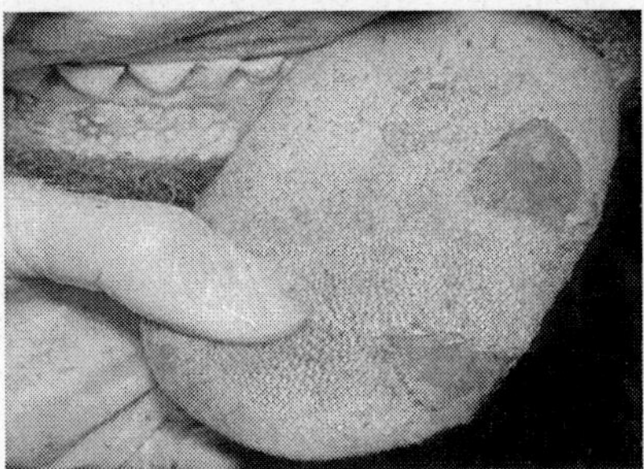

Fig. 3: Tongue leasions in FMD

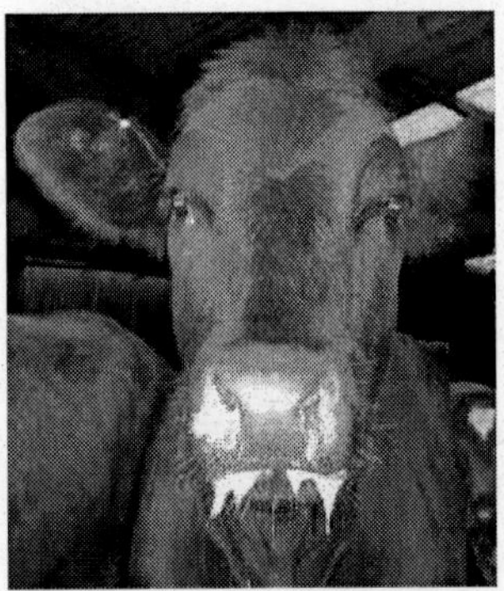

Fig. 4: Salivation in FMD affected cattle

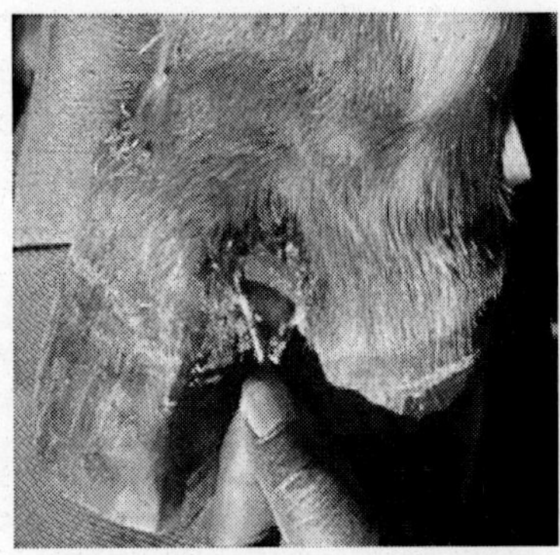

Fig. 5: Lesions in interdigital spaces

The Indian Zebu cattle is susceptible to this disease but mortality is not significant in this disease. However, the after effects of this disease, such as stunted growth, reduction in milk yield. Production of "Panters" especially in working bullocks and temporary "flattening" of semen, etc. are the most disastrous menifestations causing much economic loss.

The breeding animals show loss of fertility to varing extent. The working bullocks are unable to carry out the ploughing and carting operations at normal efficiency after affection with the disease any more.

All the above mentioned points mean to indicate that FMD bring about irrecoverable economic loss. The dairy buffaloes also show the disease symptoms similar to the dairy cattle and suffer severe economic loss. FMD in calves and piglets can bring about severe mortality with peculiar heart failure syndrome upto the extent of 25 to 50 per cent. This was observed in Taiwan outbreak in 1997 (Dunn and Donaldson, 1997). The FMD outbreaks in sheep and especially in goats are more obscure and need differentiation from Blue tongue disease and Rinderpest / PPR (*Peste des petits ruminants*) as well as vescicular stomatitis virus infection and lesions are milder or non distinct. FMD is also present in wild ruminents which often become reservoirs or carriers of the virus.

Mode of disease transmission

FMD is tramitted by a variety of methods between herds, countries and continents but spread from one animal to another is by inhalation or by ingestion. In endemic areas, susceptible animals coming in direct contact with migrating animals affected with FMD moving across the state and national boundries as trade or nomadic cattle can be a source of infection.

In non-endemic areas like Europe, the disease can get its first entry via pigs which contract infection by ingestion of infected meat scraps imported from foreign country and further spread from these pigs to cattle is via movement of people, abattoire waste or animals. Further spread from cattle to cattle may be due to airborne means as the virus can persist in aerosol form for long periods in temperate or subtropical climates. In most favourable circumstances, virus transmission can be wind borne as far as 250 k.m. distance. The speed and direction of wind as well as humidity can be other factors which are important in aerosol spread of infection. The pigs are the most potent excretors of air borne virus and cattle are the most susceptible to airborne infection.

In cattle the first site of virus infection with subsequent multiplication is "Naso-pharynx" which results into general viremia within few days. The virus appears in milk and saliva for upto 24 hours before appearance of vescicles in mouth. Other excretions like urine, faeces and semen follow the same suit before development of clinical symptoms. Period of maximum infectivity of saliva is until the vescicles are discharging the fluid. Generally, animals are infective for about 4 days post appearance of clinical signs but few animals become "Carriers" and spread disease in the field.

(Salt, 1993). The vaccinated animals (upto 50%) exposed to infection become "carriers" as the virus gets established in pharynx and is slowly excreted through naso pharyngleal discharge under the homologous antibody pressure. The pharyngeal virus go on mutating slowly and surviving variant sub-type may become a source of new focus of infection in animals coming in contact with the excreted virus after some period (upto period of 2 years).

African buffaloes are a known carrier of "SAT" types of FMD viruses. In these buffaloes, clinical disease is absent but they become a source of FMD infection to cattle in South Africa (Darve. *et al.* 1993). As virus is excreted in semen before appearance of symptoms of FMD in cattle, the semen collected from the breeder bull under incubation period of FMD and included in frozen semen bank can become a source of infection in outbreak of FMD in a herd (Mebus and Singh, 1991).

The FMD virus can survive in infected meat / pork and their products which are "quick-frozen" as this process suspends development of lactic acid formation of rigour mortis of animal carcasses. This is one important source of occurrence of sudden FMD outbreaks in FMD free countries. Meat pickled in brine or salted or smoked may also remain infective. Some outbreaks in Europe have been associated with vaccine virus either accidently escaping from the laboratory or that was incompletely inactivated (Bartling and Vreeswijk, 1991).

In endemic areas a "Six year epidemic cycle" is described for occurrence of FMD outbreaks involving one specific sub-type of virus. This is probably due to the fact that natural immunity developed post FMD outbreak lasts for about 1 to 5 years and after waining of this immunity fresh infection can flare up again in animals which have become "susceptible" again (Sharma. *et al.* 1993). In countries where yearly vaccination is practiced regularly, outbreaks are usually caused by different strain imported in "carrier" animals or infected meat.

Pathogenesis

The incubation period of FMD virus usually varies from 1 to 21 days (average 3-8 days) in most species. Viremia occurs thereafter at 17th to 74 hours and hyperthermia almost simultaneously. Clinical signs namely serous nasal discharge, salivation and buckle / feet lesions occur at the end of viremia. After the recovery of the clinical signs, virus may persist in pharyngeal area of convalescent animals.

Laboratory Diagnosis and Differential Diagnosis

In cattle, clinical diagnosis based on specific clinical symptoms is easily possible. However, identification of type and sub-type of FMD virus is needed for undertaking proper preventive vaccination in surrounding areas, if new sub-type of virus is involved in any fresh outbreak. Collection of fresh tongue epithelial material from vescicle alongwith vescicular fluid in 50 per cent Glycerine phosphate buffer solution for reproduction of the disease in suckling baby mice litters by its intracranial or intramuscular inoculation. Infected mice show typical leg paralysis within 48-72 hours post inoculation. Subsequently, CFT is done on 10 per cent suspension of the mice carcass material in PBS treated with chloroform, against type O, A,C Asia-I, SAT-I, SAT-2 and SAT-3 reference antisera for gross typing of FMD virus is done for virus typing. Calf kidney, goat kidney and BHK-21 cell cultures have been used for initial isolation and typing of virus. In case of sheep goats and pigs differential diagnosis against vesicular stomatitis, vesicular exanthema and swine vesicular disease is necessary.

Complement Fixation Test

Complement fixation test using Brooksby's technique, Macro-CFT in small test tubes or micro-CFT using epindorf micro pipettes and microplates can be standardized in FMD typing laboratory and typing as well as sub-typing of virus isolates can be undertaken. This requires raising of type, sub-type and even variant strain sera in guinea pigs against reference types or sub-types and even variant strain sera in guinea pigs against reference types or sub-type virus isolates or field isolates. Virus isolate can be serotyped, sub-typed and classified under specific "sub-type group" by calculating the cross fixation ratios and working out their products and comparing the same. This information is useful for development of suitable vaccine virus strains for optimum coverage of variant sub-type strains existing in the field (Davie, 1962).

An improved Complement Fixation (CF) technique was developed by Schjerning and Thiesen (1979) in which, consideration was given to the established presence of an antigen excess phenomenon as well as to the linear relationship between amounts of immune serum used and of complement fixed. The increased accuracy of the technique enables more precise and rapid detection of even minor serological differences. This technique was being followed by State FMD. Vaccine production Institute of Denmark at Lindholm, where in author (Dr. S.V. Pandit worked for 3 months in 1974).

Virus Infection Associated Antigen (VIA antigen)

As the virus infection associated antigens (VIA) are identical immunologically regardless of the virus type, a decision about whether an animal is "infected with FMD" can be made quickly without the need to include a large number of serotypes in a test screen. An antibody against VIA is detectable serologically in infected and recovered animals but not in FMD vaccinated animal with inactivated virus. VIA antibody test in imported vaccinated animal, harboring FMD virus sub-type not prevailing in the country, can detect the carrier state in the imported animal during the quarantine period which is helpful in not allowing this animal to be mixed in fresh farm animals.

ELISA Test

An "ELISA test" using special "monocloanal" antibodies against O,A,C sub-types is more sensitive for sub-typing of FMD strains as compared with CFT. An indirect ELISA using monovalent antibodies against A, O and C antigens can be used to detect type specific FMD virus in tongue epithelial samples (Pattnaik and Venkatraman, 1990). Similar test using "Polyvalent FMD serum against types O,A,C" is used in Mexico for routine diagnosis of FMD (Alonso. *et al.*, 1992).

Treatment of the Diseased Animals

Treatment is followed only in endemic areas where slaughter and irradiation policy is not employed. Use of mild disinfectants like Glycerine, sodium bicarbonate, etc. is made for cleaning of mouth lesions and further dressing of oral ulcers with turmeric powder / catacheu power is useful. Use of sodium carbonate/lime powder foot baths for feet lesions treatment is also useful. Paracetamol and similar antipyretic drugs are used to treat the febrile attack during the course of the disease. Broad spectrum antibodies like tetracyclines and sulpha drugs are used to address the secondary bacterial complications including mastitis.

Control measures

Many factors govern the FMD control procedure in a given area. Commonly employed procedures are: 1) Control by eradication 2) Control by vaccination 3) Control by combination of eradication and vaccination strategies. Control by eradication is seldom possible in "endemic" areas while it is logical only where only occasional outbreaks occur.

Control by eradication

Eradication programmes were undertaken in early and middle part of the twentieth century in North America, Britain, France and Italy and large member of "affected" and "incontact" cattle, sheep, goats and pigs were slaughtered during occurance of field outbreaks. Animal were either burnt or deeply buried, using lime in the burial trenches. The meat and meat products of these animals from affected areas were destroyed. The farm equipments, abattoir equipments, farm/premises were thoroughly disinfected and abbatoir restocking of farm promises was prohibited until the declared affected areas were again declared to be free from the disease.

To afford support to the eradication procedures in affected area, the surrounding areas were used as buffer zones where in FMD vaccination was undertaken, which is known as "Ring vaccination". Movement of live animals and animal products was stopped "to" and "from" the affected zones from outside.

These eradication programmes costed billions of Dollars/Pounds/ Kroners to the countries where such programmes were operated. So, some of those countries are now giving more stress on strict "Vigilance and Vaccination" programmes. For vigilance of outbreak situation, those countries had to strengthen their FMD typing and sub-typing facilities and vaccine production facilities wherein they have to stockpile the "concentrates" of inactivated FMD sub-type varients which are "predicated" to cause outbreak in the country in near future.

Control by vaccination

It is a well known fact that the animals vaccinated with FMD inactivated vaccine exposed to the field virus infection as well as unvaccinated animals after affection with FMD become carriers of the virus and remain so, for varing period for years but still FMD vaccination policy is followed by large number of countries. Where FMD is endemic, as control of FMD by eradication or by slaughter is a very costly proposition. Moreover, the modes of spread of FMD virus in nature are multiple and beyond physical possibility. Especially in countries which are vast in area and airborne spread, are beyond control or control of wild ungulates is not practicable. Only small countries / continents where physical barriers like "water surrounding the islands" can afford to use stamping out policy for FMD control.

Live attenuated vaccines

Even though, inactivated vaccines are now in practical and commercial use, the history of initial vaccine development began with live modified (attenuated) vaccines in early part and middle of 20th century (even during early sixties).

Animal Virus Disease Research Institute, Pirbright was engaged in development of live attenuated vaccine virus strains against various types of FMD by serial passages in adult mice for protection of cattle, sheep, goats and pigs. Since Mid-fifties of 20th century, Anon (1961) described a large scale field trial of such mice brain adapted polyvalent vaccine in East and South Africa undertaken in 4670 cattle in 1959, in which 70% cattle showed protection out of which 0.3% cattle showed mild oral lesions after vaccination (Report of Annual report of Pirbright Institute for 1956-1960 pp.52). Galloway (1962) described a big field trial of 2 live attended mice strains RHO-I (SAT-2 type) and RV-II (SAT-I type) in over 8,40,000 cattle in South Africa with successful prevention of field strains of different sub-type varients of these sub types.

Mackowiak *et. al.* (1955) of IFFA Lab France used passaged type C of FMDV for 60 times in Bovine tongue epithelial culture and 174 times in adult mice and found good results in loss of pathogenicity and increase of immunogenicity for cattle.

Mowat. and Prydie (1962) used RHO-1 (SAT-2) live modified mice adapted strain in 2000 Zebu and 50 low grade cattle for successful immunization in Keniya. On intradermal challenge with virulent field strain of homologous virus strain be observed 63% protection in zebu and 26% protection in low grade cattle. Mowat *et. al.* (1978) demonstrated successful propogation and production of large scale brews of above mentioned live modified mice adapted virus in BHK-21 cells in suspension for vaccine production. Rao *et al.* (1971) adapted type O, A, C, and Asia-1 strain to multiply in adult mice. These adapted strains were shown to be safe, when used for vaccination (live attenuated vaccines) but the VN test/results challenge test were variable. Noble *et al.* (1963) described neuroparalytic and hyper exitability reactions in sheep in various parts of Israel in about 5-10% animals after use of SAT-1 type live mice adapted vaccine.

Kane and Taylor (1963) also experienced mild transient in 14 out of 8,391 cattle vaccinated with live monovalent FMD vaccines, from

Pirabright (type A & SAT-1, Kernron's type O & ASIA-i) with 0.9% deaths in 4 month old calves. Fontaine *et al.* (1961) described development of live modified Type C, FMD vaccine strain by 80 serial egg embryo passages with loss of pathogenicity for cattle. Lutsevich (1961) recorded field trials of VIE lapinised FMD vaccine with successful immunity results.

Live mice passaged attenuated vaccines proved useful in control of FMD in South Africa and Venezuala while Lapinised live vaccine was largely used for control of FMD in Russia. Live vaccines were in use in the above mentioned countries during sixties and seventies of 20th century. However, live vaccines could not keep their promise of disease control for long time, as there is a need for strict vigilance on disease situation arising out of the possible mutations and reverting back to virulence of the vaccine strains during their natural spread in the susceptible population of animals.

Inactivated Vaccines

History of use of Inactivated FMD virus vaccine goes as long back as 1938 in continental Europe. Waldmann and Kobe (1938) used Bovine tongue tissue virus obtained from slaughter house for adsorption on aluminium hydroxide gel and he further inactivated the same by treatment with formaldehyde. This vaccine was found to be safe and most potent, as it is prepared from original bovine field virus. However, there were limitations for its production in large volumes.

This difficulty was solved by production of the vaccine virus grown in Bovine tongue tissue, grown in culture tanks containing Tyrode's Balance Salt Solution with nutrient protein hydrolysate by Frenkel. (1947). The author (Dr. S.V. Pandit) personally handled similar facility at Lindholm, Denmark at Danish FMD vaccine production Institute during his training in FMD vaccine production during 1974.

Dhanda *et al.* (1957) prepared monovalent, Bivalent and Polyvalent FMD vaccines using one, two or all 3 types (O,A and C) of viruses by using blood from "infected" bovines mixed with 2 to 5 per cent infected epithelial tissue from tongue. This suspension was treated with 0.03% crystal violet stain and was incubated at 37°C for 10 days for inactivation. This vaccine was proved to confer reasonable grade of immunity. These vaccines were used only experimentally but were never taken to the commercial large scale production stage.

Frenkel type vaccines produced on surviving Bovine tongue epithelium culture and adsorbed on alhydrogel before formalin inactivation and further adjuvanted with saponin (an alkaloid from quallaja saponiria a plant from South American Continent) was in use in Denmark, Netherlands, France and Britain in Italy during fifties sixties and seventies of 20th Century for effective control of FMD outbreaks. However, the haemolytic factor present in Saponin was giving rise to local inflammatory edematous swelling reactions in the vaccinated animals. This problem was addressed by development of saponins fractions free from "haemolysins" by treatment of dailysis through semi-permiable membrane (Lie and Dalsgard, 1974, from Lindholm Laboratory, Denmark). This fraction of saponin was further used for production of Iscomes "micro vasciles which were developed for "antigen delivery" as modern Adjuvants for "Subunit" vaccines in human and veterinary use.

Aluminium hydroxide gel used for adsorption of FMD virus in Frenkel type vaccine requires specific treatment for production of proper gel form which was specially developed in Denmark by the original manufacturer "M/S Danfos" which is based on "maturation of the gel" by special treatment of autoclaving and through "washing" of gel by repeated quick sedimentation in cold temperature or using "canvas bags" for gel and water separation for frequent changing of distilled water in washing of gel. Such specially treated gel has optimum capacity to adsorb FMD virus in vaccine production.

Castagnoli *et al.* (1959) describes protection of cattle for 13 months using vaccine produced on calf kidney culture inactivated with formaldehyde after adsorption on aluminium hydroxcide gel. Sellers (1960) demonstrated factors affecting formation of plaques produced on Pig kidney monolayer. Capstick *et al.* (1962) of described cultivation of 4 FMD virus strains on pig kidney monolayer cultures for vaccine production by adsorption on alhydrogel and its treatment with 0.05% formaldehyde for inactivation for 4 days at 26°C temperature. This vaccine could successfully protect guinea pigs by challenge test.

Patty and May (1961) describes a method for rapid production of FMD virus with high C.F. antigenicity in bovine kidney pig kidney and lamb testis cells grown on glass surface with high titres. Borgen *et.al.* (1964) grown 4 procine strains of FMDV from Denmark, Germany, Italy and Netherlands and 4 bovine strains from these countries in Calf kidney culture. Frederiks H.H. J and FAO expert from Netherlands and Dr. N.S. Datt of IVRI, Mukteshwar and Kumar

U.P. in the year 1966, developed FMD alhydrogel adsorbed seponin adjuvanted formalin inactivated quadrivalent (O,A,C and Asia-I strains) vaccine using Bovine Calf Kidney mololayer cultures grown in Povitzski flasks (Rectangular bottles) and Rouse flasks. This developmental work was carried out in late sixties and vaccine batches on moderate scale were available for field use during early seventies. The does of this vaccine was 20 ml which used to afford adequated protection to adult cattle but the vaccine had a disadvantage of having severe side reaction including local painful oedematous swelling due to non-purified saponin being used as adjuvant. The production of this vaccine had limitations of production scale for want of adequate availability of calf kidneys for production of vaccine with considerable bigger size of vaccine dose volume. However, due credit should be given to this vaccine, as this was a "small beginning" of modernization of vaccine production technique in India.

Ubertini *et al.* (1967) described BHK-21 cells (Baby hamster kidney cells) of commercial cell line propogated in deep suspension cultures used to prepare monolayers in roller bottles on large scale. The suspension culture was produced in 150 litter vessels with viable cell density of 2.2 to 2.5 million cells per ml. The source of BHK-21 cells was deep Frozen liquid nitrogen stored cells which remained viable for 2 years. FMD virus antigens produced in BHK monolayers in roller bottles or deep suspensions were both compared favourably with Frankel type surviving Bovine (Tongu epithelium cultures or calf kidney monolayer culcured antigens.

Even though intact viable BHK cells produced tumours in hamsters, no carcinogenic reaction were observed with BHK cell grown formalin treated (inactivated) FMD virus suspensions free from BHK cells with chloroform extraction treatment. Capstick *et al.* (1967) from Pirabright FMD laboratory described production of FMD vaccine in deep BHK-21 cells suspension cultures in fermentor vessel with temperature control range between 34.25^{0}C to 35^{0}C and at pH 7.2 with a cell concentration of 2.5 million cells/ml for optimum antigen concentration production. Peak virus yield could be obtained at input "virus/cell ratio" between 1:1 to 1:3. BHK cell production with 10% FMD antibody free serum medium and virus production at 5% FMD antibody free serum medium improved FMD virus yield.

Frederiks (1969) reported production of 2 million doses of monovalent FMD vaccine on BHK-21 cells suspension culture using simples Hanks medium containing Lactalbumin hydrolysate in Thailand, using BHK 21 cells produced from Brescia Institute, Italy, IFFA, France (Teheran Branch) and Virus Research Institute, Bankok. Report from Istituto Zooprofilattico Sperimentale, B rescia, Italy (1969) describes in details production of FMD vaccine by methods 1) using calf kidney monolayers in Roller bottles, 2) using BHK-21 all monolayers in Roller bottle, 3) using BHK-21 cells on semi-continuous suspension cultures (150 litre tanks) and then in Roller bottles 4) using BHK-21 cells in complete continuous suspension in Tanks of 500 litre capacity and virus grown in suspension culture.

Scenario of Foot and Mouth Disease and its Control in India

Indigenous cattle breeds were known for their draft capacity and were being mainly used for carting and ploughing operations. The milch cattle breeds in India like Gir, Sahiwal, Red Sindhi and Rathi and Indian buffalo were capable of producing about 3000 to 3500 litres of milk per season after calving while average Indian cow was unable to produce more than 100 to 500 litres of milk per season. This situation was existing in India upto early fifties to the beginning of sixties of 20th century. These indigenous draft and milch cattle breeds and buffaloes were known for their sturdiness and resistance against foot and mouth disease.

Foot and mouth disease is prevailing in India since ancient times but its economic loss was not much in "light" due to the fact that "draft" animals were producing only temporary lameness due to mild foot and mouth lesions while indigenous cows buffaloes being poor "milkers" were even though loosing temporary milk production after FMD out break the loss of "original low milk production" was not felt much by the farmers as milk production was not treated by Indian farmers as "commercial commodity" during these days.

However, after early fifties, after beginning of "Artificial Insemination Programme" post independence, the Indian Farmers who were engaged in "Buffalo milk production" business started "feeling bad" about considerable loss of buffaloes / milking cows milk loss after FMD outbreak. It is during this early period of fifties that Research on FMD began at IVRI, Mukteshwar and Development of "Waldman type" FMD vaccine (Crystal violet FMD vaccine) was carried out by Gopalkrishnan (1951) on experimental basis to combat FMD losses" due to loss in milk production" as described earlier.

FMD control Research Programme gathered momentum during mid-sixties, when IVRI undertook crossbreeding programme through artificial insemination using imported Jersey and Holstein Frezian (HF) bulls for improvement in milk production. During this period, N.S. Datt and Sharma developed polyvalent and monovalent FMD vaccine against, O, A, C and Asia type strains by adapting respective "local type strains" isolates to calf kidney cultures and using these seed viruses for cultivation of vaccine virus on calf kidney monolayers. Dr. Fredriks and FAO expert helped them in this project. This vaccine was based on adsorption of these viruses on aluminium hydroxide gel before inactivation by Formalin 0.05% and addition of glycerol for preservation and saponin with alhydrogel as adjuvant.

During late sixties, Behring Institute (Hoechst) of Germany importing FMD inactivated polyvalent vaccine in India and subsequently Hoechst (India) started FMD vaccine production in India in early seventies. They were having "monopoly" of commercial scale FMD vaccine production until BAIF started their FMD vaccine production in 1978, when FMD vaccine cost was drastically brought down to less than half. The cost of vaccine was further reduced significantly due to cut throat competition by commercial vaccine producers after arrival of NDDB in this picture. This helped in milk production costs which are one major factor in brining "operation flood" in milk production movement in India.

NDDB'S FMD vaccine production plant at Hyderabad started producing BHK-21 cell cultured FMD virus, adsorbed on alhydrogel and inactivated it using Acetyl Elethylene Immine (AEI) using Burrows welcome technology. This AET is a better inactivating agent for FMD virus inactivation as compared with Formaldehyde. Formaldehyde has a "tailing effect" on FMD virus as the viral Nucleic acid in the genome is not completely inactivated in early phase of inactivation in case of Formaldehyde inactivation process. Hence, if this formalin inactivated vaccine is accidently frozen during storage in refrigerator and then thawed during usage. Freezing and thawing can release the "live" virus particles and may induce FMD disease in the vaccinated animal. AEI has no such "tailing effect" but it has a possible "Carcinogenic" effect. Now-a-days, BEI (Biocetyl Ethylene Iramine) is used for inactivation of vaccine virus which is less carcinogenic and has no "tailing effect" on inactivation of vaccine virus.

FMD typing and sub-typing programme was also undertaken at IVRI Mukteshwar during 1964-65 for monitoring the FMD situation in the Field. Author (Dr. S.V. Pandit) sent one sheep virus isolate originally suspected for Bluetongue virus, during his working on this disease at Virus Research Station, ICMR, Pune during 1966 and type C FMD virus was got confirmed.

ICAR allotted Regional FMD virus typing centre to Disease Investigation Section, Aund, Pune of Maharashtra State in 1972 under All India Co-ordinated Project for Epidemiological Studies on FMD (Author Dr. S.V. Pandit worked as Assistant Virologist in this project). Complement fixation test using tissue culture (BHK-21 cells/calf kidney cells) for obtaining field isolates and their typing was developed under this programme and valuable epidemiological observations were recorded, including spread of FMD virus through bullock cart movement from peripheral villages to the central sugar factory and from there to surrounding villages from where sugarcane is procured for sugar production during sugarcane crushing season from October to January every year.

At FMD regional typing centre, Pune it was observed that out of 71 viable isolates of FMD virus during the report period 1972-73, 24 isolates were subjected to CFT, out of which 18 were typed as "O", 3 were typed as "A" and 2 were typed as "C" while only 1 was typed as Asia-I. Then indicating predominance of type "O" virus incidence (>75%).

At the end of 1975, Poona centre recorded isolation of 126 FMD virus isolates, out of which 65 (51.6%) were typed as "O" 8 (6.4%) were typed as "A" 38 (30.16%) were typed as "C" and 11 (8.7%) were typed as Asia-I, while 4 isolates were "cross reacting" type (for period from 1972 to 1975). BAIFS FMD vaccine production centre, recorded occurrence of sub-type A22 for the 1st time in India which was presumed to have come from middle east during the year 1979-80. Monovalent sub-type A-22 inactivated allydrogel adsorbed vaccine was immediately produced from the field virus isolate to combat against this new sub-type.

BAIF FMD typing laboratory also recorded a new sub-type variant of type "C" virus and sub-type variant of type Asia-I virus from the field samples which were demonstrated to have immundogical varience from "reference" C and Asia-I type viruses from IVRI, Mukteshwar, by conducting "Cross protection tests" in guinea pigs. The necessary monovalent vaccines were prepared from those isolates to protect the valuable herds of cattle surrounding those incidences.

Similar regional FMD typing centres were established by ICAR at Bengaluru, Guahati, Hisar, Chennai (Madha Varan) for study of FMD virus epidemiology in various parts of India for undertaking definite steps for control of FMD in India during mid seventries of last century.

For boostering milk production in the country, Mr. Manibhai Desai established Bharatiya Agro Industries Foundation in 1967 at urulikanchan near Pune (Maharashtra) (BAIF) wherein cross-breeding programme in cattle was undertaken in early seventies. Similar programme of Buffalo breeding was undertaken by Mr. Kurian at National Dairy Development Board (NDDB) at Anand in Gujarat. Both of these programmes were responsible for white (milk) revolution in India, in early and mid-seventies of 20th century. FMD infection was supposed to be a great hurdle in this revolution, as it is No.2 enemy of "Dairy Cattle and Buffaloes". Hence, FMD vaccine production programmes were undertaken at both of these institutions during mid-seventies and FMD vaccine production started at BAIF, Wagholi in 1978 and at NDDB, Hyderabad in 1979 -80 NDDB, Hyderabad used FMD vaccine production technology from M/S. Burrows Welcome Laboratory at Pirbright. Similar project of FMD vaccine production was completed by IVRI at its regional centre at Bengaluru (Karnataka). Both BAIF'S FMD production centre and IVRI'S FMD vaccine project centre and IVRI'S FMD Vaccine Project started using funding received from Danish International Development Agency (DANIDA) and "Danish Technology" from Danish Govt's FMD vaccine production centre at Lindholm, Denmark.

DANISH TECHNOLOGY was based on cultivation of FMD vaccine virus strains on BHK cells grown in deep suspension culture in 100 and 300 litre capacity fermenter vessels with arrangements for control of incubation temperature (36.5^{0}C) and pH control (pH 7.0-7.2) using aeration through automatic pH titrator (controller). Treatment of vaccine production virus with 1% chloroform for precipitation and centrifugal separation of serving BHK cells/debris before adsorption of the same on aluminium hydroxide gel and the inactivation of adsorbed vaccine virus with 0.05% Formalin were some important steps in vaccine production of Danish Technology. Use of Polyetheline Glycol (PEG) for separation of FMD antibody ganama globulin from serum before using in BHK cell/FMD virus growth media, use of "Canvas bag" technology for concentration of FMD vaccine virus brews for separation of water portion from virus adsorbed gel or use of this technology for quick separation of water portion of gel for quick frequent washing of alhydrogel for improving the quality of gel, etc. were the points developed by our team additionally at BAIF, Wagloli Project (Author Dr. S.V. Pandit was R & D manager at this project for above 12 years). Large scale availability of FMD vaccine produced by more than 3 commercial vaccine producers in India brought down FMD problem in animals and currently FMD has no more remained as big obstacle in animal industry in India.

Currently, alhydrogel or even oil adjuvanted FMD Trivalent Vaccine (only type O,A and Asia I strains in activated by BEI) (Type C is declared as absent in the field now) is under use by Govt. of India's FMD control programme. Since 2008-2011 in Kerala, Tamil Nadu, H.P., Maharashtra, Gujarat, Haryana, Punjab and U.P. and ELISA Test is used for typing of FMD virus isolates cultivated as Baculovirus expressed antigen for safety (Ref. V.A. Srinivasan, R & D of Indian Immunologicals Ltd., Hyderabad).

Suggested Reading

Alonso, A., Martins, M.A., Gomes, M.P., Allende, R. and Sondahl, M.S. (1992). Foot and Mouth disease virus typing by complement fixation and enzyme-linked immunosorbent as say using monovalent and polyvalent antisera. J. Vet. Diagn. Invest. 4: 249-53

Bartling and Vreeswijk (1991). Developments in foot-and-mouth disease vaccines. Vaccine. 9(2): 75-88.

Capstick, P.B., Tetling, R.C., Champman, W.G. and Stewart, Doreen. (1962). Growth of cloned strain of hamster kidney cell in suspended cultures and their susceptibility to the virus of foot and mouth disease. Nature, London, 195: 1163.

Dawe, P. S., Sorensen, K., Ferris, N. P., Barnett, I. T., Armstrong, R. M. & Knowles, N. J. (1994). Experimental transmission of foot and mouth disease virus from carrier African buffalo (Syncerus caffer) to cattle in Zimbabwe. Vet Rec 134: 211–215.

Davie, J. (1962). The classification of sub-type variants of the virus of foot-and-mouth disease. *Bull. Off. int. Epiz.* **57**: 962.

Dhanda, M.R., Gopal Krishnan, V.R. and Dhillon, H.S. (1957). Studies on foot and mouth disease vaccination in India. II. A concentrated crystalviolet vaccine. Indian Journal of Veterinary Science 27: 127.

Dunn, C. S. and Donaldson A. I. (1997). Natural adaptation to pigs of a Taiwanese isolate of foot-and-mouth disease virus. Vet. Rec. 141: 174–175.

Frenkel, H.S. (1947). La culture de virus de la fievre aptheuse sur l' epithelium de lax langue des vovides. Bulletin Office International Des Epizootics, 28: 155.

Galloway, I. A., Henderson, W. M. and Brooksby, J. B. (1948). Strains of virus of foot and mouth disease recovered from outbreaks in Mexico. Proc. Soc. exp. Biol., N.Y., **69**: 57.

Galloway, I. A., (1962). Results of the use of two live attenuated strain vaccines, Rho. 1 (SAT 2 type) and RV. 11 (SAT 1 type), in controlling outbreaks of foot-and-mouth disease. Bull. Off. int. Epizoot. 57: 748.

Mebus C.A. and Singh E.L. (1991). - Embryo transfer as a means of controlling the transmission of viral infections. XIII. Failure to transmit foot-and-mouth disease virus through the transfer of embryos from viremic donors. Theriogenology, 35(2): 435-441 .

Mackowiak C., Girard H., Camand R. and Hirtz J. (1955). Recherches sur la multiplication du virus aphteux en culture de tissu. I. etude biologique des cultures de longe dude. Rev. Immunol. 19: 426.

Mowat G. N. and Chapman W. G. (1962). Growth of foot-and-mouth disease virus in a fibroblastic cell line derived from hamster kidneys. Nature. 194: 253-255.

Mowat G N, Garland A J, Spier R E. (1978) The development of FMD vaccines. Veterinary Record 102: 190–193.

Pattnaik B, Venkataramanan R.(1989) A sandwich enzyme linked immunosorbent assay for subtype analysis of foot-and-mouth disease virus isolate. *Indian Journal of Animal Sciences*. 59: 1363–1368.

Patty R. E. and May H. J. (1961). The production of high concentrations of foot-and- mouth disease virus in cultures of cells on glass. Am. J. Vet. Res. 22: 926-931.

Salt, J. S. (1993). The carrier state in foot and mouth disease–an immunological review. *Br Vet J.*, 149: 207–223.

Sellers R. F. (1960). The growth and antigenicity of the virus of foot-and-mouth disease in pig kidney tissue cultures. Arch. ges. Virusforsch. 9: 621-636.

Schjerning and Thiesen K. (1979). Survival of foot-and-mouth disease virus in milk and cheese. In Report of the Session of the Research Group of the Standing Technical Committee of the European Commission for the Control of Foot and Mouth Disease. Lindholm, Denmark, 12-14th June. Food and Agriculture Organisation (FAO), Rome, 68-71.

Traub, E. & Möhlmann, H. (1946). Untersuchungen über immunologische Varianten der Typen A und B des Maul-und-Klauenseuchevirus. *Berl. Münch. tierärztl.*

Waldmann O. and Kobe K. (1938). Die aktive Immunisierung des Rindes gegen Maul- undKlauenseuche. Berl. tierdrztl. Wschr. 46: 317.

□□□

Chapter 2

Rinderpest (Cattle Plague)

Rinderpest is an ancient acute viral disease of cattle, buffaloes, wild ruminants, sheep, goats and swines are also rarely affected. Historically, it was a most devastating disease, spread from Asia to Europe, the Middle East and Africa, usually as a sequel to wars. The need to combat this disease was instrumental in the establishment of the first veterinary school in Lyon (France) in 1762.

Robert Koch was the first person who tried to evolve a vaccine against Rinderpest in early eighties of 19th century (Round about 1883) consisting of glycerinated bile which failed to afford considerable lasting protection against Rinderpest. However, this induced others to evolve formal inactivated/chloroform inactivated Rinderpest (RP) vaccine using lymph nodes and spleen from affected Bovines (Daubney, 1937).

It is on recommendation of Indian Cattle Plague Commission that Imperial Bacteriological Laboratory was established at Poona, in 1890 to combat against this dreadly disease which was later on shifted to Mukteshwar (Kumon, U.P.) where the epoch making work on the manufacture of Anti Rinderpest serum began in 1898. It was this Imperial Bacteriological, Laboratory, which later on received the name Indian Veterinary Research Institute (IVRI). Complete eradication of this malady is possible and its geographical distribution has been shrinking steadily since beginning of 20th century. Rinderpest was eradicated from southern Africa, Europe and China by 1950s and from East and West Africa by 1960s but due to Slackness in vaccination efforts; there was dangerous resurgence in this area after 10 years (1970s).

North America was free from this disease since ancient times and in South America and Australia occasional outbreaks were observed but were quickly eradicated. Rinderpest was endemic in India in 20th century. All ruminents and pigs are susceptible to the disease. Sheep and goats do get infected and show clinical signs. European pigs show only mild transient fever but do not spread the disease. Pigs from Thailand and Malaysia are highly susceptible to the disease and are also spreaders of the same. Sheep and goats do act as "spreaders" of the disease to cattle. There is a belief that RP became prevalent in small ruminants in Africa and Asia only after the introduction of Goat adopted RP vaccine from which the virus of PPP (*Pestis de Petit Ruminants*) probably mutated.

Virus strains of low pathogenecity cycle in wild ruminants and giraffe, deer and wildbeasts even in absence of disease in cattle (Rossiter *et al*. 1983).However, wildlife often get affected during cattle outbreaks. After independence (1947) during the first five year plan period, the Govt. of India launched a programme for eradication of Rinderpest from India since 1954. The centres for R.P. vaccine production have been established at IVRI, Izatnagar (Bareily) UP, Hisar, Mhow, Lucknow, Calcutta and Rainpet and latest equipments for lyophilizations of R.P. vaccines including Goat Tissue Vaccine (GTV) i.e. goats. Lapinised R.P. vaccine and Lapinised avianised vaccine had been procured. During the 1st five year plan areas in South India and South of River Krishna had been covered (80% animals in this region) and during second five year plan period, Andhra Pradesh, Maharashtra, Odisha, West Bengal, U.P., Punjab, Delhi, J&K, M.P. Rajasthan, Himachal Pradesh and Assam were covered by R.P. eradication progrmme and R.P. vaccinations with these live freeze dried vaccines was undertaken. It was contemplated that the whole country will be covered under this scheme by the end of 3rd five year plan.

However, it was observed in Maharashtra that inspite of completion of R.P. eradication programme by 1965 and temporary stoppage of occurrence of R.P. outbreaks after the completion of vaccination campaign, "R.P. like outbreaks" started reoccurring sporadically. It was initially thought that Bovine Virus Diarrhoea (BVD) or mucosal disease is creating these outbreaks. Dr. Sapre, Dy. Director In-charge Disease Investigation Section M.S., Poona reported occurrence of new disease which he called "Ajanta Disease" which was further got confirmed by him as "Mucosal Disease" by sending sera samples to Veterinary Disease Diagnostic Laboratory at Waybridge, Surrey, U.K. Swine fever lapinised virus antigen was used for confirmation of Mucosal Disease by agar gel diffusion precipitation test (AGPT) on basis of "lines of identity" between viruses of swine fever and mucosal disease (MD). Even though some outbreaks were certainly due to MD virus, majority of "R.P. like outbreaks" seems to have been due to "Rinderpest virus" only due to the failure of proper immunization of some animals with R.P. vaccine (improper storage/ reconstitution procedure of vaccine/negligence in proper cold chain maintenance during vaccination programme, etc.). This fact was further confirmed by the work under MDC–BT scheme at DIS, Pune (during 1967-70) using cross protection tests in buffalo calves and by development of AGP technique for differentiation of Rinderpest and mucosal disease. As it was evident that Rinderpest was still prevalent in Maharashtra and some other states in the country, even in the last stretch of the 1960's Govt. of Maharashtra strengthened its efforts against occurrence of the disease by establishment of "check posts" at the entry points of the inter-state borders and carried out R.P. vaccinations in animals (buffaloes cattle their calves, which were routinely transported from the other state and which were found to be frequent source of outbreaks of R.P. (1967 to 1973).

During 1967-70, tissue culture based freeze dried R.P. vaccine production using calf kidney monolayer culture and kebete "O" strain R.P. vaccine virus (TCRV) was undertaken at IVRI and the same was also produced at IVBP (Pune) in 1970-74. However, the production capacity was very limited.

BAIF undertook production of freeze dried TCRP vaccine using Kebete "O" strain initially on calf kidney monolayer culture and later on "VERO" cell line during late 1979-80's. During 1980-82, significant number of Rinderpest outbreaks in cattle and buffaloes in Andhra Pradesh, North Gujarat & Kathiawad were recorded wherein migration of cattle population due to drought conditions in Gujarat was incriminated as cause of spread of R.P. incidences. These outbreaks occurred inspite of use of BAIF'S TCRP vaccine in those areas.

Prevalence

In the absence of an outbreak, prevalence of the disease in endemic areas was low. In India, it was less than 10 per 100000 cattle before 1963-1974 and 2 per 1,00,000 cattle in 1974-1988 as a result of great expansion of the number of vaccinated cattle (*Ramachandran S.* and *Scott G.R., 1974)*. India was declared to be free from Rainderpest by the end of 20th century, thanks to the eradication programme undertaken by Govts. of Tamil Nadu, Kerala and Karnataka.

About the virus

Rinderpest is caused by a morbilivirus which is RNA containing virus and belongs to the family *Paramyxoviridae* which is antigenically related to "Measles" virus of human being, Equaine Influenza (Pink eye) disease virus of horses and Canine Distemper virus of dogs. It is also antigenically related to *Peste-des-petit ruminants* (PPR) virus of small ruminants (sheep and goats) which was supposed to be evolved by mutation of Rinderpest virus after adaptation of the same in goats by serial passaging artificially of cattle virulent virus for goat tissue virus vaccine (GTV) production, due to the accidental escape in goats in nature after cattle vaccination in endemic areas.

Even though Rinderpest virus does not show haemagglutination property directly either with goat/cattle/sheep/human/dog's Red Blood Cells (RBCS) as shown by the other *Paramyxoviridae* family members like "Measles virus" with human RBC, the Rinderpest vaccinated/convelenscent R.P. affected animal sera have got property to inhibit haemagglutination of "Measles virus" with human "O" RBCS. This property was used by Dr. Ramchandran of IVRI, Mukteshwar (1965) for the development of "Measles Haemagglution Inhibition Test" for diagnosis of Rinderpest in cattle by using paired sera (acute stage and recovered stage sera) from suspected R.P. affected animals or for sero-servillance of Rinderpest antibodies in R.P. vaccinated animals.

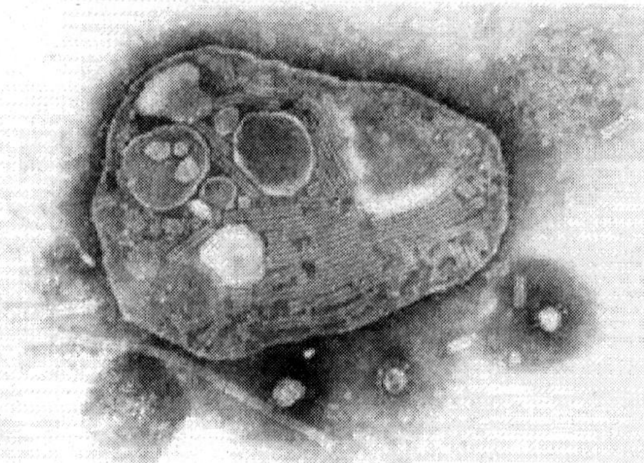

Fig. 1 : The Rinderpest Virus, *Source :* Food and Agriculture Organization

Mode of spread / transmission of the disease

Close contact between infected and susceptible animal is necessary for the disease transmission, as the virus is very fragile and can not survive for long outside the animal. The virus is excreted by infected animal through urine, faeces, nasal/eye discharge and perspiration. Inhalation of aerosol and injection of contaminated feed from affected animals are responsible for transmission and spread of the disease. At low humidity, infected aerosol can last for 30 minutes. The animals in incubation period without showing symptoms can act as spreaders of infection. Aborted bovine foetuses can contain communicable infective virus. Zebu cattle of all ages are susceptible for infection unless they are vaccinated or recovered from previous infection or in case of calves received colostral immunity. In India, "hill bulls" i.e. hill cattle from "Kumaun" area were known for their higher susceptibility while buffalo-calves and plain cattle were less susceptible. The imported Holestein frezian and Jersy cows were highly susceptible for infection and mortality and milkloss was very severe in them.

Extensive nomadic cattle movement from Kathiawad to South Gujarat especially during drought was responsible for most devastating outbreaks of R.P. in India during 1980's. Yearly routine transport of Milch buffaloes and calves from Meerut, Rohtak and Mehsana to Array Milk Colony (Bombay) by rail wagons was found to be a constant source of outbreaks of R.P. in Bombay suburban district during 1958 to 1965 period as observed by Veterinary Disease Investigation Section, Poona.

Rinderpest virus is most fragile and is actively shed during febrile stage of the disease and is not seen in discharges, when temperature comes to normal. The virus is destroyed in the carcass within 24 hours after death, due to pH changes and putrefaction. The infected premises get rid of virus easily as it is destroyed by heat, drying and most of the disinfectants. However, the virus remains infective in blood kept under refrigeration as long as one month. This is the reason why disinfection of the premises using appropriate sanitary measures and other control measures can minimize the risk of transmission of the disease.

Pathogenesis

The virus is inhaled in infected droplets and penetrates through the epithelium of the upper respiratory tract and then multiplies in tonsils and regional lymph nodes, from where the virus enters the blood in mononuclear cells and viremia is thus induced throughout the body. The virus has high affinity for lymphoid tissues and alimentary mucosa. Virus replication takes place in mononuclear cells (monocytes), lymphocytes and epithelial cells (Joshi *et al.*, 1984). Severe destruction of lymphocytes in tissues results in significant leucopenia; focal necrotic stomatitis and enteritis are direct results of viral infection. Death is usually due to dehydration in acute cases but it is due to severe immune-suppression due to leucopenia followed by secondary parasitic or bacterial infection in less acute cases.

About the Clinical Disease

The Clinical Disease is characterized by erosive mouth lesions after initial hyper pyrexia (Temp. 40.5 to 41.5^{0}C) followed by shooting diarrhoea which may result in death.

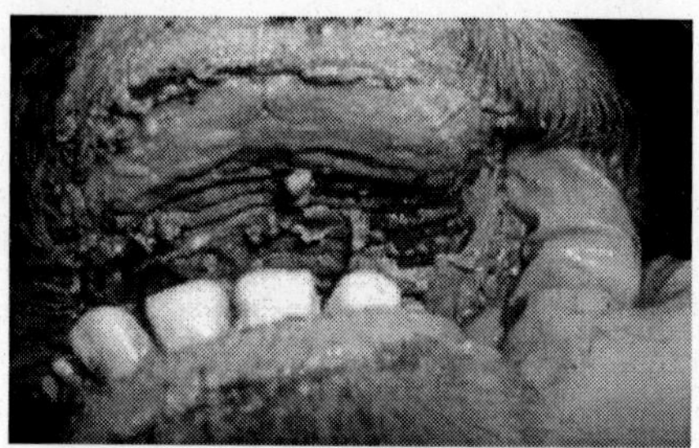

Fig. 2 : Oral legions from Rinderpest, Source : www.vet.uga.edu

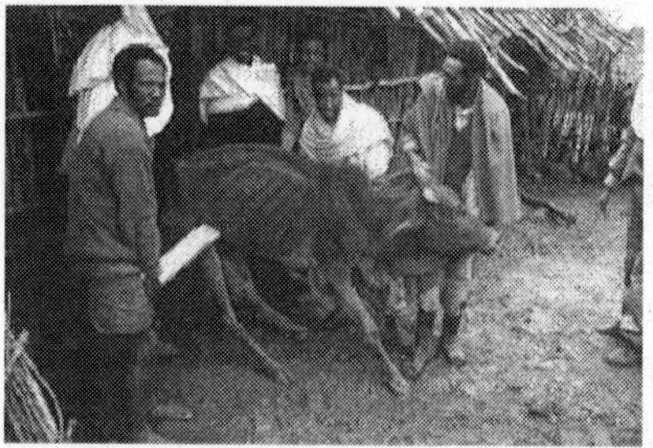

Fig. 3 : Emaciated cow infected with Rinderpest. Source : FAO

Erosive mouth lesions result into "Wheat Bran" like deposition on minute ullerative lesions which are distinctly different than large "Vescicular" lesions of Foot and Mouth disease.

In buffaloes, in endemic areas less acute disease may result into "Skin lesions" in the form of small pustules developed on neck, over the withers, inside the thighes and on scrotum. In such chronic form, diarrhoea may be insignificant or absent and temperature reaction may be mild or absent.

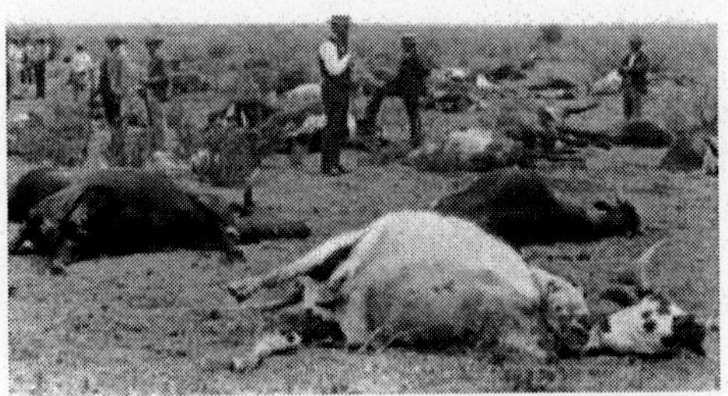

Fig. 4: Dead cattle from a rinderpest outbreak, Source: Food and Agriculture Organization

In acute cases, severe Anorexia, a fall in milk yield, lacrimation, harsh and staring coat accompany the fever. Nasal congestion and inflammation of buccal, nasal and conjunctival mucosal, hyperemia of vaginal mucosa and swelling of vulva may be seen.

Due to lympholysis, immune suppression can occur which may result into flaring up of unicellular blood parasitic infections like "Anaplasmosis" (*Anaplasma marginal's*).

Postmortem Lesions

The carcass is emaciated, dehydrated and soiled with foetid odoured faeces. Sharply walled ulcerations with branlike depositions are observed on oral mucosa which extends even upto pharynx, upper oesophagus and abomasum. Peyer's patches are swollen, haemorrhagic and necrotic on small intestinal mucosa. Severe zones of haemorrhages and erythema running transversely across the colon gives appearance of "Zebra Markings", which is a pathogenomic lesion of Rinderpest.

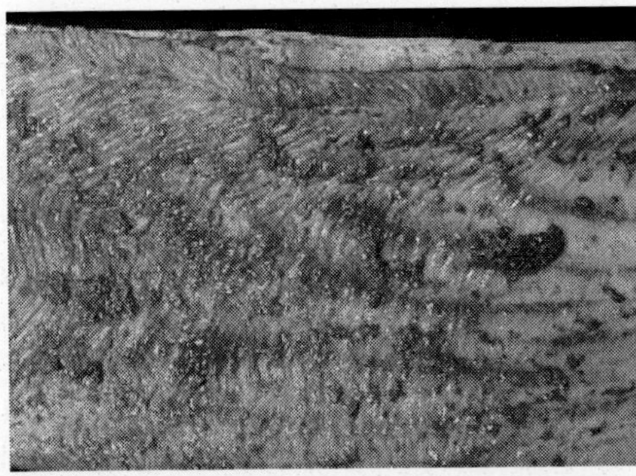

Fig. 5: Haermorrhagic congestion of large intestine

The nasal turbinates and septa are coated with mucopurulent exudates below which are erosive ulcerations. Lesions of errosive nature upto upper tracheal area in respiratory tract may be observed but not beyond that area, swelling of vulval lips and hypercemia and erossive lesions of vulval mucoca may be evident.

Mesenteric lymph nodes may be oedematous and microscopic lesions of necrotic lymphotytes may be observed in lymphnode sections. All lymphnodes show presence of "AGP" antigen (R.P. Specific), including cervical lymph-nodes which can be used for diagnosis of R.P., during affected stage in live animal by cervical lymph node biopsy.

Diagnosis of Rinderpest

Agar Gel Precipitation Test (AGPT) using 1% Nobel Agar gel semi-solid medium for diffusion of "lymph-node antigen" from R.P. infected animal (suspected) prepared as 10% tissue suspension in Phosphate Buffer Saline (PBS) and hyperimmune R.P. serum prepared in rabbit as known antiserum and lapinsed R.P. Virus (Lymp-hnode antigen) as known reference R.P. antigen was described by Scott and Brown (1961) for confirmation of field cases of Rinderpest .This test was standardized for diagnostic use by the author (Pandit, S.V.) at Disease Investigation Section, Pune for differentiation of R.P. from Mucosal Disease (Swine fever antigen produced in rabbit and hyperimmune rabbit serum against swine fever was used for AGPT against mucosal disease). Paper on this test was presented during Summer Institute in Immunology held at IVRI, Mukteshwar in May-July, 1971. Moghe R.G. and Author (Pandit, S.V.) also designed cross immunity test in buffalo calves above 6 months of age for differential diagnosis of Rinderpest and Mucosal Disease and proved presence of "Rinderpest" in 6 different outbreaks in cattle and buffaloes in Maharashtra during 1967-1970 (Report on MDC-BT scheme at D.I.S., Pune, ICAR Project).

Rinderpest needs differential diagnosis from Bovine Virus Diarrhoea and Mucosal Disease as mentioned above as well as from FMD, Blue tongue and Vesicular Stomatities. However, clinically the lesions can be differentiated and final virus isolation and AGPT can be used for confirmation of diagnosis. Yokobor first described Complement Fixation Test (CFT) using bovine lymph-node antigen and bovine sera as a diagnostic test for Rinderpest in the year 1916 (Nakamura, 1958). Mizuki used heated antigen in CFT for differentiated strains "O" and "K" of Rinderpest virus.

Nakamura (1940) demonstrated R.P. antigen in rabbit lymph-node tissues infected with Lapinised R.P. virus using boiled lymph-node antigen. Nakamura J. and Miyamoto T. (1954) demonstrated R.P. virus in chick embryo tissue after boiling and extraction (Bull Off. Intern Epiz 42: 692). Nakamura *et al.* (1955) demonstrated antibody response in cattle vaccinated with Lapinised vaccine in Korea.

The virus can be detected immunohistochemically in lymph-nodes and tonsils despite marked putrefaction of carcass (Brown, 1997). Using specific cDNA probes, isolates of Rinderpest and PPR viruses now can be differentiated (Diallo *et al.* 1989). Fluoroscent Antibody Test (FAT) and Immunoperoxidase test for detection of R.P. antigen in tissue sections. ELISA seems to be the most accurate test for detection of virus and its differentiation between R.P. and PPR (Diallo *et al.* 1995). Plowright (1986) described all aspect of Rinderpest in detail including diagnostic aspects and its control by vaccination.

Treatment

Treatment of Rinderpest is not desirable in previously disease eradicated areas as desimination of disease from affected but recovering animal through excretion of virus and its spread to susceptible animals in contact is possible. However, treatment was being undertaken past in endemic areas like India, wherein use of anti Rinderpest hyperimmune serum by subcutaneous or intravenous route was successful. Use of sulpha drugs and antibiotics for control of secondary bacterial infection adjuncted with antiserum treatment was also found successful. Author (Pandit S.V.) used Rinderpest hyperimmune serum prepared in buffaloes using formaline inactivated spleen and lymph-node material from R.P. affected animals for serial immunization subcutaneously of serum obtained from such hyperimmunised buffaloes for treatment of Rinderpest affected buffaloes during some Rinderpest outbreaks round about Pune during 1963-64 while working at Vety. Disease Investigation Section, Pune and obtained very good results of recovery of these animals from Rinderpest.

Control of Rinderpest

Stamping of policy : Control of Rinderpest is comparatively easy as survival of virus in infected animals is short-lived after the recovery of animal and virus excretion is limited only for a week or so and survival of virus in carcass is low after putrefaction. Moreover, the virus is destroyed easily by common disinfectants like Lysol and Caustic soda. Eradication programme include slaughter of affected and in contact animals, rigid disinfection of affected premises and deep burial of slaughtered animals in addition to complete halting of movement of animals and animal products from affected areas and stoppage of re-stocking of animals from outside to affected zone until disappearance of the disease are some of the preventative measures if undertaken religiously, the eradication of the disease is possible.

In North America and Australia, R.P. had never appeared but there have been single outbreaks (sporadic) which were quickly eradicated using "Slaughter and Stamping out" policy mentioned above.

Control by Vaccination

In endemic areas, control is carried out by Annual vaccination and surveillance policy. The use of efficient vaccination procedure and disease surveillance at national, regional or continental level is done. For example, the Organization of African Unity successfully initiated the Joint project 15 of 1962-1976 in Northern equatorial Africa and is currently (during the year 2000) implementing Pan-African Rinderpest Campaign (PARC) to rid the whole continent of the disease. The initial step was to vaccinate all animals in each national herd annually until the immune status exceeds 90 per cent. Thereafter, calves were vaccinated annually and re-vaccinated the following year until there are no more outbreaks for at least 5 years. Periodic surveillance (using tests like CFT, AGPT, ELISA or cDNA probing, etc. described previously) to monitor the immune status of the national herd and to deal quickly with any new outbreaks by control of animal movement and ring vaccination of all the surrounding herds was undertake effectly to get success. As mentioned earlier, India also resorted to undertake Rinderpest eradication programme by undertaking mass scale Rinderpest vaccination programme in various states during the first and second five year plan period (in October, 1954 to 1965). Accordingly, IVRI, Izatnagar (B.P. Division) and subsequently many of the State Govt. Biological product centres (Lucknow, Hisar, Mallo, Rainpet, Calcutta) designed production of Goat tissue adapted R.P. Vaccine also known as "Goatis". The following is the historical background of development of "GTV" freeze dried vaccine at IVRI narrated by Seetharaman and Sinha in their book on Biological production: ICAR, Publication, 1962.

Initially, living R.P. virus contained in the spleen of infected bovine has been used as a vaccine in conjunction with the serum (serum simultaneous method of vaccination). Later on, modified viruses were evolved for use as vaccine. Schein (1926) reported marked attenuation of R.P. virus in goats. Edwards (1928) announced replacement of serum simultaneous method of R.P. vaccine with goat adapted virus vaccine in Nagpur conference (Trans, for East Assoc. Trop. Med 3699). Following years (Daubney, 1937), Krishnamurthy (1945), Pfaff (1938), Saunders and Iyyar (1936), Bawa (1939), Starling (1932), Minett and Seetharaman (1950). The GTV was tried extensively with success (As referred to by Seetharaman in his book on Biological Production mentioned above). The work on this caprinised R.P. virus was pursued and the line "W" strain has been used as a seed virus for production of a Potent Vaccine for cattle immunization in years to come (Datta *et al.* 1951). Haddow and Idnani (1947), Sitaraman and Sinha (1957-58), Uppal *et al.* (1959) as quoted by Sitaraman & Singh as above. The immunity of this vaccine lasts for 14 years as reported by him.

However, caprinlised GTV strain was found to induce Rinderpest disease itself in Himalayan cattle and crossbred or imported European cattle and hence, Nakamura *et al.* (1938) and later on Edwards (1927 and 1952) reported successful infection and adaptation of cattle virus in rabbits to get lapinised vaccine virus. Haddow and Idnani (1947) reported usefulness of lapinised virus vaccine in combating Rinderpest. The modified lapined virus was distributed by FAO in various countries which became known as "Nakamura III strain". However, there were moré susceptible cattle stocks and hence, further modified "Lapinised - avianised RP vaccine virus was evolved (Shope *et al* 1946) as narrated by Seetharaman in his ICAR book mentioned earlier.

The spleen tissue from goats infected with seed as soon as to passage level was used for vaccine production, which was freeze dried after making its pulp while spleen, messentric lymph-nodes and infected blood from healthy rabbits infected with lapinised (41 serial passage level) Nakamure III strain was used for vaccine production after blending in wearing blender for freeze drying while some 41 rabbit passage levelled lipinised virus further passaged for 77 passages in chicken embryos was used for seed production of lapinised avianised vaccine production. Initially, intravenous inoculation of this seed virus was used for production of vaccine brew harvest embryo material. Later on, yolk sac method was used for getting infected embryos for vaccine production.

The most important problem associated with Rinderpest vaccination is the activation of existing latent infections including protozoal infections like Anaplasmosis and Theileriosis, especially after use of old attenuated vaccines including freeze dried GTV, lapised for lapinised avianised Rinderpest vaccines (Scott, G.R., 1985) due to the immune suppression caused by these vaccine by necrotizing effect on lymphoid cells.

Moreover, mass scale use of GTV was presumed to be responsible for natural "cycling" of goat adapted RP virus in sheep and goats to produce occasional Rinderpest outbreaks in those species and even this cycling is incriminated to have caused accidential mutation of GTV into *Peste-des-petit Ruminants* (PPR) virus in Africa and Asia (including India) which has become an "endemic disease" in these small ruminants in recent past. This fact made FAO to advise banning of production of Freeze dried Rinderpest G.T. vaccine that is why IVRI, Izatnagar, Bareily, U.P. and all the State Govt. Vet. Vaccine Production Laboratories had to stop R.P. goat tissue vaccine production by mid of 1970's and hence, they resorted to produce calf kidney adapted Kebete "O" strain freeze dried Rinderpest vaccine production.

The calf kidney adapted vaccine needs "good cold chain" maintenance for its effective storage which has posed a problem of big cost in developing countries during their eradication programmes. Moreover, primary calf kidneys can pose a problem of BVD virus contamination in cell cultures used for vaccine production (Scott, G.R. 1985 referred previously). This problem can be addressed by use of "Vero cell line" for vaccine production (Singh, S.N. 1992, DAE symposium DHE symposium on vaccine production Animal Cell Biotech, Pune current status and future Direction Feb. 22-24, 1992, pp 16). This vaccine is comparatively stable at ambient temperature after freeze drying (Groocock, C.M. 1992 which is referred to earlier). However, authors (Pandit, S.V.) personal observation at BAIFS vaccine production laboratory at Wagholi, Pune indicates possibility of interference of R.P. vaccine virus multification by intranuclear inclusions (dormant cell line virus) of vero cells.

Measles vaccine is also reported to have protected calves at the age when ordinary Rinderpest vaccines are ineffective due to interference from colostrums antibody. It is also an efficient vaccine for adult cattle (Provost A. *et al.*, 1986; Vet. Microbiol. 22: 119).

Recombinent vaccines against R.P. are being developed and clinical trials will be required to assess the claims of success. Yilma, T.D. (1989) claimed development of highly attenuated vaccine virus, a double recombinant that expresses both F and H genes of Rinderpest virus which was found to protect cattle against experimental R.P. virus infection and did not cause pox lesions and calves can be vaccinated at any age, even in the presence of colostral immunity (vaccine 7 : 484). The author had a lecture on this subject at Institute of Immunology, New Delhi (Dr. Talwar's Institute) from Dr. Yilma during 1988. However, there was a general feeling amongst the scientists that Recombinent vaccines pose of problem of very high costs which can be instead spent on development of cold chain system for classical vaccines equally effective in control of the disease.

Suggested Reading

Brown C.C. (1997). A review of three pathology-based techniques for retrospective diagnosis of Rinderpest, with comparison to virus isolation. Res. Vet. Sci., 63: 103–106.

Daubney, R. (1928). Observations on Rinderpest. J. camp. Path. Ther. 41: 228-48. 263-97.

Diallo A., Barrett T., Subbarao S. M. and Taylor W. P.(1989). Differentiation of Rinderpest and *peste des petits ruminants* viruses using specific cDNA clones. Journal of Virological Methods, 23: 127–137.

Diallo A., .Libeau G.,Couacy-Hymann E. and Barbron M.(1995). Recent developments in the diagnosis of Rinderpest and peste des petits ruminants. Vet. Microbiol. 44: 307-317.

Edwards, J. T. (1928). Rinderpest: active immunization by means of the serum simultaneous method; goat virus. Agric. J. India, 23: 185.

Joshi R. C., Sharma B., Bandopadyay S. K. and Bansal R. P. (1984). Detection of Rinderpest antibodies. Trop Anim Health Prod. 16(3): 167-70.

Nakamura J. (1940). On the experimental infection with Rinderpest virus in the rabbit. III. Neutralisation experiment. Jap. J. vet. Sci. 2: 567–578.

Nakamura J. (1958).Complement-fixation reaction in Rinderpest study. Guide for technique and application .International Office of Epizootics.

Plowright W. (1986). Rinderpest in the world today. State vet. J., 40, 44 70.*Ramachandran, S.*and *Scott, G.R.(1974) Rinderpest* in sheep, in

Andhra Pradesh and its control by vaccination. Indian Vet. J. 51: 439–450.

Rossiter, P.B., Jessett, D. M., Wafula, J. S., Karstad, L., Chema, S., Taylor, W.P., Rowe, L., Nyangi , J.C., Otaru, M., Mumbala, M. and Scott, O. R. (1983). Re-emergence of Rinderpest as a threat in East Africa since 1979. Veterinary Record 113: 459-461.

Schein, H. (1926). Experiences sur la peste bovine. Bull. Soc. Path. Exot. Paris. 19: 915-928.

Scott, G.R. & Brown, R.D. (1961). Rinderpest diagnosis with special reference to the agar gel double diffusion test. *Bull. Epiz. Dis. Afr.*, 9: 83-120.

□□□

Chapter 3

Mucosal Disease Complex/Bovine Virus Diarrhoea

A disease model involving 3 phases of immune mechanism, namely immunotolerance, immune suppression and immunocompetance together in single entity.

Mucosal Disease complex/bovine virus Diarrhoea is a disease entity caused by Bovine Pesti virus, with several different disease menifestations including: 1) Benign infection of bovine virus diarrhoea (BVD) which is usually subclinical, 2) Fatal mucosal Disease, which occurs in persistently viremic animals which are specifically immunotolerant as a result of an infection acquired in early foetal life, 3) Peracute, highly fatal diarrhoea, 4) Thrombo cytopenia and haemorrhagic disease, 5) Reproductive failure, 6) Congenital abnormalities in calves as a result of faetal infection in mid-gestation, 7) Manifestation of immune suppression. The mucosal disease was first recognized in 1946 and for the next 35 years, it was assumed that the disease was a result an infection prior to the onset of illness (Radostits *et al.*, 2000).

It is now clear that mucosal disease occurs only in persistently infected (PI) animals as a result of a congenital infection (from infected mother cow via placenta) with non-cytopathic strain of virus acquired in early foetal life. These animals remain specifically immune tolerant to the homologous strain of BVDV throughout post-natal life and total mucosal disease is precipitated by a super infection with a cytopathic strain of the BVD virus occurring usually at 6-24 months of age or older (Rodostits *et al.*, 2000).

In the late 1980s and early 1990s, a peracute enteric form of the disease and thrombocytopenia in young and adult immune competent animals infected with highly virulent non-cytopathic Type II strains of the BVD virus were recognized which occur as a result of post-natal infection (Taylor *et al.*, 1995; Ridpath *et al.*, 1994).

About the virus

Bovine Virus Diarrhoea Virus (BVDV) is one of the 3 Pesti viruses including Classical swine fever virus (European origin) and Border disease virus of sheep, which are closely related antigenically. BVDV belong to the family "*Flaviviridae*" and is a member of genus Pestivirus.

There are two biotypes of BVDV, designated as non-cytopathic (NCP) and cytopathic (CP), depending on their effects on tissue cultures. The NCP virus is most common and important which crosses the placenta of the infected mother cow and invades foetus and establishes the Persistant infection (PI) in the foetus as a result of

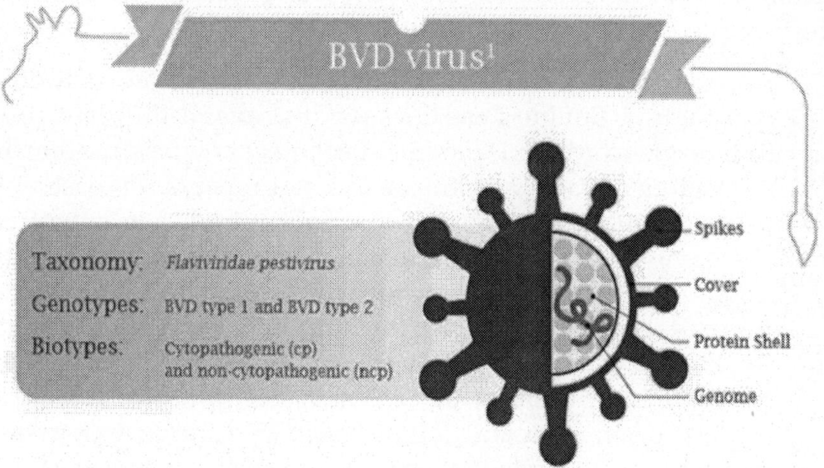

Fig. 1: Structure of BVD Virus

immunotolernce, when mother gets infected CBKDV in early stage of pregnancy (upto 3-5 months of pregnancy). The BVDV antigens get recognized as "self" and hence, no antibodies against the homologous BVDV are produced in the post-natal life of the foetus and hence, BVDV infection become "persistent" throughout the life of newborn calf. Such persistently infected (PI) calves either do not show clinical disease at all or may remain unthripty and stunted and show chronic mild diarrhoea but do not die of BVD disease. Such PI calves in BVD endemic areas can form only small percentage of population (1.9%) but they can become a source of acute or sub-acute mucosal disease in remaining immunocompetant MDC seronegative cattle population (herds) the age between 6 and 24 months of age and rarely beyond both the sides of this age range (Radostits *et al.*, 2000).

Cytopathic virus of BVD (CP virus) is usually associated with only mucosal disease in animals already persistently infected (PI) with non-cytopathic biotype and appears to arise by mutation from "NCP" virus bio type within PI animals. It was postulated that super infection of cytopathic (CP) virus from the field in persistently infected (PI) calf/adult animal carrying homologus non-cytopathic (NCP) virus results into precipitation of fatal clinical mucosal disease. However, there is strong evidence that cytopathic viruses (CP) are derived from non-cytopathic (NCP) viruses by mutation within the animal rather than introduction into the herd (Bolin, 1995).

Blood feeding flies, contaminated A.I. equipment and rectal examination gloves can be important sources of spread of infection. Infection can remain persistent in herds from generation to generation successively through Trans-placental infection from PI cow to the foctus which becomes neonatally infected newborn calf persistently remaining infected throughout its life. Unvaccinated animals, improperly vaccinated animals or animals whose immunity has waned, are the most susceptible to infection and potential for clinical disease. Even the vaccinated animals may be susceptible, if the field strain of the virus of BVD is district from vaccine strain and persistently infected (PI) animals can develop mucosal disease, when they get superinfected with cytopathic virus. P.I. calves are infected during early foetal life and are born sero negative and immunotolerant to the specific strain of the virus in their tissues but they will respond immunologically to other pathogens.

Pathogenesis

The consequences of infection with BVDV depend on the status of the animal:

i) In immunocompetent sero-negetive, non-pregnant animals; sub-clinical BVD occurs after the waning of colostral immunity. There is no clinical manifestation of the disease and SN antibodies develop, which eliminate the disease virus or there can be evidence of mild disease with slight fever and diarrhoeal symptoms. Sometimes, severe disease is observed clinically in such animals at the later stage at the age of 6 months to 1 year. Non-cytopathic type II isolates may cause peracute bovine virus diarrhoea with high fatality in herds of animals with inadequate vaccination progrmme in which P.I. animals are introduced recently.

Thrombocytopenia and haemorrhagic syndrome is quite common in this category of animals, in which Type II cytopathic virus strain is associated. There is evidence that post-natal BVDV infections of cattle can cause immune suppression and enhance the development of other infections disease (Potgieter, 1995). The lesions of BVDV in cattle suggest immune suppression because of lymphoid depletion and neutropenia, even some live BVDV vaccines are immune suppressive in calves or may potentiate concurrent infections. Primary post-natal infections cause a transient reduction in the absolute numbers of T and B lymphocytes and in percentage of T-lymphocytes. In outbreaks of respiratory disease of calves and adult cattle by multiple viral infections including Pasturella haemolytica, Infections, Bovine Rhinotracheitis (IBR) and PI-3 influeza infection, BVDV is also associated which is incriminated as playing immunosuppressive role. It is postulated that BVDV precipitates secondary bacterial and viral infections in lungs of calves which is responsible for high mortality due to pneumonia caused by these infections.

ii) In immune competent seronegative pregnant cattle, BVDV can cause significant early reproductive loss including failure of fertilization, embryonic mortality and abortion. Infection of foetus between 42 and 125 days may result into persistently infected (PI) foetuses which are carried to terms and calf may be born a live thrive normally or be unthrifty.

Clinical findings : The following clinical findings may be apparent in this disease in various forms occurring in different situations mentioned in the paragraphs contained under "Pathogenesis" as below:

a) In case of subclinical form of BVD mild disease with high morbidity and low fatality is observed. Mild fever, leucopenia, inappetence and mild diarrhoea followed by rapid recovery is observed. This form is observed in immune competent seronegative cattle affected in post-natal life. This is referred to in literature as "Bovine Virus Diarrhoea".

b) Peracute bovine virus diarrhoea is highly fatal enteric form of the disease in which seronegative unvaccinated or inadequately vaccinated cattle of all age-groups from calves to adults were involved and the outbreaks were caused by highly virulent isolates of Type II virus. Disease occurred in

Quebec and pensylvania in USA (1998) and Ontario in Canada (1992) and Britain (1994). The source of virus in all these outbreaks was importation of animals from abroad with the common history of unvaccinated herds. The outbreaks were slowly progressive and lasted for several weeks with severe depression, respiratory distress, anorexia, profuse watery diarrhoea, dysentery, high fever, conjunctivitis and loss of milk production. Oral erosions are inconsistent and abortions occur in late pregnancy. Morbidity of 40% and mortality rate upto 25% was observed. Persistently infected (PI) calves were born several months following the outbreaks.

iii) **Acute mucosal disease :** This form of the disease occurs in animals from 6-24 months of age, which were infected during early foetal life. Morbility is low (5-25%) but fatality is high (over 90%), sporadic cases may occur over several weeks or months (Lee, S.C. *et al.*, 1994). It is the P.I. animals in the herd which develop mucosal disease. After the outbreak in the herd, No. of P.I. animals decline in the subsequent years and the breeding females develop acquired immunity.

Anorexia, drepression, drooling saliva and high fever (40-41^{0}C), absence of ruminal contractions and profuse watery diarrhoea after onset of clinical illness are major symptoms. Mucous and blood in faces which are foetid smelling are seen.Straining during defaecation with fibrinous intestinal contents is common. Shallow erosions inside lips, on gums, dental pad, hard pallet and comminssures of mouth as well as on tongue occur which become confluent afterwards, are quite common. Mucopurutent nasal discharge, lacrimation and corneal ocdema are usual symptoms. Deaths with in 5-7 days may occur.

iv) **Thrombocytopenia and Haemorrhagic disease :** This is associated with BVDV but wheather animals in this case are previously P.I. or not are not certain. The disease is characterized by bloody diarrhoea, patechial or echymotic haernorrhages on mucous membranes, prolonged haemorrhages from infection sites or from insect bites are common. In some cases epistaxis is also seen. Thrombocytic (platelets) counts are low with fever, diarrhoea and ruminal stasis is common 25% case fatality is seen.

v) **Chronic mucosal disease :** Some acute cases turn chronic and may show intermittent bouts of the disease with diarrhoea, inappetence, progressive imanciation, rough dry hair coat, chronic bloat, hoof deformities, chronic mouth and skin erosions especially around scrotum, perineum, preputied orifice and vulva as well as between legs and skin horn junction/inter digital cleft and at heels, which do not heal easily.

vi) **Unthrifty P.I. calves :** Calves born P.I. may be dwarf as compared with their normal contemporaries. They show curly hairs on their body and survive for long time, when finally they develop fatal mucosal disease after several months (Larsson *et al.* 1991).

vii) **Reproductive failure and Neonatal disease :** BVDV infection of susceptible breeding females result in conception failure, increased embryonic mortality, foetal mummification, abortion, premature births, still births, birth of stunted calves and P.I. calves which may develop mucosal disease subsequently.

Diagnosis : For confirmative diagnosis, virus isolation and serological tests are needed.

Bovine kidney cultures can be used for virus isolation attempts. Generally BVDV is non-cytopathic and it can be identified by indirect immune peroxidase staining of the infected cell cultures in micro titration plates (Brock, 1995). The diagnosis of acute infections must be done as early as 3 days after infection to 8-10 days after infection. Whole blood sample is used for separation of "Buffy coat" of WBC which contain virus. This is used for virus isolation in cell cultures.

Paired sera samples (from acute and convalescent stage samples) collected 30 days after infection are used to detect the rising antibody titers against BVDV, using serum Neutralization test in cell culture by using cytopathic BVDV for confirmative diagnosis. Thymus, Thyroid, Payers patches, spleen, lung or mesenteric lymph-nodes are used for virus isolation by using FAT, PCR or *insitu* hybrid probing tests. ELISA is used for sero diagnosis which co-relates well with SN test. Nasal swabs, buffy coats are used for acute and peracute case diagnosis.

In abortion, the dam may have already sero converted before abortion and hence, there may be no sero conversion between acute and convalescent sera However, some aborted females may be serologically positive which confirms intrauterine infection in the later part of foetal life. If dam is negative, BVDV as a cause of abortion can be ruled out. Calves born with congenital defects may have antibodies but blood sample must be taken before ingestion of colostrums. Persistently Infected (PI) calves can be identified by collection of sequential buffy coat samples, 30 days apart for showing virus by isolation in cell cultures. Most PI animals are seronegative after waning of colostral immunity but they may develop SN antibodies to heterologous strains of BVDV.

Control and Prevention of BVD – MDC

Success of control and prevention depends on:

1. Prevention of introduction P.I. animals in herds as well as their elimination, if already present in herd.
2. Prevention of introduction of infection through fomites.
3. Vaccination of breeders before breeding.

P.I. animals can be detected by sequential blood (Buffy coat) testing as described earlier. These P.I. animals should be eliminated from herd by destruction. After elimination of P.I. animals, whole herd should be vaccinated and when ever fresh animals are introduced, they should be tested for P.I. status. A.I. units should also test their bulls for P.I. status before introduction for use.

Important strategy for successful control is to vaccinate breeding females at least several weeks before breeding (Bolin, S. 1995). All females in breeding programme should have antibodies to BVD before they become pregnant in order to prevent the foetus from natural infection for the entire gestational period. Modified live vaccines (MLVS) usually contain a single strain of attenuated cytopathic virus, such as BVDV NADL, BVDV-Singer and BVDV-C24C. While most inactivated vaccines contain cytopathic or non-cytopathic strains.

Above mentioned live vaccines have capacity to replicate restrictively with reduced virulence and shedding. They are less expensive; as small dose is needed being live and only single vaccination is sufficient for immunization and takes care of wide range of antigenic varients. Duration of immunity is more than one a year or several years in many animals.

Disadvantages of MLV vaccines are:

1. The attenuation of vaccine virus may not be sufficient which may be responsible for some mishaps like outbreaks.
2. MLVS are facto pathogenic and hence, should not be used in pregnant animals especially between 51 to 190 days of pregnancy which may result into transplacental infection and consequences like abortions, congenital abnormalities, growth retardation of calves and P.I. animals may be the end result due to immunotollerant status.
3. Immunosuppression and genetic recombination are other potential risks with MLVS.

A temperature sensitive BVDV vaccine is now available with no clinical signs of the disease and no side consequences like leucopenia in experimental animals. Disadvantages of inactivated BVDV vaccine are high cost and need for booster vaccination.

Vaccination strategy

Based on above mentioned knowledge the following vaccination strategy can be adopted:

1. Use of MLV vaccine in all calves above 4-6 months of age for prevention of foetal infection in dairy herds.
2. Immunization of heifers before breeding so that the virus does not reach the foetus before 120 days of gestation (i.e. immunization 3 to 6 weeks before breeding). This will avoid immunotollerance and P.I. in their foetuses.
3. Immunization of pregnant animals will have to be undertaken to take care of recently reported peracute form of the disease described earlier in Britain, Canada and U.S.A. by using inactivated BVD vaccines as live vaccines are dangerous at that stage.

Immunization without vaccines

Controlled exposure of non-pregnant heifers to a P.I. carrier animal for 12 days on pasture results in sero conversion by about 20th day (Cook *et al.*, 1990). Subcutaneous, intranasal or conjunctival inoculation of infective blood from known P.I. animal into yearling heifers also results in sero convertion without any clinical illness. This practice is used for successful immunization of dairy herds in Australia where BVDV vaccine is not available. This practice is based on the scientific fact that P.I. animal is only harmful for transmission of infection and clinical disease to foetuses of non-vaccinated pregnant heifers.

Eradication of BVD infection

This is now being considered in some Scandinavian countries like Finland and Denmark. The success will depend on: 1) Detection of P.I. animals and their elimination from the herds, 2) Identification of non-infected herds using antibody detection tests and then monitoring their disease free status by continuous antibody testing programme. Testing of bulk milk for antibody is useful to indicate the "infection status" of the herds and 3) Prevention of the infection of non-infected herds.

The Danish programme of Eradication of BVDV (Pasman *et al.* 1994) has recommended following steps:

1. Bulk milk testing of individual herds at intervals of 6-9 months, using indirect ELISA test for antibody detection from Bulk herd milk samples.
2. Random blood testing of nine animals (3 cows, 3 pregnant heifers and 3 calves above 8 months of age) each from each herd.
3. Random blood testing of 3 young animals older than 8 months for virus and antibodies.
4. Individual testing of animals in suspected P.I. herds to identify than (by using ELISA for virus detection in P.I. animals).

The measures of prevent introduction of infection into herds include:

1. Only tested P.I. negative animals are admitted to be introduced in herds.
2. Antibody positive pregnant animals introduced into herd should be isolated at calving and their progeny not admitted to the herd unless test is negative for P.I.
3. Newly introduced animals should be kept isolated for at least 3 weeks.

4. On pasture, animals are not allowed to come in contact with P.I. animals.
5. Animals sent to exhibition or auction sales should be blood tested for P.I. before accepting them back to the herds.

Mucosal Disease Complex: Indian Scenario

BVD/MDC was unknown in India upto late fifties of twentieth century. However, Rinderpest disease which has some similarities in the symptomatology with BVD/MDC was prevailing in India on a wide scale before fifties and it was taking a heavy tole of dairy cattle and buffaloes. As described in a chapter on Rinderpest, Govt. of India undertook an eradication programme for control of Rinderpest in the country post independence under first five years plan and wide scale Anti-Rinderpest vaccination programme using live attenuated goat tissue freeze-dried vaccine was undertaken throughout the country with an aim to eradicate this disease by 1965. This step was quite effective and by 1959-60, Rinderpest outbreaks were fully under control in most parts of the country.

However, during 1959-60, Disease Investigation Section of Maharashtra Govt. received some reports of Rinderpest like disease outbreaks in Maharashtra State in cattle and buffaloes inspite of R.P. Vaccination. Dr. Sapre, S.N. (Dy. Director, DIS,Pune) reported 1st R.P. like outbreak in cattle at Village Shewagebahal near Ajanta caves in Aurangabad District which, he designated as "**Ajanta Disease**" as even though the disease symptoms were simulating mild Rinderpest like, the incidence of the disease occurred in certainly known R.P. vaccinated animals.

He reported outbreaks in cattle with symptoms of anorexia, rough body coat, high fever upto 104^{0}F followed by severe diarrhoea with foetid odour, mucous, blood and enteric casts in faeces. The mucopurulent nose and eye discharge, branlike deposits on shallow mouth erosions and valvo-vaginitis were other symptoms occurring in these cattle with history of known R.P. vaccination. He described occurrence of erosive lesions on mucosa of abomasum, at illiopyrolic junction and presence of longitudinal haemorrhages (unlike horizontal haemorrhages described as Zebra markings in case of Rinderpest) in rectum, swelling of mescentric lymph-nodes with haemorrhages, during postmortem examination.

Sapre, S.N., Chaudhari, P.G. and Kulkarni, S.G. of D.I.S., Pune described in their outbreaks reports described similar R.P. like outbreaks during their working at later on during 1961-62 in both cattle and buffaloes. They developed AGPT test in Petriplates, using Noble Agar 1% in normal saline with merthiolate as preservative for production of gel used in the test known hyperimmune serum against swine fever (lapinised) virus sapinised swine fever vaccine virus (Payer's patch, spleen and pancreas pooled material from rabbit infected with swin fever vaccine virus) as known Antigen for diagnosis of Mucosal Disease in unknown antigenic material from suspected Mucosal disease (So, called "Ajanta Disease") from cattle/buffaloes. They could demonstrate line of "identity" between swine fever antigen and unknown lymph-node/spleen antigen samples from affected field cases suspected to be died of mucosal disease and thus, arrived at diagnosis of Mucosal Disease in those field cases as per method described by Derbyshire (1962). Sapre, S.N. also sent some sera samples (Paired) to Animal Disease Research Laboratory (Reference Lab for mucosal disease) weybridge, Surrey England (UK) and received confirmation of Mucosal Disease antibodies in the same which confirmed the diagnosis of Mucosal Disease in those particular outbreaks, establishing existence of Mucosal Disease in India.

The Author (Pandit S.V.) and Apte V.H. while working at Disease investigation section, Maharashtra State, Pune during 1964-66 also investigated some outbreaks of R.P. like Disease in buffaloes near Arey Milk Colony, Goregaon, Bombay and at Ambad near Aurangabad, in which the mild chronic type of R.P. like disease with unusual skin lesions, vulvo vaginitis and lesions on scrotum, preputial sheeth, etc. were observed. These lesions had a close resemblance with the lesions of Chronic Mucosal Disease described under Clinical findings in this chapter.

In view of recording of good number of R.P. like outbreaks in buffaloes especially at Arey Milk Colony and round about buffaloes stables in Bombay suburban district and in Pune, inspite of R.P. vaccination programme, Govt. of Maharashtra established two units for Mucosal Disease Control under Disease investigation section M.S. Pune, one at Goregaon near Arey Milk Colony and one at D.I.S., Pune. These units started production of hyperimmune serum in buffaloes by serial inoculation of spleen and mesenteric lymph-node material suspension (source of material was those tissues from buffaloes died due to suspected mucosal disease) inactivated with 0.5% formaldehyde and collection of hyperimmunised serum by bleeding of these animals 20 days after last (3rd) inoculation. This serum when given along with 10% glucose saline (Serum quantity 100 ml and glucose saline 1 to 5 litres) by intravenous route was found to cure the animals ailing with suspected Mucosal Disease (showing R.P. like symptoms including diarrhoea & fever). However, the diagnosis of MDC was based symptomatically and prior R.P. vaccination history in them. Large number of such affected animals were saved by this empirical treatment from the disease and deaths during the period from 1964-67.

Even though large number of outbreaks of R.P. like disease suspected to be due to Mucosal Disease were being detected during our field investigations at Disease Investigation Section, Maharashtra State, Pune the confirmation of Mucosal Disease/BVDV in the same was lacking due to the absence of availability of confirmatory diagnostic test with known reference antiserum and antigen for BVDV at D.I.S., Pune. Moreover, the known susceptible animals or cell culture system for isolation of BVDV/RP was not available at D.I.S., Pune for confirmative diagnosis in mid-nineteen sixties.

ICAR sanctioned a combined scheme for Diagnosis of MDC and BT diseases which worked for 3 years during 1965-67 at D.I.S., Pune. During this period, we at DIS screened 6 outbreaks of R.P. like disease suspected as "Mucosal Disease" by cross immunity test in buffaloes calves above 6 months of age and proved that at least these 5 outbreaks were that of "Rinderpest" and were not due to mucosal disease. However, this evidence was not considered as enough to finally prove the presence or absence of mucosal disease in India, as number of outbreaks screened were only five, out of which only a small part of total number of outbreaks in India being recorded yearly as R.P. like disease outbreaks.

During 1994-95, workers at BAIF'S vaccine production unit at Wagholi near Pune, came across acute type of Mucosal Disease in an exotic herd near Pune showing typical mucosal disease symptoms including high fever, mouth lesions and severe diarrhoea with foetid odour containing mucous and blood, nasal discharge and mucopurulent eye discharge, few pregnant animals aborted. They could isolate a cytopathic virus in MDBK cell line (Bovine kidney cell line) with typical inclusion bodies on inoculation of the whole blood / serum from mother cow and still born foetus. From circumstantial evidence, it seems that there were no new introductions of fresh calves / animals in the recent past in the herd and hence, it seems likely that the herd was having persistently in infected (P.I.) old animals without showing any clinical disease for few generations after their importation in past and non-cytopathic BVD infection in these P.I. Animals might have undergone slow mutation into cytopathic virus which might have produced "Super infection" and resulted into acute Mucosal Disease.

Disease control

Experimental inactivated (formation killed) autogenous vaccine was produced which was adjunvanted alhydrogel adsorbed vaccine using this cytopathic cell cultured virus (identified as BVD by AGPT using swine fever hyperimmune serum in rabbits and swine fever lapinised virus known as positive antigen). This vaccine was reported to have given good protection to other in contact clinically unaffected herd and avoided further losses due to this disease (Personal communication).

In India, even though various manifestations of BVD including Acute Mucosal Disease, chronic skin form of Mucosal Disease and existence of P.I. animals, etc. were reported /observed, proved evidence of immune suppression due to BVD has not yet come forth. However, if we fish out old literature and our own old observations, it is sure that many reports of neonatal mortality in crossbred exotic cattle as well as high bred buffalo calves due to multiple bacterial infections of respiratory and alimentary tract (pneumonia and enteritis) have been recorded which includes pathogenic *E. coli*, *Salmonella* and *Pasturella multoceda/haemolytica*, strepto-staphylococcal infections as well as rotavirus and cornavirus infections (Pathak *et al.*, 1992). As crossbred cattle and buffaloes have been shown to have suffered from Mucosal Disease Complex/BVD, under the literature referred to in this chapter in previous paragraphs, it seems that it is quite likely that these bacterial/viral causes of neonatal calf mortality might be only secondary causes of calf mortality. The original precipitating cause might be the neonatal BVD which might be responsible for immune suppression which results into flaring up of bacterial/viral infections and subsequent calf mortality as the crossbred, exotic cattle and buffalo herds harbour BVDV PI infection. This needs further detailed investigation to know the real truth.

Suggested Reading

Bolin S.R. (1995). Control of bovine viral diarrhoea infection by use of vaccination. Veterinary Clinics of North America: Food Animal Practice. 11: 615-625.

Brock, K.V. (1995). Diagnosis of bovine viral diarrhoea virus infections. Vet Clin North Am Food Anim Pract. 11: 549-61.

Cook, L.G., Littlejohns, I.R., Jessep, T.M., (1990). Induced sero-conversion in heifers with a field strain of bovine pestivirus—a comparison of methods and doses. Aust. Vet. J. 67: 393–395.

Darbyshire, J.H. (1962). Agar Gel Diffusion Studies with a Mucosal Disease of cattle, Res. Vet. Sci. 3: 118-120.

Pasman, E.J., Dijkhuizen, A.A. and Wentink, G.H. (1994). A state-transition model to simulate the economics of bovine virus diarrhoea control. Prev Vet Med 20: 269-277.

Potgieter L.N. (1995). Immunology of bovine viral diarrhoea virus. Veterinary Clinics of North America: Food Animal Practice; 3: 501-520.

Radostits, O.M., Gay, C.C., Blood, D.C. & Hinchcliff, K.W. (2000). Veterinary Medicine: A Textbook of the Diseases of Cattle, Sheep, Pigs, Goats and Horses, 9th.W.B. Saunders Company Ltd. 1173-1184 pp

Ridpath, J.F., Bolin, S.R. & Dubovi, E.J. (1994). Segregation of bovine viral diarrhoea virus into genotypes. Virology 205: 66-74.

Taylor L.F., Van Donkersgoed J., Dubovi E.J., Harland R.J., Van den Herk J.V., Ribble C.S. and Janzen E.D. (1995). The prevalence of bovine viral diarrhoea virus infection in a population of feedlot calves in western Canada.Can J Vet Res. 59(2): 87-93.

❑❑❑

Chapter 4

Cow Pox, Buffalo Pox and Pseudo-Cow Pox Infections

Cow pox is a virus disease of cattle and is characterized by pox lesions on skin especially on teats and udder (lower part), which may spread to insides of the thighs and rarely to perineum, vulva and mouth. Suckling calves may develop lesions around the mouth and bulls may develop lesions on the scrotum.

About the virus

Cow pox is a member of the genus *Orthopox* virus in the family *Poxiviridae*. Other members of this genus include horse pox, small pox and vaccinia virus. All orthopox viruses are extremely similar antigenically but can be differentiated by phenotypic and genetic tests. Buffalo pox virus is also related closely to cow pox antigenically (Iwad P.I. *et al.* 1981). However, the Buffalo pox virus experimental infection in buffalo calves has a shorter course of progress of the disease as compared to cow pox virus course. In January, 2009, few human cases of pox lesions were noticed in Kolhapur district. It was from buffaloes, that the infection was traced. Vaccina virus i.e. small pox vaccine virus is antigenically close to the cow pox virus but is different virus. All these orthopox viruses can be grown on chrioallantoic membrane of embryonated hens eggs, which show similar morphology of pox lesions on the chorio-allantoic membrane but when subjected to AGPT against homologous and heterologous hyperimmune sera, they exhibit common precipitation lines which indicates sharing of common antigen but also exhibit separate precipitation lines which prove their identity as separate "species".

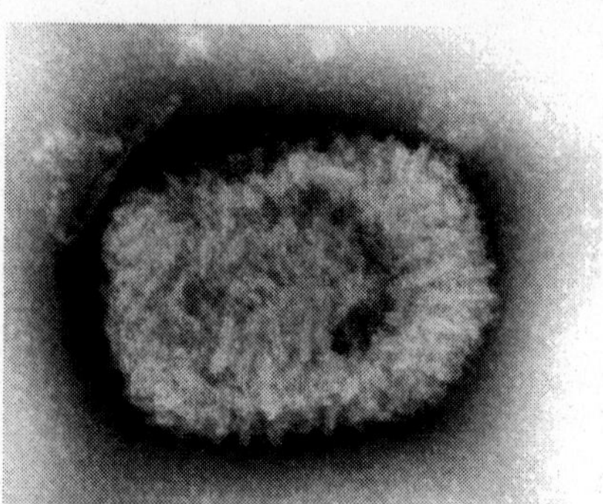

Fig. 1: Structure of Cow Pox Virus

Preudo-cow pox is a separate virus belonging to a genus *Parapox* virus of the family *Poxviridae*. The other viral diseases of the genus are Pustular dermatitis (Orf) virus of sheep (contagious ecthyma) and viral pustular dermatitis of horses are the other members. This virus even though causes similar clinical disease with very close resemblence to cow pox in the cows; it is antigenically very distinct from cow pox vaccinia-virus group. It is possible that para pox virus may be a single virus adapted to different species of ruminants.

About the disease epidemiology and transmission

Spread of the disease from herd to herd may be through introduction of infected animals but spread from animal to animal is generally through milker's hands or through teat cups during milking. The virus enters the skin of the teat through minute injuries. The virus can fly through flies least to another cow from cow to cow.

Pathogenesis

A total of 5 stages of typical pox eruption can be observed. After 3 to 6 days of incubation period, roseolar erythema is followed by light coloured firm raised papules with a zone of hyperemia around the base. This is followed by yellow blister like vesciculation which subsequently develops into pustule topped with a thick red tenacious scab. The lesions are essentially hyperplastic.

Clinical findings

The vesicular lesions get ruptured during the milking. True cow pox scabs are 1-2 c.m. in diameter and are thick, tenacious and yellowish brown to red in colour. But in milking cows, typical scabs do not form but get ruptured and are replaced by deep ulceration. Lesions spread from teats to lower part of udder. Milk let down is interfered due to soreness of the lesions by handling during milking. Secondary infection of lesions lead to spread of bacterial infection from soiled flooring to the glandular tissue of udder via teat canal which leads to mastitis. Pox lesions may take 2 to 3 weeks to heal or even it may take a month or more to complete the course due to secondary spread of the pox. Lesions can spread to skin between the two thighs and perineum. Sucking calves may get mouth or lip lesions.

Diagnosis

Scab material or swabs from sour cow pox lesions can be used for virus isolation in egg embryos by chorioallentoic inoculation and by use of bovine kidney cultures and demonstration of intracytoplasmic inclusion and subsequent AGPT or electron microscopy.

Control

Treatment of affected cows and their isolation from herd. Milking them to the last and use of disposable paper towels for udder washing and disinfection of teat cups, if machine milking, etc. can be preventive for further spread of disease in herd. The prevalence and significance of the disease in cattle is to warrant the development of vaccine.

Zoonosis

Milkers nodulesis a clinical manifestation of the disease Pseudo-cow pox in human beings. Few pox lesions can develop at milker's hands due to true cow pox. Small pox vaccination using cow lymph origin vaccine virus can spread accidental infection to cows through freshly vaccinated milkers. It was the milk maid Sarab Nelms who is reported to have uttered "I have cow pox, so need not worry small pox". This reply led Edward Jenner to evolve epoch making world's first ever vaccine against small pox (May, 1878). It can be recalled that milkman's immunity to small pox led Jenner for epoch making discovery of development of vaccinea virus for using vaccine against small pox for human.

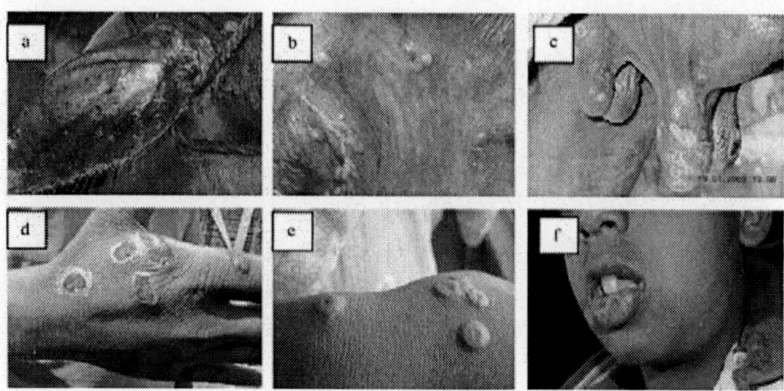

Fig. 2: Pox lesions

Cow / Buffalo pox: Indian Scenario

Buffalo pox is a highly contagious acute viral disease of buffaloes, with 80% morbidity in affected herd population (Bhanuprakash *et al.*, 2012). The first recorded incidence of buffalo pox was reported in Lahore of undivided part of India in 1934 (Sharma, 1934). Only sporadic outbreaks occur in cow herds throughout India with no much economic significance. However, Chaudhari, P.G. (1963-65) from Disease investigation section, Maharashtra State, Poona reported few outbreaks of buffalo pox from Jalgaon district and Bombay (Goregaon) with significant losses in milk (personal communication).Use of experimental Autogenous formalin inactivated vaccine produced by egg embryo chorio-allantoic membrane grown virus suspension controlled the disease spread effectively as reported by him and was followed by frequent reports of outbreaks from various states of India (Sehgal *et al.*, 1977). Disease also reported from Nepal, Bangladesh, Pakistan and Egypt (Singh *et al.*, 2007a). In buffaloes, the disease outbreaks may be allied with elevated morbidity rate and loss of production (Chandra *et al.*, 1987; Singh *et al.*, 2006a, 2006b, 2006c, 2007a). The severity of the infection ranges from localized mild form to the infrequent severe generalized form. The infection poses economic impact due to reduced milk yield resultant from mastitis in milch animal and reduced working capacity in draft animals (Bhanuprakash *et al.*, 2010c). Although buffaloes are commonly infected, cattle and human beings are infrequently get infection. Transmission potential of BPXV includes cattle, buffaloes and humans imply the potential re-emergence of the infection in Indian subcontinent as like VLV outbreaks observed in other countries in recent years (Singh *et al.*, 2012).

Suggested Reading

Bhanuprakash, V., Venkatesan, G., Balamurugan, V., Hosamani, M., Yogisharadhya, R., Gandhale, P., Reddy, K.V., Damle, A.S., Kher, H.N., Chandel, B.S., Chauhan, H.C., Singh, R.K. (2010c). Zoonotic infections of buffalo pox in India. Zoon. Public Health. 57(7–8): 149–155.

Bhanuprakash V., Hosamani M., Venkatesan G., Balamurugan V., Yogisharadhya R., Singh R.K. (2012). Animal poxvirus vaccines: a comprehensive review. Exp. Rev. Vaccines. 11(11): 1355–1374. http://dx.doi.org/10.1586/erv.12.116.

Chandra, R., Garg S.K., Rana U.V.S., Rao V.D.P. (1987). Pox infection in buffaloes. Farm Anim. 2: 57–59.

Iwad, F.I., Saber, M.S., Amin, M.M. and Yousuf, H.M. (1981). Some epizootiological studies on buffalopox in Egypt. *Acta Veterinarica Yugoslavia* **31**: 41–47.

Sehgal C.L., Ray S.N., Ghosh T.K., Arora R.R. (1977). Investigation of an outbreak of buffalo pox in animals and human beings in Dhulia District, Maharashtra. J. Laboratory Studies J. Comp. Dis. 9: 171-176.

Singh R.K., Hosamani M., Balamurugan V., Satheesh C.C., Shingal K.R., Tatwarti S.B., Bambal R.G., Ramteke V., Yadav M.P. (2006a). An outbreak of Buffalopox in buffalo (Bubalus bubalis) dairy herds in Aurangabad, India. Sci. Tech. Rev. O.I.E. 25: 981–987.

Singh R.K., Hosamani M., Balamurugan V., Satheesh C.C., Rasool T.J., Yadav M.P. (2006b). Comparative sequence analysis of envelope protein genes of Indian Buffalo pox virus isolates. Arch. Virol. 151: 1995–2005. http://dx.doi.org/10.1007/ s00705-006-0761-8

Singh R.K., Balamurugan V., Hosamani M., Satheesh C.C., Rasool T.J., Yadav M.P. (2006c). Comparative polypeptide profiling: isolation, propagation and purification of Indian isolates of buffalo pox virus. J. Anim. Vet. Advs. 5: 260–265.

Singh R.K., Hosamani M, Balamurugan V, Bhanuprakash V, Rasool T.J., Yadav M.P. (2007a). Buffalo pox: An emerging and re-emerging zoonosis. Anim. Health Res. Rev. 8(1): 105–114. http://dx.doi.org/10.1017/S1466252307001259

Singh R.K., Balamurugan V., Bhanuprakash V., Venkatesan G., Hosamani M. (2012). Emergence and re-emergence of vaccinia-like viruses: global scenario and perspectives. Indian J. Virol. 23(1): 1–11. http://dx.doi.org/10.1007/ s13337-012-0068-1

□□□

Chapter 5

Sheep Pox, Goat Pox and Sheep & Goat Pox Infections and Contagious Ecthyma (Orf).

Pox disease of caprines including sheep and goats is generally species specific in nature but in Kenya, the same viral agent causes disease both in sheep and goats naturally. The sheep pox, goat pox and Kenyan sheep and goat pox disease are collectively called as *Capripox* infections (Carn, 1993). All members of the genus *Capriox* virus are closely related on the genome mapping and can cross species barriers in experimental infections (Bhat, 1993). Recombinations may occur naturally between isolates from different host species (Gershon *et al.*, 1989).

Disease occurrence

Sheep pox and goat pox is wide spread in Africa, Middle East and Israel,all countries of old Soviet Union, China, Indian Sub-continent (India, Bangladesh and Pakistan) occurring as endemic disease. Sporadic outbreaks occur in South European countries. U.S.A. Canada, Australia, South America is free from the disease. Sheep and goat pox are the most serious out of all the pox disease in animals with outbreaks causing mortality upto 30 to 50 per cent of the affected animals.

Epidemiology and transmission

The disease is highly contagious and occurs by contact with infected animals and contaminated articles. Virus can also spread by inhalation of dust and dandruff from affected animals by the susceptible animals. Even flies of the species *Stomoxys calcitrans* can spread the infection through biting of the skin of animals.

Imported exotic sheep, such as Merinos from disease free countries to the endemic countries may result into a very severe sheep pox disease with very high mortality. Young lambs are also highly susceptible to sheep/goat pox. In India and Middle East including Israel, sheep pox and goat pox are host specific but Kenyan sheep and goat are affected with the same capripox virus.

Pathogenesis

After the inhalation of the virus through nose, viremia takes place through respiratory tract mucosa and virus spreads in respiratory organs, esophagus, nasopharynx, abomasum, body skin and reproductive tract, etc. and this produce specific lesions (Pock lesions), the incubation period is between 7 to 14 days, when highest viremia is observed. Pox lesion develops from initial papular stage of nodular stage which becomes vesicular, pustular and finally scab formation takes place. Nodules may become tumour like masses (Afshar. *et al.* 1986).

Disease Symptoms and Postmortem findings

In lambs, the disease takes a malignant form with marked depression and prostration. They show high fever with eye and nasal discharge and may die before development of typical pox lesions. In adult sheep, skin lesions appear on unwooled skin and on buccal, respiratory, digestive and wrongenital tract mucosae, with mortality upto 50%. In benign form more common in adult sheep, pox lesions occur only under the tail and without any systemic reaction.

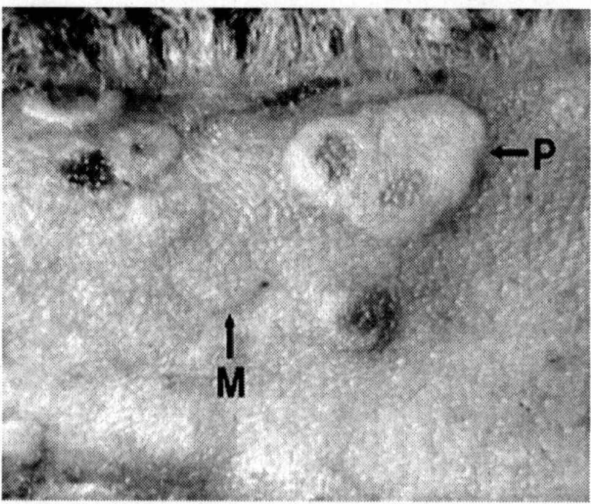

Fig. 1: Sheep pox lesions

Goat pox in sheep is some times more severe than sheep pox in sheep and lesions may occur on lips, oral mucosa, teats and udder. Goat pox in goats exhibit similar symptoms as sheep pox in sheep. Sheep pox and goat pox in the respective species may result into secondary bacterial infection of glandular tissue of the udder, as bacteria can get easy access into udder through wounds created on teats due to pox disease.

In the malignant form of the disease, pox lesions are extended into the mouth, pharynx, larynx, vagina, abomasums, arches with catarrhal pneumonia haemorrhagic enteritis may also develop.

Diagnosis / Differential Diagnosis

The scabs and ordema fluid swabs from pox lesions can be used for isolation of sheep/goat pox virus in cell culture (sheep or goat kidney culture). The intranuclear inclusion bodies can be demonstrated in Leighton tube cover slip cultures by May grunwald giema staining. The specificity of inclusions can be proved by fluorescent antibody staining of these smears. Indirect fluorescent antibody test or Agar Gel Immune Diffusion (AGID) test are the preferred serological techniques for detecting rising antibody titres in paired sera samples for confirmation of sheep/goat pox but cross reaction occurs in sera from para pox (contagious pastuler dermatitis orf-virus infection. However, virus specific analysis of antibody response by western blot analysis can differentiate these infections specifically (Chand, *et al.*, 1994).

Control of Sheep / Goat pox

In disease free countries, ban/restriction on importation of sheep or goats along with quarrantine measures are followed strictly and if disease occurs, stamping out and complete disinfection programme on affected premises is followed for successful control of the disease. Such programme is quite successful in countries like Australia, Newzealand,USA and Canada. Sheep/Goat pox in endemic countries is controlled by vaccination with single capripox (either sheep pox or goat pox strain) strain vaccine which gives protection across all the species of sheep and goats (Carn,1993) against both sheep pox and goat pox viruses.

Most of the capripox vaccines are attenuated live vaccines and appear to give excellent protection for a period of over one year.

Vaccinations are carried out in lambs/kids above 6 months of age after waning of maternal immunity due to colostral feeding, which interferes with vaccinal protection (Carn, 1993 and Kitching *et al.*, 1987).

Indian Scenario

In India, sheep pox and goat pox infections are endemic since ancient times. There is an excellent review on sheep pox by Singh *et. al.* (1979). Contagious Pastular Dermatitis (CPD or Orf) with 100% morbidity and 1% fatality is recorded in goats with scab lesions on commissures of lips and mouth lesions in Madhya Pradesh (MP) by Sharma and Bhatia (1959) and Kumar *et al.* (1974). They also reported high fever (105^0 to 108^0F) and presence of macopurulent nasal discharge. Joshi *et al.* (1996) isolated virus from scab lesions material by CAM inoculation of embryonated eggs.

Rao (1938) described development of sheep pox vaccine at Imperial Bacteriological Laboratory (IVRI) at Mukteshwar using scabs of the stock sheep pox which forms the seed in preparation of sheep and goat pox vaccine. 10% stock scabs of sheep pox virus suspension were inoculated linearly on scarified portion of belly of susceptible sheep, previously depilated. The scabs from the lesions developed 6 days postinoculation are collected dried and powdered and put in 0.3 gm quantity in ampoules. This vaccine is used for prophylaxis against sheep and goat pox after trituration in glycerine saline.

Sheep pox vaccine using Orya strain of sheep pox was being manufactured at IVBP, Pune IVRI, Izatnagar and some other state vety. biological production units during sixties and early seventies of twentieth century. However, it was found that the virus of sheep pox is lost by continuous serial passaging of the seed and only staphylococcus culture has remained in the vaccine and hence, this vaccine production was discontinued.

Sheep pox, in organized farms, was more serious due to the presence of imported exotic merino and other sheep and sanen goats which were more susceptible to sheeps goat pox viruses. For example, at Central Sheep and Wool Research Institute, Avikanagar (South East Rajasthan), 6 outbreaks of sheep pox were recorded in a period of 25 years (1969-1993) with major outbreaks in 1969; 1975-76 and 1980-81 with interval of outbreak being 5 years. At Bikaner Centre (North Rajasthan), 5 outbreaks were recorded in 19 years (1975-93) with interval of 1-2 years between the outbreaks. The annual vaccination of sheep with attenuated cell cultured vaccine of sheep pox (Ranipet strain) from 1982 onwards at Avikanagar and from 1988 onwards at Bikaner resulted into no outbreak at Avikanagar and disease incidence of only one flock in 1992, at Bikaner (M.M. Sharma *et al.*, 1994; Report on XIV Annual Conference & National Symposium of Ind. Asso. Vet. Microbiologists and Immunologists and Specialists Inf. Dis. At NCL, Pune, pp. 52, 1994). Bakshi *et al.*, 1994 (same report on symposium at NCL, Pune 1994 pp. 52 mentioned above) reported successful control of sheep pox in field trial of BAIF'S live tissue cultured sheep pox vaccine using Ramiyar strain of sheep pox live attenuated virus received from Razi Institute (Experimental Vaccine field trial).

Bhattacharya and Nagi (1994) reported studies on BPL inactivated aluminium hydroxide gel adjuvanted vaccine prepared from virulent "Uttarkashi" strain of Goat Pox Virus produced at Deptt. of Vet. Microbiology, B.C.K. Vidyapeeth Mohanpur, Nadia (West Bengal) in Black Bengal goats with successful sero convertion without side effects (same report on symposium at NCL, 1994, pp. 51 mentioned above).

Atteri *et al.* 1992 from IVRI, Mukteshwar reported studies on cell line (Vero, MDBK and BHK-21) adapted (40 passages for attenuation) goat pox virus as a candidate vaccine virus strain with possible good results. It could be seen from above that various workers were engaged in development of sheep and goat pox vaccine virus strains (attenuated or inactivated) by cell culture cultivation for production of sheep/ goat pox vaccine, as earlier sheep/pox goat vaccines were not found satisfactory for successful immunization.

Suggested Reading

Afshar, A.; Bundza, A.; Myers, D.J.; Dulac, C.C. and Thomas, F.C. (1986): Sheep pox: Experimental Studies with West African Isolate. Candian. Vet. J. 27 (8): 301-306.

Bhat, PP (1993). Molecular characterization of pox (viral) DNA. Indian Journal of Animal Sciences 63: 857–862.

Carn, V.M. (1993). Control of capripox infections. Vaccine. 11(13): 1275-1279.

Chand, P., Kitching R.P. and Black D.N. (1994). Western blot analysis of virus specific antibody responses for Capripox and contagious pustular dermatitis viral infections in sheep. Epidemiol. Infect., 113: 377.

Gershon, P.D., Ansell, D.M. and Black, D.N. (1989). A comparison of the genome organization of capripox viruses with that of the orthopox viruses. Journal of Virology 63: 4703–4708.

Joshi, R.K., Garg, S.K., Chandra, R. and Sharma, S.N. (1996). Growth behaviour of Sambalpur strain of goat pox virus on chorioallantoic membrane of developing chicken embryo. Indian Journal of Virology 12: 109–111.

Kumar, P.N., Pachalag, S.V., Chattopadhyay, S.K. (1974). A note on fatal contagious ecthyma in recently imported adult Russian merino sheep. Indian Vet. J. 51: 725-728.

Rao (1938), cited by Singh, I.P. (1979). Sheep pox: a review. The Veterinary Bulletin 49(3): 147.

Singh, I.P., Pande, Y.R, Srivastava, R.N. (1979). Sheep pox: a review. Vet. Bull., 49: 145-153.

□□□

Chapter 6

Rabies

Paris is proud of both the world famous "Eiffel" tower, and of Dr. Louis Pasteur, the towering celebrity from the world of Preventive Medicine.

Mankind was all "dumb" before the furious Rabies. Nothing positive was known about the aetiologic agent. Against this back-drop, 'men of letters' regard 6th July, 1885 as the 'red letter' day, when a lad of 9 years, Joseph Meister, was given, by Dr. Pasteur, the first post-bite Antirabic Treatment (PBARVT). Second 'trial' child 'Jupile' also survived, his statute, now adoring the entrance gate of Pasteur Institute, Paris. Out of 350 cases, 349 cases were successful at the hands of L. Pasteur and many Pasteur Institute were opened in all parts of the world, one such being at Connor in Southern India.

With his bold experiments, Dr. Louis Pasteur had opened "new vistas" for further experiments/trails and new vaccines. The story of evolution of antirabic vaccine during the past century is as engrossing as it is enchanting. It is expedient, therefore, that before one tries to know how to prevent the disease, one should get acquainted with, the disease to be prevented.

Aetiology and Transmission

It is known, for certain, that rabies affects all warm-blooded animals all over the world from colder Arctic to hotter equatorial region. With the "bullet – shaped" virus in infective saliva (Zinke, 1804), the furious dog runs amuck on all the longitudes and latitudes of the globe. Is dog the only animal infecting man? Is bite the only way of infection? The replies are replating with references. The dog is the carnivores like jackal foxes, wolves, hyenas, cayotes, skunks, raccoons, mongoose, wassels, and bats of all varieties contribute to the sylvan cycle. Besides, bite wounds near head, face, fingers are regarded as more serious. Oral (Fischman and Ward, 1968) and inhalation routes have been recorded as portals of transmission. Aerosal transmission has also been recorded by (Constantine, 1962). From bat-caves and also from a laboratory, where, by accident, fixed rabies brain suspension was being blended (Winkler, 1973).

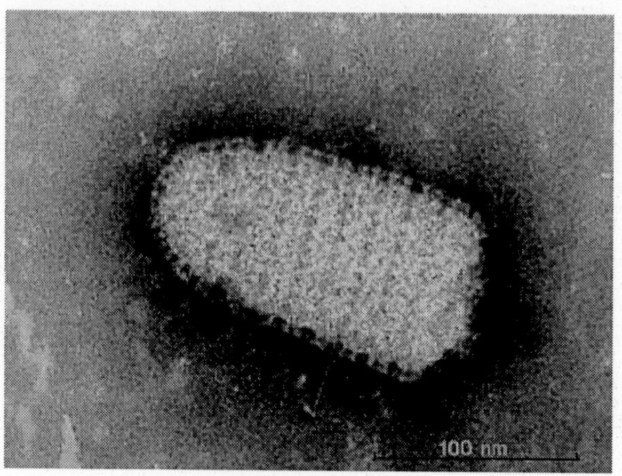

Fig. 1: Rabies virus

Incubation Period

The incubation period in various species is variable as also in dogs but on an average, it is 4-10 days to 4-6 months. Dr. Veer Raghavan has recorded few cases in dogs as asymptomatic carriers. As stated earlier, 80% of the human cases are through dog bites and children that too, male children under 15 years are more vulnerable for the disease; frankly for their love for pets, and for their inability, to easily shun away from the rabid dog. The vulnerability of children should not be confused with their susceptibility.

Epidemiology

The variable incubation period in different species, the bat-transmitted rabies in wild and domestic animals, and the stray dogs are the strong links to perpetuate the virus. Sulkin and Allen (1974) has shown that brown fat tissue of bats can maintain the virus in infective stage for one hibernation period. Experimentally, the virus has been shown to be transferred transplacentally in the bat progeny (Sims *et. al.*, 1963). One case of human rabies in Andhra Pradesh is reported in India by Veer Raghavan (1964). Wild animals, like Foxes and Jackals, can infiltrate at the out skirts of the villages and trigger up a wave of rabies from rural to urban areas. This has been observed from countries like Germany, France and America. From Chiplun area of Maharashtra too, 105 cases in animals were seen with some deaths from the village Agwe. Negri bodies were observed in few brains submitted for histo-pathological examination. Wolf and fox-wounds were of severe nature and saliva from these animals was stated to contain more connection of virus, as it is copious in quantity also, as compared to that of dog. Thomas *et al.* (1965) have mentioned correlation between bat-inhabited caves and fox rabies. If the bat number per sq. ft. exceeds 300 bats, the caves and atmosphere thereof has been found to be vitiated and Constantine opines that Aerosol infection is likely. Thus, it is clear that, if animals as well as bats conglomerate, the disease can be triggered thereby confirming Cowan's statement, that, "infection of rabies is density related." The foxes and dogs are supposed to contribute more rabies cycle during their respective breeding seasons.

Pathogenesis

Soon after the bite, the virus is supposed to travel centripetally @ 3 mm. per hour, and later it is seen to have reached the brain tissue. Much more has to be known about the complete sojourn of the virus from the wound to the brain and from the brain to the salivary glands.

Spectrum of Symptoms

The symptoms in dogs are too well known for veterinarians. The symptoms in man are equally well-described. The most agonizing sight is that of hydro-phobia. The patient has intense thirst and he has the utter inability to gulp the water, two paradoxes seen synchronously in the same patient. The bite, from whatever the species of animal, in man can be fatal once the symptoms have started exhibiting themselves. The prognosis is precarious and the imminent death is all but inevitable. Man to man transmission has not, so far, been recorded.

Diagnosis

Negribody detection, FAT (Jean *et al.*, 1973) would help for positive diagnosis, coupled with biological tests in mice.

Treatment

Among the 9 recovered cases so far, only one case of Ohio-boy (America) is well-documented to have recovered from even the paralysis of the disease (Hattawick *et al.* 1972). WHO in their Sixth report (1973) had catagorized wounds and advised regimen for treatment as well as prophylaxis. The age-old advice of washing the wounds with soap and water, (even upto 48 hours after the bite as per Haffkine Institute recommendation) and treating the wounds with tincture of iodine has been accepted even today.

Prophylaxis in Dogs

Since bat rabies and sylvatic rabies pose many problems for their control, initially, the dog rabies has got to be controlled. Tierkel (1975) has reiterated that if dog rabies is minimized by disposal of dogs and by vaccination of pets, the incidence of human rabies would, decidedly, be minimized. He was supporting the statement by statistical data from America (CDC, 1966).

Year	Dog rabies cases	Human rabies cases
1938	8452	47
1965	412	1

Not only the incidence in dog is minimized but also by such methods, few countries like Australia, Denmark, Fiji, Ireland, U.K., Spain, Japan, Malaya, etc. have virtually eradicated rabies from their territories and in order to prevent re-entry of infection these countries are enforcing strict quarantine measures. The quarrantine period is usually of four months with a lease of 2 months more (WHO Expert Committee on Rabies, 1973).

In India, the statistical picture of incidence and mortality in domestic animals as well as in human beings is too very sketchy (Steel, 1975). As per available reports, every year, over 3 lakh people in India are subject for post bite anti rabies treatment, as compared to the figure of the world, of 1.5 millions. Deaths due to rabies in the country figure to 15,000 cases per year. Such figures for the state of Maharashtra and Pune are respectively 525 and 202. Figure of post bite anti rabies treatment in animals in Pune District alone is 2,000 cases. Considering the magnitude and severity of the disease. Govt. of India, have diverted their finance, energies and expertise towards the control of this dreadful disease. At the cost of 13.8 million rupees, 30 centres are to be established in various cities in the country. The centres will be established with a view to eliminate the stray dogs and to help effective vaccinations in dogs. It is hoped that religious sentiments of benevolence will not impede the progress since elimination of stray dogs, as these are the animals responsible in dissemination of the infection. Maharashtra State too is having two centres, one at Disease Investigation Section, Pune-7 and another at Aurangabad.

Sylvatic rabies also has to be considered in detail as to the population control of foxes, wolves and other wild animals by baiting, trapping, gassing, poisoning, etc. The oral vaccination for wild life is on experimental scale in other countries, hence our country will like some more time to implement it.

Vaccine

Vaccinations in dogs need priority. Vaccines in animals can be broadly classified as live attenuated and inactivated, derived from: 1) Nervous, 2) Avinised, 3) Tissue culture origin. Nervine origin vaccines are manufactured by using Pasteur's fixed virus in ovine or caprine brains and further the brain suspensions are treated with phenol (Semple, 1911), UV light, Ether, Chloroform Semple type phenolised brain tissue vaccine is being used on large scale till today. Umeno and Doi (1921) have conducted potency trials in dogs and have used with advantage the semple type vaccine. For post bite anti rabies treatment now, BPL treated 5% brain suspention is being utilized (Table 1).

After the initial work from Kliglet and Bernkof (1939) of developing fixed ARV in Chick Embryo, further improvement was made by utilizing the Flury strain (derived by Dr. Johnson from twelve years old girl named Flury), for adaption to chick embryo the product is freeze-dried. The Avinised Vaccine (Flury LEP) engenders immunity in dogs for a period of three years. Flury strain vaccines are both of LEP (49-50) and HEP (180-200) both useful for dogs and in other animals (Table 2). Kelve Strain (Komorov *et al.*, 1953) is similar to flury and is utilized in Israel for dog immunization.

Tissue culture based vaccines are utilizing canine kidney, porcine kidney, ERA, Chick embryo fibroblast, Hamester Kidney, with Flury and Vnukowa 32 strains (Table 3).

In Africa, particularly polyvalent rabies vaccine with inclusion of Lagos, Bat, Makola and such virus strains, would be more suitable. In veterinary practice, rabies vaccine is coupled with other components, such as canine Hepatitis virus, Distemper Leptospirosis, etc. i.e. in one vaccine dose, respective disease, including rabies, is protected. Newer tissue derived vaccines are both live and inactivated. Live vaccines have now been asked by WHO to be discontinued. Amongst the inactivated vaccines, Sir David Semple's method is as yet time honoured one and in those years also had only 0.19% mortality with 2009 Europeans subjected by him for PBARVT. The Coonoor Institute reports testify the use of this vaccine as per 1970 report.

Nerve Tissue vaccines have not been unequivocal. Webstar (1942) concludes; "Never Tissue vaccines can be said to be effective, as well as non-effective, both the conclusions being too very disturbing" Brain tissue vaccines for humans are poor antigens, and also contribute, though rarely (1:22000) for post-vaccinal Neuro-Paralytic accidents and reactions. This encephalitogen factor is more observed in adult brain and hence, suckling mice brain vaccine (Fuenzalida and Palacios 1955), suckling rat brain tissue vaccines were used in Netherland (Gispen *et al.*, 1965). Even the suckling animal brain tissue vaccines were not without untoward reactions. Duck embryo vaccines were not elicting the desired response.

Hence, the researches yielded tissue cultured vaccines. Of all the tissue culture vaccines, the safest vaccine for human use is that from Human Diploid Cell System (HDCS) (Viktor *et al*, 1964). The HDCS are the cells, with normal karyotype. Their freedom from microbial contamination, karyotype-stability absence of spontaneous transformation and absence of oncogencity have been demonstrated and proved for each batch. The HDCS used is WI 38, now known as MRC 5. Rabies virus strain used is Pitman Moore PM-38-1503-3 M. The product is BPL or UV inactivated and is lyophilized. There are no chances of heterologous infections or of some occult viruses creeping in. The product is highly safe and non-neurotoxic. So far over ten lakh doses of vaccine have been utilized and trial shows HDCS derived vaccine to be superior to any brain tissue, avinised or Tissue Culture vaccine in all respects. The vaccine is innocuous and elicits antibody response as early as in 10 days and the immunity so developed lasts upto 3 years. Total quantity to be injected is just 6 ml. as against the quantity of 70 ml. of brain tissue vaccine and moreover, the protein content is minimum. Tomorrow subunit vaccines by genetic engineering and cloning would be developing (Crick, 1978) but, as of today, HDCS vaccine holds the promise. Immunity in rabies by interference or by interferon or by both has been argued. There are other hypotheses of humoral or cellular type of immunity but all these hypotheses need to be studied further.

Biological challenges for estimation of vaccine potency pose variety of problems. Hence, based on Webstor's (1935) investigation of intracranial inoculation of mice. Habel (1945) had developed indirect potency test for estimation of potency of vaccine viruses. NIH test also is in vogue (Fox, 1958).

WHO expert committee's sixth report, 1973 had delineated and elaborated the outlines for areas of research in rabies, right from antigenic complex, pathogenesis treatment, propylaxis both in donor and recipient animals, epidemiological studies at Urban/Sylvan/State/ National/International levels meaning thereby, that, while much has been learnt since Pasteur, much still remains to be explored and investigated.

Meister, Jupille, Ohoi-boy are representatives of our human race, awaiting yet another 'Pasteur' or his creed who, in the coming 21st Century, would offer measures and means, to solve the "riddle of rabies" and thus, would help the animal species and human race to live without rabies.

Selected References

Editor / Author	Title	Publisher
1. Geroge M. Baer	The Natural History of Rabies Vol. I & II (1975)	Academic Press
2. Joint WHO/IABS Symposium	Standardization of Rabies Vaccines (for human use) produced in tissue cultures (1977)	S. Karger Basel
3. M.M. Kaplan & H.Koprowski	Lab. Techniques in Rabbies III Monograph (1973)	WHO GENEVA
4. D.D. Banker	Modern Practice in Immunization * 1980)	Bombay Popular Prakashan III Ed.

Other authors have been quoted mostly from Ref. (1) above.

Table 1 : Nervous tissue Vaccines

Sr. No.	Name of Vaccine	Author	Man	Dog	Cat	Cattle	Horse	Sheep & Goat	Remarks
1.	Fixed virus on Nervous tissue Lapinised, Live dried cord	Pasteur, 1885	+	-	-	-	-	-	These vaccines are now discontinued
2.	Dilution of Live CNS	-- -	+	-	-	-	-	-	
3.	Mature CNS partly inactivated	Fermi, 1908	+						
4.	Mature CNS (Ovine, Caprine inactivated)	Semple, 1911	+	+	+	+	+	+	
5.	Suckling Mouse Brain tissue vaccine (inactivated)	Fuanzalida and Palacio, 1955	+	+	-	-	-	-	
6.	Suckling Rate Brain tissue vaccine (inactivated)	Svet Moldacki *et al.*, 1965	+	-	-	-	-	-	
7.	Suckling Rabbit Brain tissue Vaccine (Inactivated)	Gispen *et al.*, 1965	+	-	-	-	-	-	

NB =1) + = Used for 2) – = Not used for

Table 2: Avian Embryo Vaccine to be used in

Sr. No.	Name of Vaccine	Author	Man	Dog	Cat	Cattle	Horse	Sheep & Goat	Remarks
	LIVE VACCINES								
1)	Chick Embryo origin flurry vaccine (LEP)	Kopreowski & Cox, 1948	-	+	-	-	-	-	
2)	Chick Embryo origin flurry vaccine (HEP)	Walker & Crawley, 1959	+	+	+	+	-		
3)	Kelve Strain vaccine	Komorov & Hornestein, 1953	-	+	-	-	-	-	
	INACTIVATED VACCINES								
i)	Duck Embryo vaccine	Powell & Culbertson, 1956	+	-	-	-	-	-	

NB =1) + = Used for 2) – = Not used

Suggested Reading

Constantine, D.G. (1962). Rabies transmission by non-bite route.Public Health Rep. 77(4): 287-289.

Fischman, H.R. and Ward, F.E. (1968). Oral transmission of rabies virus in experimental animals. American J. Epidemiol. 88(1): 132-138.

Jean, S., Pamela, A.,Yaager and Baer, M.(1973). A rapid reproducible test for determining rabies neutralizing antibody. Bull. World Health Organ. 48(5): 535-541.

Sims, R.A., Allen, R. and Sulkin, S.E. (1963). Studies on the Pathogenesis of Rabies in Insectivorous Bats: III. Influence of the Gravid State. The Journal of Infectious Diseases, 112(1): 17–27.

Sulkin, S.E. and Allen, R. (1974). Virus infections in bats. Monogr Virol. Basel, Karger. 8: 10-26.

Tierkel, E.S. (1975). Canine rabies. In: The natural history of rabies. G.M. Baer Ed. Vol. 11. New York: Academic Press, Inc., pp. 123-137.

Thomas J.B., Ricker A.S. Baer G.M. and Sikes R.K. (1965). Purification of fixed rabies virus.Virol. 25: 271-275.

Winkler, W.G., Fasinell, T.R., Leffingwell, L., Howard, P. and Conomy, J.P. (1973). Airborne rabies transmission in laboratory worker. JAMA. 1973; 226(10): 1219-1221.

Zinke, G.G. (1804). Neue Ansichten der Hundswuth; ihrer Ursachen und Folgen, nebst einer sichern Behandlungsart der von tollen Thieren gebissenen Mensch; C.E. Gabler: Jena.

❑❑❑

Chapter 7

South African Horse Sickness

South African Horse Sickness (SAHS) is an infectious but non-contagious arthropod borne virus disease of equines including horses, mules and donkeys, endemic to South Africa, however, the enzootics occurred in past in the middle east (Turkey, Iran) meditarian coasts (Cyprus) and Indian subcontinent including India, Pakistan and Bangladesh.

SAHS is also recorded in dogs as a clinical disease and only as subclinical infection in zebras, elephants and perhaps in other wild-life.

About the virus

SAHS is caused by an *Orbiviurs* (family *Reoviridae*) of which 9 antigenic strain with varience in virulence are recognized "Compliment fixing activity" can be induced in SAHS virus by treatment protamine sulphate as the inducing agent and this C.F. technique can be used for typing of SAHS virus in 9 different types (Anderson, R.M. and May, R.M., 1991) Indian isolate of SAHS virus was typed as type IX virus using this CF technique SAHSV is an arthropod borne (Arbour) virus and it is truly transmissible by the vector Midges, namely *culicoides* species including *C. Varipenis, C. Pulicaris* and *C. Obsoletus,* etc. *Culicoides* are not only mechanical carriers of the virus but the virus "multiplies" in this "Vector". However, transovarin transmission of infection between generations of these midges does not occur. The virus persists by cycling between the mammalian host and vectors year round in enzootic areas (Skowronek, *et al.,* 1995). The virus is transmitted by the bite of haematophagus insects including midges (*Culicoides* species), ticks (nyaloma and brown) dog ticks as well as mosquitoes. However, the virus does not persist over the winter months when viremic animal recover after infection in rainy season is over and the "vectors" culicoides species die due to cold weather, in the areas in which the disease is not endemic.

Horses, donkeys and mules which when become "viremic" after the infection are able to infect "vectors" during febrile episode of the disease as the source of the virus in blood and body fluids of infected animals. (Zebras can be viremic for 28 days and horses are viremic for 18 days and horses are viremic for 18 days and are, therefore, prone during these periods for becoming source of the virus though vector bites). (Skowronek, *et al.*, 1995).

Dogs are infected by eating infected animals or by infected "tick" bite. Transmission of the virus to "new areas" takes place by movement infected animals like zebra or by midges getting transported by wind even upto 700 k.m. distances (Sellers, 1980).

Pathogenesis

The virus affects vascular endothelium. The virus serotypes have differences in their tissue tropisum which determines the "form" of the disease they can produce, such as "Dikkop" i.e. "Cardiac form" or "Dunkkop" i.e. "Respiratory Form" e.g. In India, SAHS virus of type-IX was responsible for cardiac form (Dikkop) as quoted by Dutt, N.S. *et al.* (1960) during outbreak at cavalry unit Jaipur. After infection, the virus multiplies in lungs, spleen and gets bound to erythrocytes in blood (Viremia) for upto 18 days in horses. Fever and viremia are simultaneous secondary viral multiplication occurs in endothelium of target organs which causes the disease. Natural incubation period of virus is 5-7 days.

Clinical Disease Picture

The acute or pulmonary form "Dunkkop" is characterized by "fever" with laboured breathing, severe paraoxysms of coughing and profuse nasal discharge of straw coloured serous fluid and froth. Stagery gait is followed by recumbency. Death occurs after 4-5 days of illness. Severe respiratory distress persists for several weeks in surviving animals. This form occurs in horses as well as dogs too in natural cases.

The subacute or cardiac form (Dikkop) of the disease occurs most commonly in horses in enzootic areas. The incubation period in this form is upto 3 weeks with more of protracted course of the disease. The oedema of head, especially of temporal fossa, swelling of eyelids and lips as well as that of chest after febrile course of the disease for a week occurs. Mild abdominal pain, paralysis of oesophegus with inability to swallow and regurgitation of food and water through nose is quite common. Fatal course is for about 2 weeks and recovery may take place after a long period. A combination of above 2 forms can also be observed in some outbreaks. Some cases may show only fever and no other symptoms.

Postmortem findings

The classical old book entitled as "Animal Diseases in South Africa" by Henning should be worth reading for complete account of clinical and postmortem findings in SAHS. Gross necropsy findings include severe hydrothorax and pulmonary oedama and moderate ascitis with straw coloured serous fluids in these cavities which may be also blood tinged. Oedama of small and large intestines and acute congestion of liver is also evident. The pharynx, trachea and bronchi are filled with yellow serous fluid and froth. Marked cardiac form in characterized by severe hydro pericardium and epicardial as well as endocardial haemorrhages and fluid filled in supra orbital fossa.

Diagnostic tests

Laboratory confirmation of the disease by serological tests in acute deaths may not be possible (Martinez–Torre cuadrada, *et al.*, 1997) AGID, Indirect FAT, CFT, VN and ELISA tests are all useful diagnostic tests for antibody detection while viral antigen can be demonstrated by ELISA or Reverse Transcriptase Polymerase Chain Reaction (RT-PCR) Zientara *et al.* (1993).

Control

The control of the disease in non-enzootic areas can be aimed at by preventing introduction of the diseased or infected animals by proper quarantine measures and eradication by "stamping out" the disease, if it gets introduced accidentally i.e. by slaughter and ring vaccination policy. Early attenuated virus vaccines were able to prevent the disease but were associated with side effects, such as encephalitis.

These early vaccines were prepared by attenuation of virulent SAHS virus strains isolated from viremic infected horses blood collected in Oxalate carbolic acid glycerine (OCG) solution and passaging serially in adult mice / mice litter by intracranial injection until the virus isolate looses the pathogenicity in horses but showing encephalitis symptoms in adult mice only. Such mice brain adapted vaccine virus isolates show satisfactory immunogenicity in vaccinated equines against homologous virulent SAHS virus strain only and hence, polyvalent vaccines were prepared against the existing virulent SAHS typed isolates from the particular areas/continents in those days. These vaccines were able to protect the horses for about one year and hence, annual re-vaccinations were required to be undertaken. Vaccinations of foals were being undertaken, when they were 3-4 months age (progeny of non-vaccinated mothers). However, foals from immune mothers were vaccinated, when their maternal immunity was waned after at least 8 months old (Blackburn and Swanepoel, 1988).

SAHS Incidence, Indian Scenario

India was free from the SAHS until reporting of 1st outbreak of the disease in India, in 1960, which was reported by Indian army's 61 calvalry unit at Jaipur. This outbreak was investigated by Dr. N.S. Dutt and his two pathologists colleagues including Dr. S. Kumar. They carried out postmortem examinations of large number of ponies from this cavalry unit and isolated the SAHS virus which was then revealed by C.F. test, as type IX. They also passaged this virus isolate serially in adutt mice as well as in the developing chick embryos via yolk sac route to get vaccine strains of type-IX. They produced freeze-dried SAHS vaccine which was used in the field as well as in the laboratory at IVRI, Mukteshwar.

The author (Pandit, S.V.) was working in Rinderpest eradication scheme in Dhulia district during June-July, 1960, when Govt. of Maharashtra Animal Husbandry Directorate informed the arrival of SAHS in village horses and Tanga ponies and directed the field veterinarians under RP Eradication scheme to undertake postmortem of the suspected deaths of SAHS, if found within their areas of working jurisdiction and report. The author happened to carryout few such postmortems and could find postmortem lesions simulating "Dickkop" i.e. cardiac form of the disease.

The author also could take part in conducting CF tests against type IX SAHS "Protamine sulphate " treated CF antigen on suspected field equine sera under VRC'S survey programme received at VRC, Now known on National Institute of Virology (NIV) (ICMR'S Arbor Virus Research Centre), Pune under the guidance of Dr. (Miss)

Khurshid M. Pavri during his training progrmame on deputation from DIS, Pune during 1963-65.

VRC, Pune also conducted some programme of Arthropod survey including collection of culicoides and mosquito samples for study of epidemiololgy of Horse sickness under the guidance of Dr. V.M. Dhanda and Dr. K.P. Singh during early/mid-sixties.

However, it is interesting to note that even though IVRI, Mukteshwar/Izatnagar developed mice-adapted type IX SAHS vaccine and VRC, Pune developed CFT for serological survey of horses mules and donkeys against SAHS, the South African Horse sickness surprisingly disappeared from Indian Scenario not to return back up-to-date, the reason for which is obscure.

Suggested Reading

Anderson, R.M. and May, R.M. (1991). Infectious diseases of humans: dynamics and control, Oxford University Press, Oxford.

Blackburn N.K., Swanepoel R., African horse sickness in Zimbabwe, 1972 to 1981, Trop. Anim. Health Prod. 20(1988): 169-176

Martinez-Torrecuadrada, J.L., Diaz-Laviada, M., Roy, P., Sanchez, C. & Vela C. (1997). 'Serologic markers in the stages of African horse sickness virus infection', *Journal of Clinical Microbiology* 35: 531-535.

Sellers R.F. (1980). Weather, host and vector - their interplay in the spread of insect-borne animal virus diseases. J Hyg (Camb) 85: 65-102.

Skowronek, A.J., Lafranco, L., Stone-Marschat, M.A., Burrage, T.G., Rebar, A.H. and Laegreid, W.W. (1995). Clinical pathology and haemostatic abnormalities in experimental African horsesickness. Veterinary Pathology, 32: 112-121.

Zientara S., Sailleau C., Moulay S., Cruciere C. (1993). Diagnosis and molecular epidemiology of the African horse sickness virus by the polymerase chain reaction and restriction patterns, Vet. Res. 24: 385-395.

❑❑❑

Chapter 8

Hog Cholera (Classic Swine Fever)

Hog cholera which is also known as classic swine fever is a highly fetal but sometimes chronic infectious disease of pigs, caused by "*Pestivirus*" with manifestations attributable of involvement of the body as a whole generally, but sometimes exhibiting a persistant congenital infection in newborn piglets infected during foetal life. This multiple phase exhibition of symptoms has a relation with a phenomenon of "Immuno tolerance" against swine fever virus shown by the pigs, when infection occurs during the early period of pregnancy. This type of virus behaviour seems to be a characteristic of Pestiviruses and is also shown by antigenially related another pestivirus, namely "BVDV"

About the virus

Swine fever is caused by a *Pestivirus* which is a member of the family "*Flaviviridae*". The virus is antigenically related with BVD virus. It is interesting to note that in Denmark, BVDV (Bovine Virus Diarrhoea Virus) antibodies were found in 6.4% pig sera which were totally negative for classical swine fever virus antibodies. Classical swine fever virus is totally different from African swine fever virus antigenically, but symptoms of both the diseases have very close resemblance.

Epidemiology and Transmission

All age groups of the pigs are susceptible to this infection. The disease originated in U.S.A., but is presently occurring almost worldwide with the exception of Canada, Australia, Newzealand and South Africa. However, mild form of the disease was experienced by Australia in 1960-61 (Kamolsiriprichaiporn, *et al.* 1992,) U.K. and USA were free from the disease except during the periods 1963 to 1967 and 1978 to 1986 respectively after which outbreaks were recorded in those countries time to time. Epidemics occurred time to time in

Germany (1982 & 1984), Belgium, France, Italy and Greece. Ireland, Denmark, Norway, Sweden, Finland and Switzerland were free as of 1985 but currently the disease is endemic in most countries of continental Europe, South America and far East. In Philippines, it is endemic. Morbidity in epidemics is often 100% with the mortality almost approaching 100%, when a virulent strain affects susceptible population of swine. However, in recent years, mild strains are spreading widely with the disease going almost unnoticed in growing and adult pigs but exhibiting perinatal mortality, abortions and mini field fetuses more preminontly.

Infected pig or its products are almost always the source of infection which is acquired by either injection or inhalation which serves as portal of entry of infection. In areas free of the disease, introduction of infected pig under incubation period or feeding of garbage containing uncooked pork scraps is responsible for precipitation of outbreaks. Disease can be transmitted inadvertently by veterinarian. Classically, infection of hog cholera rapidly results in clinical disease due to sort incubation period. However, it is now recognized that less virulent strains are emerging which produce a "Carrier state and exhibit" less overt" disease which results into more spread of the disease, then such animals in long incubation period move the newer area with susceptible pig population.

Susceptible pregnant sows, if exposed to less virulent virus strain may remain clinically healthy but infection (transplacental) of their fetuses may result in utero and virus may be introduced into susceptible herds by way of these infected offsprings (Persistently infected (P.I.) piglets, being immunotollerant remain as healthy carriers and become spreaders of the infection and perpetuation of the infection occurs in herds (Terpstra,1987). If the sows are exposed to inadequate vaccination or antiserum treatment at the time of their infection (exposure) even virulent clinically expressing virus can be transmitted through placenta in utero resulting into piglets supporting a virema for long periods after their births.

Pathogenesis

After oral exposure virus invade tonsils where primary multiplication of virus occurs, followed by passage through lymphatic and then to general blood circulation through blood capillaries resulting in viremia in 24 hours, when virus is present in spleen, perferal and visceral lymph-nodes, bone marrow and payer's patches.

The virus attacks endothelial cells, lymphoreticular cells and macrophages and epithelial cells. Most significant patho immunological consequences of acute swine fever infection are lymphocyte deficiency due to viral destruction of germinal centres of lymphoid organs (Susa, *et al.*, 1992). Hydropic degeneration and proliferation of vascular endothelium results in the blood vessel occlusion which brings about characteristic lesions including congestion, haemorrhages and infarction in the organs affected with the virus, such as lymph-nodes, spleen, kidneys and gastro-intestinal tract in which thrombosis of small and medium-sized arteries also occur. Thymic atrophy and depletion of lymphocytes in peripheral lymphoial tissue in their germinal centres also occur resulting in early leucopenia which is characteristics of swine fever infection, followed by leucocytosis later on. Thrombo cytopenia and anaemia also occur (Sussa *et al.*). Secondary bacterial infections including salmonella choleriae suis also occur in number of instances resulting into lesions of ulceration and enteritis.

Transplacental infection of porcine foetus with either milk field strains or vaccine strains of the virus may result into a spectrum of foetal abnormalities including hypoplasia of lungs, malformation of pulmonary artery, firrsures in renal cortex multiple septa in gall bladder and malformation in brain, etc. which induces retarded growth and growth reduction of brain. Earlier the infection during gestation period of embryo the more severe, the embryonal abnormalities likely to occur. Sequelae of transplacental virus infection is a congenital persistant virus infection (PI) with a runt like syndrome during first few months of life of young piglets which may appear normal.

Clinical Symptoms

Young pigs may die without symptoms in peracute form of the disease. In acute form, depression, inapetanance and standing in dropped position with hanging tails, disinclination to move and showing of swaying movement of hind quarters, if forced to move, lie down and burrowing into bedding or often piling one on top of others are some signs of the disease prior to showing other characteristics symptoms. High temperature (105^0-107^{0}F), constipation followed by diarrhoea and vomiting, diffuse purplish discolouration of the abdominal skin, small areas of necrosis on the edges of the ears on the tail and lips of vulve are seen conjunctivitis with sticking of eyelids by dried purulent exudates is observed in some animals. In co-ordinated movement, muscular tremors and convulsions are some of the nervous symptoms seen. Diarrhoea due to secondary bacterial infection due to salmonella coleraesuis in generally developed as simultaneous infection which results into high mortality. A nervous form of the disease with brain symptoms described above occurs due to a variant strain of swine fever virus.

Low virulent strains produce a chronic form of the disease with longer incubation period, pigs may apparently recover following a short period of illness but subsequently relapse and die, if stressed. The affected animals with low vireulent strains appear more susceptible to salmonella infection and may die due to secondary bact, infection.

Reproductive failure can be a significant feature and may occur without other clinical evidence of the disease within the herd. This type of the disease occurs, when the pregnant sows inadequately protected (substandard vaccines) are exposed to virulent virus infection or susceptible pregnant sows are vaccinated with live attenuated vaccines or exposed to low virulent field strain. This may result in mild pyrexia but high incidence of abortion, low litter size mummification, still birth and anomalies of piglets (Trautwein, 1988). Live born piglets, although carriers may be week or clinically normal. Persistent congenital infection is characterized by persistent viremia, continuous virus excretion and late onset of disease with death occurring 2-11 months after birth. No specific antibodies are produced inspite of Persistent Infection (P.I.) but pigs have normal immune response to other infections.

Postmortem Lesions

In peracute deaths, no postmortem lesions are observed. In acute form of the disease submucosal and subserosal haemorrhages are observed which may not be constant in all animals. Subcapsular haemorrhages on the kidneys are characteristic Haemorrhages are also present in the cortical sinuses of lymph-nodes, the illio-caecal valve, bladder and larynx which may be usually petechial and rarely ecchymotic. Enlargement of lymphnodes and spleen with marginal infarcts is common. Infarctions of gall bladder mucosa, though not seen in every case is a pathognomic feature. Congestion of lungs, liver and bone marrow is also observed, circular raised button ulcers in the colonal mucosa are usual but may also be due to salmonella infection.

Non-supportive encephalitis is a histopathological feature on chronic swine fever. Fibrinoid necrosis of tunica media with hydropic degeneration and proliferation of vascular endothelium causing occlusion of blood vessels. Ulceration of mucosa of large intestine and secondary pneumonia is a feature of chronic swine fever.

Foetus infected with immunotolerant persistent infection is non-cytotic without cell necrosis or without inflammatory reaction.

Aborted factuses show non-diagnostic patechial haemorrhages and ascitis. Antibodies against swine fever do not occur in foetal blood, when infection occurs early in foetal life. In pigs showing signs of myoclonia congenital, cerebellar hypoplasia is highly suggestive of hog cholera infection.

Diagnosis

Detection of marked leucopenia is valuable in differentiation from bacterial sepicaemias in only early stage of disease is leucocytosis occurs in later part of the disease Hog cholera. Virus isolation on cell cultures is not effective method of diagnosis, as CPE may be minimal and slow.

Animal inoculation tests provide excellent method for diagnosis of Hog cholera and involve challenge of susceptible and known immunized pigs with suspected material (tymphnode/spleen material), followed by subsequent challenge at a later date with highly vireulent hog cholera virus. This is used for final confirmation.

More rapid diagnosis can be arrived at by detection of swine fever antigen using fluorescent antibody (FAT) technique. Antigen capture ELISA & AGPT are other tests which are useful in diagnosis. PCR technique is used for differentiation of swine fever from Bovine pesti virus infections in pigs i.e. BVDV in pigs.

Control

For control of newly detected swine fever outbreaks in disease free areas, slaughter and stamping out policy adjucted with disinfection of utensils, vehicles and infected premises is used, 5% cresslic acid is used for the same. Entry to and Departure from infected premises must be carefully controlled to avoid spread of the disease virus on footwear, clothes and automobile tyres. Prohibition of feeding of infected garbage or boiling of garbage before feeding must be practiced.

In disease free countries, when fresh outbreak occurs, vaccination of pigs in not permitted, as it induces carrier stage and development of mild and chronic forms of the disease. The inactivated vaccines are safe but their immunogenicity is short and in adequate. One such vaccine was produced by Ten Broeck C., 1941 (J. Exp. Med. 74 : 427) which was produced from infected blood of swine fever infected pig inactivated with crystal violet. Use of serum vaccine or serum virus simultaneous method of prevention of the disease was followed in past but now discontinued as safer vaccines are now getting available.

A mutant strain swine fever vaccine from Thiverval (French vaccine) is immunogenic and produces no clinical illness and viremia and produces immunity of 3 years duration. Vaccinated animals should be kept separated from pregnant sows. Attenuated vaccines are in wide use in Europe and Asia, such as lapinised vaccines produced by repeated rabbit passaging, such as Chinese or LPC and GPE strain vaccines.

Swine Fever Scenario in India

Swine fever outbreaks were recorded in Maharashtra, in Pune and Bombay suburban districts during early 1960's for the 1st time by Sapre, S.N., Kulkarni, S.G. and Chaudhari, P.G. and confirmed the same by conducting AGP test on spleen and mescentric lymph-node material from field cases using known positive swine fever antiserum. Author also came across outbreaks of swine fever during 1963-64 at Arey Milk Colony (Regional pig breeding centre) and Vasai Taluka in Cross bred pigs, showing typical pin point haemorrhages on kidney surface, ecchymotic hemorrhages on illio caccal valve mucosa and button shaped ulcers on rectal mucosa.

Workers at Disease Investigation section, M.S., Pune used commercial crystal violet inactivated swine fever vaccine which was made available by "Decruz Corporation", Bombay for protection of the incontact healthy animals in affected herds.

Later on IVBP, Pune brought Lapinised swine fever vaccine strain from IVRI Izatnagar (B.P. Division) and produced attenuated swine fever vaccine for undertaking preventive measures in affected herds. However, the chronic form of swine fever was not noticed by workers at D.I.S. M.S., Pune during their working.

Suggested Reading

Kamolsiriprichaiporn, S., Hooper, P. T., Morrissy, C. J. and Westbury, H. A. (1992). A comparison of the pathogenecity of two strains of hog cholera virus. 1. Clinical and pathological studies. *Aust. Vet. J.*, **69(10):** 240-244.

Susa, M., Koenig, M., Saalmueller, A., Reddehase, M. J. and Thiel, H.J. (1992). Pathogenesis of classical swine fever: B-lymphocyte deficiency caused by hog cholera virus. *J.Virol.*, **66**: 1171-1175.

Terpstra, C. (1991). Hog cholera: An update of present knowledge (special review series).*Br. Vet. J.*, **147:** 397-406.

Trautwein, G. (1988). Pathology and pathogenesis of the disease. In: classical swine fever and related viral infections, ed. Liess, B. pp. 27-54. Martinus Nijhoff Publishing, Boston, MA.

□□□

Chapter 9

Equine Influenza

Equine Influenza is caused by influenza A equine -1 (H7N7) or influenza A/equine-2 (H3N8) virus belonging to the family *Orthmyxoviridae* and is characterized by disease of upper respiratory tract, complicated usually by pneumonia and rarely by myositis and encephalitis. In susceptible population, it occurs in severe outbreak form involving almost whole population of horses in the area (about 98% morbidity) but mortality is usually absent (rarely upto <1%), the deaths occurring due to secondary bacterial complications. However, outbreak in China, in 1991 caused by H3N8 strain was associated with 80% morbidity but 20-35% mortality (Webster, *et al.*, 1992).

Incidence

The disease occurs almost worldwide except in Australia and New Zealand which is free inspite of large equine population. Widespread use of aircraft to move horses between countries in short periods has increased the spread of equine influenza virus e.g. South Africa which was previously free from this disease and in Hong Kong with infection originating from North America and United Kingdom respectively, through importation of horses (Kawaoka *et al.*, 1989; Poweld *et al.* 1995).

Epidemiology and Transmission

The outbreaks always originate from infected horse imported from outside in a susceptible population of horses or through contaminated equipment or fomites. The duration of infectivity from clinically affected animal is 3 to 8 days and incubation period is short, i.e. 2-3 days. Frequent coughing produces a very rapid new infection and characteristics explosive outbreak. Transmission of the virus occurs by direct contact, inhalation of aerosols of infected material and on formites.

Equine influenza virus in aerosols survives 24 to 36 hours i.e. longer than aerosols produced by human or porcine influenza virus strains (15 hours). Housing of large number of horses in barns and stables provide optimum conditions for facilitating contact and aerosol spread of the virus.

Formite transfer on veterinary clothing, equipment or vehicles occurs which is responsible for spread of the infection. Outbreaks occur during transportation of horses for racing and sale, and movement of show and breeding animals.

Pathogenesis

The inhaled virus attaches to respiratory epithelial cells with its haemagglutinin spikes, fuses with the cells and is released into cytoplasm, where it replicates. New virions are released from the cell surface and infect other cells or expelled into environment. Initial infection and replication occurs in nasopharyngeal mucosa but by 3-7 days, it occurs throughout the respiratory tract, which results into death of epithelial cells of respiratory mucosa, inflammation, oedema and loss of protective mucosialliary clearance. This results into proliferation of opportunistic bacteria in respiratory tract, which exacerbate the inflammation and broncho-pneumonia viremia. If it occurs (in certain strains only) is mild and causes systemic signs, such as myositis and encephalitis which occurs only occasionally (Liu, *et al* 1985).

Disease Symptoms and P.M. lesions

Disease is characterized by sudden onset and rapid spread. The disease peaks in a population in one week's time and new cases do not occur after 21-28 days in congested horse population. In vaccinated animals, disease may be clinically simulating to disease caused by EHV-1, rhinovirus or arthritis virus which show only mild disease of upper respiratory tract.

Typically, disease starts with fever (101 to 106^{0}F temperature), with dry hacking cough which lasts for 1 to 3 weeks. Nasal discharge is either absent or is watery with painful submaxillary lymph-nodes. Abnormal lung sounds including crackles, wheezes with increased intensity of the normal breath sounds. Depression, anorexia and reluctance to prove are other symptoms observed. Recovery may take 7-14 days.

More severe disease with complication can occur in worked, transported animals or those exposed to adverse climatic conditions, in which severe cough and pneumonia due to secondary bacterial infection, such as strepto coccus zooepidemicus may occur resulting into mucopurulent nasal discharge, persistent fever, pneumonia, icterus, encephalitis, in co-ordination and myoglobinuria, etc. can occur. Electrocardiographic abnormalities can also occur in some cases (Wilson, 1993).

Diagnosis

Confirmation of diagnosis of infection of equine influenza is achieved through virus isolation in avian egg embryo by choreco allantoic inoculation of nasal swab material from affected horse and conducting haemagghatination and haemagghtination inhibition test using avian RBCS and known hyperimmune serum against homologous equine influenza virus strain (H3N8 or H7N7) or the demonstration of secro convertion or an increase in serum antibody titre in paired sera samples from affected animal (3 to 4 fold increase in HAI antibody titre or doubling in antibody titre by single radial haemoly test (SRH).

Recently a rapid test that identifies influenza viral neucleoprotein by membrane bound enzyme immunoassary has been reported from human medicine to detect equine influenza in nasopharyngeal swabs (Chambers, 1992).

Rattan, B., Yadav, M.P. and Uppal, P.K. (1994) from National Research Centre on Equines, Hisar (Haryana) developed immunostick ElISA for detection of equine influenza virus antigen (directly in the nasal swab samples) and antibodies (in the serum). For detection of antigen in nasal swab, they prepared immunosticks coated with rabbit antiserum to density gradient purified A/Equi-2 virus dipped in nasal swab samples and the bound viral antigen was sandwiched with horse anti A/Equi-2 serum. For the detection of antibodies, the immune sticks coated with A/Equi-2 virus were put into the diluted test sera. Rabbit antihorse IgG-HRPO conjugated was used to detect the bound antibodies in both the cases. By this technique, antibodies could be detected as early as 5th /7th days post infection, whereas antigen was detected in nasal swabs from infected horses from 2nd to 7th day post infection.

Control

Control programme involves the fundamental aims as follows:

1. Increase the immunity of both individual animals and the horse population to infection.
2. Reduce the opportunities for the spread of infection between horses.
3. Prevent the introduction of new strain of the virus into equine population.

These aims are achieved by vaccination, hygiene and quarrantine.

Vaccines are used to limit the severity of clinical illness and morbidity during the outbreaks. It is observed that the older vaccine strains are unable to give sufficient protection against clinical disease due to the antigenic drifts which occur time to time in the field strain and hence, it is needed that the updated vaccine strain should be used every time, when antigenic drift is observed by surveillance laboratories. The current vaccines contain inactivated virus of various strains of equine influenza A-1 and A-2 sub-types which are updated time to time (Mumford and Woods, 1993).

Majority of the currently available equine influenza vaccines contain inactivated whole virus preparations along with an adjuvant such as aluminium hydroxide or oil or polymer. The vaccines generally contain at least one representative of H7N7 (Prague/56) and 1022 H3N8 (Miami/63 and either fontaineblean/79 or Kentucky/81 sub-types. The vaccines are standardized on the basis of HA content by Single Radial immune Diffusion (SRD) test and Potency test is based on attainment of optimum HI titres in guinea pigs and H1 response and/or protection to virulent challenge in horses. Single Radial Haemolysis (SRH) test gives more constant and reliable results than the conventional HI test.

The vaccines need to be updated periodically depending on variations or replacement of virus strains. As H7N7 equine influenza virus has not been isolated after 1980, its inclusion in current vaccine needs to be reviewed. Inactivated sub unit vaccines containing immunogenic proteins in an immune stimulating complex (ISCOM) induce a more sustained and greater immune response than the conventional oil adjuvated or aluminium hydroxide gel adjuvanated vaccines (Mumford, *et al.*, 1994).

Indian Scenario

Uppal and Yadav (1989) reported on outbreak of equine influenza from Ludhiana (Punjab) in 1987 from which they isolated equine influenza A/Equi-2 type virus which was designated as Equi-2 Ludhiana, 87 equine influenza isolate. Ludhiana /87 equine influenza strain resembled fontaine blean /79, whereas Bhiwani 87 strain was similar to Miami/63 (H3N8) i.e. A/Equi-2 virus. Isolation of Miami / 63 like viruses from Europe, India, Japan and Brazil between 1979 and 1992 seems to suggest "Frozen evolution" of A/Equi-2 virus. There is a need for increased surveillance and standardization and characterization of virus isolates employing gene sequencing, updating of vaccine on emergence of new varients and updating of reagents for SRD latency test. (Ref. M.P. Yadav, P.K. Uppal and A.K. Gupta, IAVMI, XIV Annual Conference and National Symposium at Pune 29-31st Jan., 1994). While virus isolate from Bhiwani (Haryana) in 1987 was designated as Equi-2/Bhiwani 87 isolate.

Regional Disease Survillence Station Laboratory located at disease investigation section, Maharashtra State, Pune recorded an incidence of Equine Influenza in horses during horse fair in October, 2008 at Nandurbar (Dist. Dhulia) in Maharashtra State, wherein source of the disease was pointed out to be from migration of equines from UP and Bihar. The virus responsible for the outbreak was Diagnosed as Equine Influenza A/Equi-2 type strain. Currently equine Influenza outbreak is reported around Pune in stud horses in 2008 (November and December) which showed rapid spread and very high morbidity (Personal communication from Private Vets from Pune).

Suggested Reading

Chambers, T. M. (1992): Cross-reactivity of equine influenza vaccines with new analysis of an equine influenza virus from China. Vet. Rec. 131, 388-391.

Kawaoka, Y., W.J. Beans, R.G. Webster (1989): Evolution of the haemagglutinin of equine H3 influenza viruses. Virol. 169: 282-292.

Liu I.K.M., Pascoe D.R., Chang L.W.S., Zee Y.C. (1985). Duration of maternally derived antibodies against equine influenza in newborn foals, Am. J. Vet. Res. 46: 2078–2080.

Mumford J.A. and Wood J.M. (1993). WHO/OIE meeting: consultation on newly emerging strains of equine influenza. Vaccine 11: 1172-1175.

Mumford, J.A., Jessett, D.M., Rollinson, E.A., Hannant, D. and Draper M.E. (1994) Duration of protective efficacy of equine influenza immunostimulating complex/tetanus vaccines. Veterinary Record 134: 158-162.

Powell, D.G., Watkins, K.L., Li, P.H. (1995). Outbreak of equine influenza among horses in Hong Kong during 1992. Vet Rec; 136: 531-536.

Uppal, M.P. and Yadav, M.P. (1989). Isolation of A/equi-2 virus during 1987 equine influenza epidemic in India. Equine Veterinary Journal 21: 364-366.

Webster, R.G., Bean, W.J., Gorman, O.T., Chambers, T.M. & Kawaoka, Y. (1992). Evolution and Ecology of Influenza A viruses.*Microbial Review*, 56: 152-179.

Wilson W.D. (1993). Equine influenza. Vet. Clin. N. Am. (equine Pract.), 9: 257–282.

❑❑❑

Chapter 10

Swine Influenza

Swine influenza is an acute zoonotic disease of pigs with significantly high morbidity but very low or negligible mortality. The disease is caused by a virus belonging to the family Orthomyxoviridae and is characterized by severe respiratory symptoms and high fever with transient viremia and occasional high mortality in pig occurring due to secondary bacterial invasion.

Swine Influenza even though not recorded in pigs uptill now (upto July, 2009) in India, has become a subject of enquiry and discussions amongst the elite Indians including Vets Since early June, 2009. When "news items" were prominently flashed on electronic and conventional news media including T.V. and newspapers regarding detection of "Swine flue" cases in human patients amongst the human travellers returning to Indian International airports including Bombay, Delhi, Kolkata, and Hyderabad from Mexico, USA and Canada, where in large scale outbreaks of "Swine flue" in human population have recently been recorded which is suspected as being the beginning of new "influenza pandemic". It is stated that the source of this human episode of "influenza pandemic" which has shown its existence in Mexico, USA, Canada, Europe and now in India with significant human to human spreading potential, originates from pigs suffering from "Swine Influenza" in Mexico (South America), which is a virus disease of pigs with "Zoonotic potential". This zoonotic disease coming from Mexican pig population has already affected significant member of human patients in Mexico, USA, Canada. Some European countries, Malaysia, Bangladesh and now in India with number of patients suffering from respiratory signs including sneezing, coughing, pyrexia and few cases with vomiting and diarrhoea. However, only 8 cases in Hyderabad were confirmed by laboratory diagnosis upto 13th June 2009 and 23 cases were confirmed by laboratory diagnosis in India by 15th June which included one case from Kolkata as per newspaper reports from "Daily Sakal". Totally more than 115 cases of this disease are now recorded by 31st July, 2009 in Pune alone while 525 cases were recorded in India. Now "Swine flue" has become a frequent visitor of urban populations in India especially in Bombay, Pune cities every year.

History

It is interesting to note that the 1st outbreak of swine influenza was recorded in Autumn of 1918 in "Middle West" in pigs by Koen (1919). An inspector in Division of Hog Cholera Control Bureau of Animal Industry), who was the 1st to recognize this new disease which was resembling "human flue". He recognized that "human flue" and "Swine flue" are caused by the same contagion (Virus entitly was not known at that time) on circumstantial evidence as this 1st outbreak of "Hog flue" mentioned above followed immediately after the pandemic of human influenza in which 21,000,000 of the global human population was killed and 25 times of the said numbers were suffered with respiratory disease symptoms during this worst ever human episode during this human Pandemic period. 1st swine influenza outbreak mentioned above also took place and millions of swine were ill while thousands of pigs died after this respiratory disease episode as mentioned by Dorset, *et al.* (1922). The discovery of virus in human flue (Smith *et al.*, 1933) very closely related to the one earlier discovered in swine flue furnished the second bit of scientific evidence supporting koen's hypothesis that both swine flue and human flue viruses have evolved from each other (Smith *et al.*, 1933).

About the virus

Swine Influenza Virus (SIV) is a type "A" orthompco virus with a segmented RNA genome. The type A swine Influenza viruses are further subdivided based on their haemagglutinin and neuraminidase glycoproteins. Sub-types of SIV that are most frequently identified in pigs include H_1N_1, H_1N_2 and H_3N_2. Other sub-types that have been identified in pigs include H_1N_7, H_3N_1, H_4N_6 and H_9N_2.

The H_1N_2, H_1N_1 and H_3N_2 sub-types that have been identified in Europe are antigenically and genetically different than those found in the United States of i) America Brown, I.H. *et al.*, 1998.

Swine Influenza Virus (SIV) is pathogenic for white mice (Andrews C.H. *et al.*, 1934 and Farrets (Smith *et al.*, 1933 and causes febrile illness and produce plum coloured oedematous pneumonia of variable extent in ferrates, with or without death but death is sure in SIV inoculated white mice. SIV is 80-120 mm in dia (Elford W.J. *et al.*, 1936, size identical with human flue virus. It is type A virus and is mildly pathogenic to swine in bacteriogically uncomplicated cases, but with presence of Haemophilus influenza bacterium, severe illness in swine occurs as in the field cases and both bacterial and viral agents are transferred from sick to normal animals by contact (Shope R.E. 1934).

Epidemiology and Virus Transmission

During the outbreak of swine influenza in pigs, swine influenza virus (SIV) is transmitted from affected pig to susceptible pig by contact with SIV containing secretions, such as aerosols created by coughing or sneezing and nasal discharge especially when the piglets or adult pigs are confined in crowded premises. Winter months of November, December and January are more favourable for swine influenza outbreaks in pigs due to cold weather which is favourable for precipitation of respiratory infections due to respiratory stress. However, the disappearance of virus between 9 months from February to October every year in enzootic areas remained unexplainable for long time.

Now it is known that lung worms inhabitants of bronchioles of lungs of swine are capable of harbouring SIV and transmitting the same from animal to animal during the interval between outbreaks (9 months between February to October) during which the disease disappears in swine, every year. As lung worms pass their 3 larval stages through earthworm during their life-cycle from swines respiratory tract to the soil via their alimentary tract, earthworm becomes important as accessory carrier of the disease. Rearing swine on concerate flooring may be able to prevent spread of swine flue virus through lung worm earth worm cycle.

As already described under history of the SIV's 1st epidemic during 1918's human influenza pandemic (Spanish flue) it was hypothesiged by Koen and further shown by experimental evidence by virological identification and physico-chemical studies on virus by Shope, Smith and Andreus, etc. that swine influenza virus of 1918 was most probably evolved from Influenza virus responsible for human pandemic of 1918.

Avian Influenza type A
Virus (AIV) strain H_1N_1
From migratory ducks

↓

Asymptomatic Swine infection } Adopted to swinethrough Several passages in swine (without symptoms of influenza in swine)

↓

This H1N1 swine adapted virus (Mild) with genes from AIV of Wild ducks passed on to the Human patients infected with Unknown human type A influenza Virus strain through swine contact (may be mild avirulent strain of human flue)

↓

Severe human disease (Pandemic flue, 1918) } Process of genetic reassortment Took place between mild human Flue virus and swine adopted Avian Virus which resulted in evolution of Highly pathogenic New pandemic Human influenza virus (1918)

↓

Severe pig disease (epidemic of swine flue) } Swine contacted with pandemic human Type A influenza virus perpetuated this Virus in swine population which resulted in swine population which resulted in swine flue epidemic, 1918

(**Ref** : Public health risk from Avian Influenza viruses – M.L. Perdue and D.E. Swayne (2005) Avian Disease 49 : 317-327.

Note : This is a classical example of zoonosis occurring from human to swine during 1918 epidemic of swine influenza.

During serological surveys of 1934 and 1935 on humans era from Influenza affected areas in the world, it was found much to everyone's surprise that the era of practically all adults (humans) neutralized the swine influenza virus while sera of almost all the children failed to do so (in case of both British and Americans era). It was also revealed that swine flue virus and pandemic human influenza virus of 1918 were antigenically similar and that (as suggested by Koen on circumstancial evidence) swines may very well have acquired the agent which we now know as the "Swine flue" virus from man at that time. Work of Davenport *et al.*, 1953 pointed out that antigenic stimulus responsible for swine flue virus neutralization i.e. SIV antibodies in humans era prevailed in human population during and following 1918 pandemic. It would appear that immunology of swine flue virus fits well with historical aspects of the disease in indicating its origin as a new virus disease in swine in 1918 (Spanish flue).

Later on it was proved through a remarkable molecular detective work on "Spanish flue" pandemic of 1918 that its responsible virus was H_1N_1 strain of type A influenza virus and full molecular sequence of this strain was also almost completely deciphered. Thus, we also now know much about the virulence contribution of several genes of this virus responsible for human and swine influenza epidemic (Pandemic) of 1918. Most of these researchers believe that these H_1N_1 virus genes are contributed by Avian Influenza (AI) virus from wild migratory ducks through a process of "genetic reassortment" by spending some time in mammals (mostly pigs) before getting adapted to human pandemic. However, the ultimate source of the 1918 pandemic strain remains a mystery, but it is now taken as certain that this 1918 human pandemic type A flue virus is a source of 1st swine flue epidemic of 1918. This above mentioned complicated situation can be suitably consolidated by the above given diagram:

In case of human influenza-A pandemic of 1957, H_2N_2 sub-type virus was responsible for the pandemic which had 3 genes (haemagglutinin (HA), Neuraminidase (NA) and Polymany (B1) from Avian Influenza Virus (AI) while the 1968 Pandemic virus (H_3N_2 sub-type) had only 2 genes for Avian Influenza virus (AI), namely HA and polymans (B1) only while neuranminidase gene was derived from existing (already circulating H2N2 season influenza human virus no gene from pig origin was present in either of 1958 or 1968 pandemic influenza A viruses but still the pig acted as the "reaction vessel" for generation of reassortment in these pandemic viruses without contribution of genes from themselves.

Pigs (swine) acting as "Reaction / Mixing Vessel"

As seen from the above mentioned epidemiological situations, it is significant to note that several type A influenza viruses from mammals including swine, human, equine and primates as well as from Avians (including LPAI of migratory/wild ducks/quils/poultry and HPAI of poultry/Ducks/Turkeys are highly mutagenic viruses are identified. These type A Influenza viruses exist with 15 haemagglutinin (HA) types (H_1 to H_{15} types) and 9 Neutranminidase (NA) types (N1 to N9). Each virus strain have specific HA and NA glycoproteins as antigenic determinants on their surface. Thus, each influenza virus strain in the field/vaccine is identified with HA & NA antigenic determinant e.g. : H_1N_1, H_2N_1, H_3N_1 or H_1N_1, H_1N_2, H_1N_3 ...., etc. Thus, influenza type A viruses of 121 combinations of HA and NA sub-types have been identified since 1976 (48 combinations are isolated from faecal samples of ducks in Alaska, Siberia, Mangolia, Taiwan, China and Japan and 73 other combinations have been generated by genetic re-assortment in chicken embryos and all these 121 combinations are stocked for use as vaccine candidates and for diagnostic use. It is presumed that all the above mentioned combinations of HA & NA sub-types influenza type viruses must be either already existing or may be possibly generated by nature primarily in migratory birds or their nesting lakes in Alaska/Siberia/ North pole areas.

Since influenza A viruses of all known sub-types are perpetuated among migratory ducks and their nesting lakes, we must accept that influenza is not an eradicable disease and its prevention and control should be the only realistic goals at present. Since it is now clear that humans, pigs, poultry and migratory ducks are associated with interspecies transmission of influenza virus and emergence of pandemics in birds, pigs/other mammals and humans, it is essential to expand global surveillance in these species.

Originally Avian Influenza (AI) viruses are considered as "avirulent", when they are present in migratory and wild aquatic duck species in polar lake areas of Alaska and Siberia and they are in the phase of evolutionary statis (Suarez, 2000). However, when an influenza A virus infects a new host species, it can quickly adapt to new host species, if given opportunity. In particular the HA protein of the virus has been shown to have a rapid rate of evolution in variety of species including pigs, humans and chicken, etc. (Schultz *et al.*, 1991). It is known that currently circulating H1N2 and H3N2 swine influenza strains in pigs, in both the USA and Asia contain Influenza genes derived from viruses that once circulated in 3 different hosts, namely birds, humans and pigs (Jung, K. *et al.*, 2004).

It is now concluded from the instances of genetic reassortment observed in newly emerging novel swine influenza/human influenza strains, swines really act as "reaction avian influenza/mixing vessels" for influenza A viruses. It seems that this is due to the fact that pigs have receptors in their respiratory tract which will bind swine, human and avian influenza viruses which undergo recombination in pigs.

Recent swine influenza incidences in the world

Swine influenza is a common infectious respiratory disease and H_1N_1 and H_3N_2 are currently the most popular sub-types of influenza viruses circulated in pigs population in China. H_9N_2 virus was detected in pigs which were imported from mainland China in Hongkong, in 1998 and extensive viral surveillance conducted since then indicated that H_9N_2 viruses are widely distributed in pig population in China. Phylogenic analysis indicated that H_9N_2 have now highly established a stable lineage in pigs in China. During the routine survillence, 2 H_5N_1 viruses from pigs in Fujia province in 2001 and 2003 respectively were isolated from pigs respectively. Molecular analysis indicated that they are originated from duck H_5N_1 viruses. Their replication in chickens, mice and pigs has also been investigated (Chen H. *et al.*, 2006). According to Richard Webi (As quoted by Dr. Ramesh Mahajan, "Daily Sakal" pp.6, dt. 31.7.2009) swine flue virus of 1998 is evolved from swines from pig breeding flue and human flue, including RNA polymerase from bird flue virus" and hence, it showed property of rapid multiplicity and spreading potential. Next few years since influenza virus with genes from all the 3 viruses (human, Avian and swine) started spreading in American piggeries and breeding centres. Present maxican H_1N_1Swine Influenza Virus is also evolved in the same way which is spreading to North-East America.

There are preliminary reports that this swine influenza virus of H_1N_1 sub-type which was prevailing in Mexico during last few years which is evolved by reassortment of some genes from Avian species with recombination of genes from swine. This hybrid swine flue virus also received some genes of human type A influenza virus which resulted in a novel swine flue virus which was picked up by human patients in Mexico. As quoted by Dr. Ramesh Mahajan (in "Daily Sakal" dt. 31st July, 2009 pp.6) Pig breeding centres which were highly studed with pig population (due to production pressure from USA for mass supply of pork and bacon products under "NAFTA" Agriment of 1994) at La guaria Municipal Area in Mexico, with highly unhygienic pig production centres is the place of origin of 1st human child patient of this present "Mexican swine flue" infection (which is also called as "NAFTA Flue" in USA & Mexico) this 1st death incidence occurred on 18th March, 2009). This noval human influenza causing "Swine flue" virus is now spreading from human to human patients very rapidly in U.S., Canada, Europe and Malaysia, South East Asia, Bangladesh and now in India (about 160 countries are affected up-to-date). In USA alone, 44000 human patients are reported to be affected from this swine flue, H_1N_1 hybridvirus with mortality of 301 patients upto July 31st, 2009 officially (unofficial estimates are about 10 lakh patients). Information about USA swine flue incidences is available at American Centre for disease control on website (cdc.gov.who.int). 1st case of this swine flue human adapted virus was reported in travellers coming fro mexico/USA to Bombay in June, 2009 with recent most tally of human patients reaching upto 306 cases in India upto July, 2009 end, as described in earlier paragraphs of this article.

It is interesting to note that the 1st swine flue epidemic of 1918 was originated from human (influenza type A virus H_1N_1 of human Pandemic of 1918) i.e. its spread was from human to swine. Converse is true in case of present swine flue 2009 which is also H_1N_1 virus but this time, it is spreading from swine population of mexico towards global human population leading for possible human pandemic of 2009. However, one phenomenon is constant in both these pandemics and that is "reaction vessel is "Pig" only, wherein there is evolution of reassortant Influenza A virus with genetic recombination of H_1N_1 genes from Avian, swine and human origin.

Disease symptoms of swine influenza in Pigs and human cases

In both swine and human cases, fever, anorexia, cough and other respiratory symptoms are prominent. A leucopenia occurred in all cases. 104^0F body temperature seldom exceeds 105.8^0F range. It reaches its peak on 3rd day upto 106.5^0F. Increase respiratory rate, peculiar dia phrygmatic breathing and clumping paroximal cough are prominent, especially when animals aroused. Anorexia, prostration and listlessness are the other important symptoms exhibited by affected animals. Death may occur in case of severe infection especially when secondary bacterial complication with Haemophilus influenza organisms in lungs and upper respiratory tract, between 3rd to 6th day of infection in pigs.

Exaggeration of respiratory symptoms and in co-ordinated delirium may occur with lying on its side or running motions with legs attempting to stand and staggering may also follow.

The morbidity may be very high reaching upto almost 100% but mortality will be restricted from 1 to 4%. Post influenza cough may last for more than 3 weeks.

Postmortem lesions : Pharyngeal and laryngeal mucosae show mild to significant hyperemia and they may be covered with white glassy tenacious mucous. Similar lesions may also be observed in trachea. Small bronchi and bronchioles may be full of mucous exudates with sago like masses embedded in it. Lungs are deep purplish in colour and line of demarcation between the affected and normal tissue is sharp. Massive atelectatic pneumonia may be present mostly unilaterally. Cervical and mediastinal lymph-nodes are enlarged and oedematous.

The liver, kidneys and spleen are normal while serofibrinous pleuritis may be present in fatal cases with frothy blood tinged mucous exudates is present in large bronchi and bronchioles.

Clinical signs and nasal shedding of virus can occur within 24 hours of infection. Two forms of the disease occur in swine, namely epidemic or endemic forms. The virus quickly moves through all phases of a swine unit with rapid recovery provided there are not complicating factors, such as secondary bacterial infections. In endemic form clinical signs may be less obvious and not all pigs may demonstrate traditional clinical signs of infection. The primary economic impact is related to weightloss resulting in an increase in the number of days to reach market weight.

Even though classical symptoms and lesions of swine influenza are related to respiratory tract, SIV infections are associated with reproductive disorders, such as abortions.

Human transmission of infection of SIV can occur with SIV containing secretions, such as aerosols created by coughing or sneezing and nasal discharges of swine, when human operators in abattoirs / swine farms/live pig markets come in contact with the animal operations. Limited number of deaths have been reported. In classical human Influenza A virus infections human patients exhibit respiratory symptoms, pyrexia headaches and malice with occasional death but during present swine flue virus infection (SIV) pandemic, additional alimentary tract involvement with diarrhoeal and vomiting symptoms are observed in human patients, as reported in the electronic news paper media and reason for which is explained as the present "swine flue" pandemic virus is derived by recombination of human, swine and bird flue (HPAI) genes, with unique amino-acid sequences of HAI genes.

Therapeutic treatment

No affordable therapueutic treatment is available in Veterinary practice for swine flue in pigs. However, the newly developed anti-flue chemical molecule generically named as "Oseltamivir (Brand names "Tamiflu" or Zananmivir") is claimed to be viricidal and highly effective against human patients of any influenza virus including swine flue or "Bird flue virus".

Diagnostic techniques

Because SIV is a potential human pathogen, all work with infections tissues, swabs, embryonated eggs and cell cultures are to be carried out in a class-II biological safety cabinate.

Isolation of SIV (Swine Influenza Virus) from field materials for identification

Swine influenza can be suspected in an outbreak in pigs, if large number of pigs/piglets show respiratory syndrome with pyrexia and few deaths occur with post mortem lesions generally restricted to respiratory tract including nasal pharyngeal tracheal and bronchial reagion and lungs (liver, kidneys and spleen not showing any lesions in general). Nasal swabs and lung tissue is collected in cell culture medium without serum or in PBSC antibiotics and transported to diagnostic laboratory.

Nasal discharge from swab is extracted by vigorous stirring on "Vortex mixer" and lung tissue is minced in morter and pasfle with neutral glass powder with cell culture medium with antibodies and 10% tissue suspension is produced following standard cell culture isolation procedure after centrifugation. Nasal swab material suspension/10% tissue suspension, thus prepared is used for seeding of Madin-Darby Canine kidney (MDCK) cell line monolayer cultures and adsorbing the same for 30 minutes by standard laboratory procedure and incubation of adsorbed cell monolayer cultures (MD bottles/legthons tube converslip cultures etc or petriplates) with/without 5% of co-tension of CO_2 incubator or normal incubator as per the case for upto 7 days till CPE is observed by periodic microscopic observation of cultures. Swine kidney/swine lung cultures can also be used for virus isolation and identification by HA/HAI tests. Virus isolation from Nasal discharge material or lung material described above can also be possible using 10-11 days old embryonated SPF chicken eggs using 0.1 to 0.3 ml inoculums into allanotic or aminio-allantoic sack inoculation (4 eggs per sample generally) 1st 24 hours mortality in egg embryos is discarded. Allantoic/amniotic fluids are collected from dead embryos after 24 hours for further identification of virus isolate. Embryo fluids are centrifuged at 1500 RPM for 10-20 minutes at 4^0C and are used for HA/HAI test for virus identification.

HA / HAI tests for SIV identification and virus typing

Chicken RBCS are generally used for detection of virus presence in infected MDCK/swine kidney/swine lung cell culture fluids or in infected chicken embryo allantoic/amniotic fluids especially for Europeon isolates. Turkey RBCS are used in USA for American swine flue isolates identification. Haemagglutination (HA) test is conducted on suspected isolates in cell cultures/embryo fluids using 0.5% RBC suspension using standard protocall for HA test, which is preformed in 96 well V or U bottom microplates (test time 30-60 minutes) for detection of endpoint of haemagglutination titration.

HAI test using 8 HA units of the haemagghtinating unknown virus containing cell culture / amnio-allantoic fluids as well as reference H1, H3 or other virus type fluids is performed using standard WHO/ OIE terrestrial manual 2004 protocol (chapter 2.11.11 of OIE terrestrial manual 2004) for typing of SIV virus isolates. This protocol uses receptor destroying enzyme (RDE) in calcium saline solution equal to 100 units per ml and 0.1 ml packed washed erythrocytes per ml for removal of non-specific haemagglutination activity from serum. Using this test SIV virus Haemaglutination Antigen (HA) sub-type is identified, such as H1,H3, H9, etc.

Neuraminidase Inhibition test

Sub-type identification based on the Neuraminidase Inhibition (NI) test is generally beyond the scope of many laboratories. Only international references labs of WHO/OIE should be consulted for Neura minidase of isolates, such as N1,N2, etc. If both HAI and NAI tests are conducted final sub type combination can be determined on suspected isolates of SIV such as H_1N_1, H_1N_2, H_3N_1 ...

Other sero-diagnostic tests on SIV

FAT (Fluorescent Antibody test) using fluorescein labbed swine influenza antibody can be used for tissue sections or cover slips/ slides of infected cell monolayer for frozen tissue sections.

Similarly immune-histochemistry procedures are performed using primary mouce anti-SIV monoclonal antibody (directed against the viral nucleoprotein and secondary antibody (biotinylated goat anti-mouce antibody) and tertiary antibody (peroxidase conjugated streptovidin) and diaminobenizidine tetra hydrochloride solution for development of brown staining in bronchiolar epithelium and pneumocytes in lung tissues (paraffin embedded formalin fixed) on microscopic slide section after counter staining the tissue section of gills haematoxalin for demonstration of SIV viral antigen in unknown sample of tissue section (chapter 2.10.11 "Swine influenza" in OIE terrestrial manual, 2004).

Similarly antigen capture enzyme linked immunosorbant assay (ELISA) and NIV (National Institute of Virology, Pune) has imported Diagnostic "RT-PCR" commercial kits for quick diagnosis of swine flue viral genome of present strain of "Mexican Swine Flue" from

Naso Pharyngial fluid samples. Real time polymerase chain Rection (RTPCR) and some other tests are available commercially for detection of SIV sub-type antigens in tissues (Fouchier, R.A. *et al.*, 2000).

Veterinary Vaccines for SIV Protection

Methods for SIV vaccine manufacture

All Veterinary SIV vaccines are produced by cultivation of SIV on swine kidney or swine lung tissue monolayer or suspension cell culture systems or by cultivation of vaccine virus is chick embryos by allantoic/ammiotic sac inoculation using SPF eggs using protocol WHO/OIE terrestrial manual, 2004.

These vaccines are produced by inactivation of vaccine virus lots using chemical inactivants including formalin or binary ethyleneimine (BEI) and after testing of the inactivated vaccine brews by standard safety sterility stability and potency procedures for inactivated viral vaccines. Thimersal (0.01%) is added as preservative and mineral oil adjuvants are used for enhancement of duration of immunity.

It should be noted that many sub-types are prevalent in the endemic areas of swine influenza, such as H1N1, H1N2, H3N2 predominantly in Europe and American continents in additional to H1N7, H3N1, N4N6 and H9N2 as described in previous paragraphs. Moreover European and American sub-types, even though belonging to the same sub-types but serologically different in their immunogenicity in-vivo due to differences in their terminal amino-acid sequences due to point mutations antigenic drifts and even antigenic shifts (development of new inter-species reassortments as described in previous paragraphs). Hence, the immunological vaccine strain behaviour varies from case to case. It is, therefore, prudent to keep continuous watch on molecular behaviour of the vaccine strains and the field strains of SIV as is done in case of human A influenza virus isolates from the field every year by WHO and change the vaccine virus seed isolate as and when required on continuous monitoring basis. This is required to take care of shedding of field virus from vaccinated animals which in fact brings about emergence of new recombinant viruses under vaccination pressures as swine is supposed to be a "reaction vessel" for evolution of both swine and human influenza viruses in nature. If the veterinary Swine Influenza Virus (SIV) vaccines are "tailor made" every time by continuous laboratory monitoring of SIV molecular structure, it will help in reduction of shedding of virus from vaccinated animals which in turn reduce the chances of development of new pandemic human influenza A viruses, as explained in chapter on Avian influenza.

Preventive measures

As evolution of new recombinant strains of swine influenza are evolved by "antigenic shifts" during inter-species transmission between birds - swine human due to confinement of swine breeding and poultry breeding operations and continuous perpetuation of the newly evolved "novel" swine influenza strain occur in so-called confined animal feeding operations (CAFOS), wherein swine breeding and feeding is carried out in highly congested and confined jigantic building, (PUEU commission appointed last year for 2008.) Suggesting recommendations for control of swine flue in USA suggested that swine and bird breeding/feeding centres/operations should be away from each other and they also suggested several effective hygienic measures which were not liked by the concerned animal/bird operating establishment in USA and hence, the said commission itself had to be abolished. But this resulted in evolution of the present pandemic of swine flue in Human population.

Suggested Reading

Dorset, M., McBryde, C.N., Niles, W.B. (1922). Remarks on "Hog Flue". J. American Veterinary Medical Assoc. 62: 162-171.

Koen, J.S. (1919) A practical method for field diagnosis of swine diseases American. Journal of Veterinary Medicine 14: 468-470.

Smith, W, Andrews C, Laidlaw P. A virus obtained from influenza patients. Lancet. 1933; 2: 66–68.

❑❑❑

Chapter 11

Bovine Papillomatosis (Cutaneous Warts) of Viral Origin

Cutaneous warts in cattle, horses, sheep and goats are benign tumours induced by host specific papilloma viruses. However, no much research on papilloma viruses of horses and small ruminants has been done but in cattle 6 types have been identified, namely BPV-1, BPV-2, BPV-3, BPV-4, BPV-5 and BPV-6. This causes true epithelial papillomas (Jarrett *et al.*, 1984).

About virus

6 cattle types of papilloma viruses show site specificity as follows:

BPV-1	:	Fibro-papillomas of teat skin and penile fibro-papilloma.
BPV-2	:	Fibro-papilloma of forehead neck and back (common cutaneous warts) and cauliflower like warts of anogenital and ventral abomen.
BPV-3	:	Cutaneous papilloma
BPV-4	:	Papilloma of oesophagus, oesophagial groove and fore stomach which may become malignant.
BPV-5	:	Ricegrain fibro papilloma of udder skin.
BPV-6	:	Epithelial papillomas of bovine udder and teats.

BPV can be typed by ELISA as well as by PCR on biopsy material or tissue scrapings.

Epidemiology and Transmission

The disease occurs all over the world. Method of shread is by direct contact with infected animals and infection gains entry through cutaneous abrasions. The virus persists on inanimate objects in live stock premises and infects animals rubbing against them (Campo. *et al.* 1994). Crops of warts occur around earotags, at branding sites or long scratches due to barbed wire. It can also spread by tattooing devices, dehorning equipment or even due to injection injuries including tuberculin testing outbreak of perianal warts is recorded spreading through rectal examination for pregnancy.

Pathogenesis

The virus infects the basal keratinocytes, replicating its genome in the differentiating spinous and granular layers causing the excessive growth that is characteristic of wart formation. The tumour contains epithelial and connective tissues and it can be papilloma or fibro-papilloma depending upon the relative proportions of epithelial and connective tissue, the former contains more epithelial tissue while the later contains more connective tissue.

Symptoms and Lesions

Warts appear on any part of the body, its distribution and nature depending on the type of the virus as detailed out in a paragraph on "About virus" mentioned previously. The most common papillomas occur in the skin of cattle under 2 years of age, mainly on head, around eyes and on neck as well as shoulders but may spread to other parts of body. Size may vary from rice grain, peanut tennis ball to a coconut size and appear as cauliflower like with dry and horny consistency. The tumours may regress spontaneously, after persistence for 5-6 months and as long as 16 to 18 months in some cases Warts can be pedunculated or in some cases they may be sessile. Teat and udder warts can be "rice grain" like elongated.

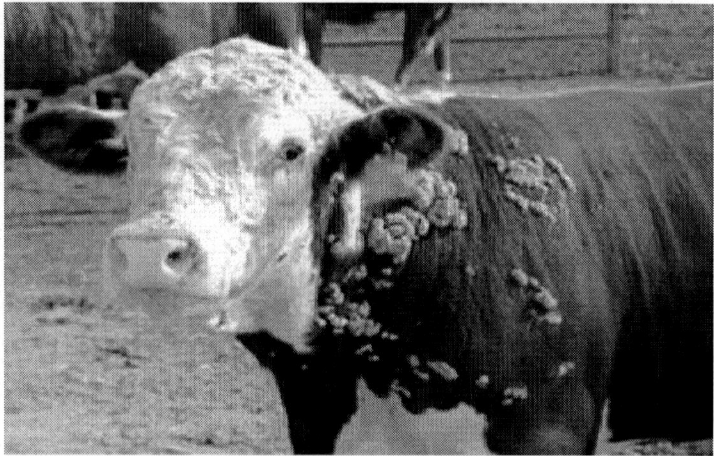

Fig. 1: Bovine papilomatosis lesions

Treatment

Surgical removal of few tumour growths may result into spontaneous regression of all the warts in the animal. Pedunculated warts can be removed by tieing the root of wart with horse hair.

Use of autogenous vaccine prepared by trituration of wart material from single animal, fittered through 9 sterile gauge and inactivated with 0.2% formaldehyde (final concentration) for intra dermal or sub cutaneous inoculation of all the individual wart affected animals may bring about regression of papillomas in all the herd due to development of immunity against virus as well as tumour antigen.

Vaccination and Control

Commercial vaccines against individual BPV type as well as polyvalent BPV vaccines are available abroad which can be used for prevention of occurance of papillomatosis in cattle. However, monvalent BPV vaccines are poor in performance as compared with autogenous vaccines prepared from single calf's tumour tissue material.

Animal to animal variation in regression following vaccination of a group of calves with a vaccine prepared from a single calf in the group has been attributed to more than one BPV type producing disease in the group. (Ndarathi and Mbuthia).

Indian Scenario

Incidence of Bovine papillomatosis in indigenous cattle of working type is not prevailing at cognisible level in village cattle. However, the author has seen very high incidence of skin papillomatosis of infectious origin in many Gir herds of Panjrapols in Maharashtra, especially Panjrapols at Nasik, Ahmednagar and Malad (Bombay). It was reported that the crops of such warts show regression spontaneously in old age after appearance of the said papillomas during calfhood or during heifer stage. Use of autogenous vaccine prepared from single animal for regression of the tumors of animals in the herd was found useful.

Suggested Reading

Campo M.S., Jarrett W.F., O'Neil W., Barron R.J.(1994). Latent papillomavirus infection in cattle. Res. Vet. Sci. 56(2): 151–157.

Jarret, W.F., Campo, M.S., O'neal B., Laird, H., Coggins, L. (1984): A novel bovine papilloma virus (BPV-6) causing true epithelial papilloma of the mammary gland skin: A member of a proposed new BPV subgroup. Virology 136: 255–264.

Ndarathi, C.M.and Mbuthia, P.G. (1994). Individual bovine specific and species-specific autogenous vaccine in treatment of bovine cutaneous papillomatosis. Indian J Anim Sci, 64: 218-221.

□□□

Chapter 12

Peste Des Petitis Ruminants (PPR) of Sheep and Goats

Peste Des Petitis Ruminants (PPR) is a virus disease of goats and sheep which is of recent origin and is caused by morbilli virus. The disease was confused with Rinderpest clinically in the earlier years.

Incidences and Geographical Distribution

Out breaks of PPR were first described in West Africa in 1942. Outbreaks were also reported from sub-Saharan Africa, north of equator, Arabian Peninshula, India and Pakistan.

The first outbreaks in Saudi Arabia were associated with importation of sheep from Africa or the return of unsold lambs from livestock markets.After the development of Rinderpest, Goat adapted spleen tissue vaccine by Edwards in 1924 by serial passaging of virulent Bovine R.P. virus in Goats, he (Edwards) declared in 1928 at Nagpur conference that serum simultaneous method of R.P. hot Bovine virus method will be replaced by "Goatis" i.e. GTV vaccine. The work on "Caprinisation" of the R.P. virus was further persued by development of the line W. strain which represents a highly modified caprinised strain which was being used as seed virus for GTV. GTV was being used under Rinderpest control and Eradication scheme since 1954 on large scale in South India and Maharashtra. Dr. Manjrekar and later on S.P. Phadke reported occurrence of "Rinderpest" or Rinderpest like disease in goats and sheep in their outbreak reports of Assistant Disease Investigation Officers (Cattle sheep and goats), i.e. ADIO (CSGS) under Disease Investigation Section (DIS) Maharasthra State, Poona during early 60's and late 50's expressing possibility of accidential goat/sheep vaccination as the source of this Rinderpest infection in goats and sheep. Now it is doubted that the "Goatis" virus, thus slipped accidently in goats and sheep might be the source of "Cycling and recycling" of R.P. virus in these small ruminants which might have resulted into natural "mutation" of R.P. virus into "PPR" virus as the close antigenic relationship of both these "Morbilli viruses" is well known (Abu-Elzein *et al.*, 1990). For many years, PPRV was considered to be a disease endemic within regions of Africa but then, during the 1980s, the virus was discovered in the Sultanate of Oman on the Arabian peninsular (Taylor, 1984) and was then later, and significantly found to be circulating in India (Shaila, *et al.*, 1989). It was the discovery and subsequent spread of PPRV across India and surrounding countries that highlighted PPRV as a disease of significant economic burden across much of Asia and the Middle East. However, serological screening of small ruminant populations across these regions suggest that the virus may have been present for a significant period of time prior to the increased disease inflicted by what is assumed to be the emergence of a highly virulent strain in India during the 1980s.

Tatvarthy *et al.* (1994) reported occurrence of Rinderpest like disease condition in goats in south Maharashtra showing respiratory involvement pyrexia and digestive tract involvement, with 44% morbidity and 64% mortality amongst morbid animals. Shaila *et al.* (1996) confirmed this outbreak as PPR, using RNA Hybridization test. This is the first confirmed incidence of PPR in goats in Maharashtra.

Etiology

PPR is caused by *Morbillivirus* (Family *Paramyxoviridae*), which is closely related to Rinderpest virus as well as the viruses of canine distemper in Dogs, Phocine distemper of seals, measles in human and equine influenza (pink eye) described in Austrelia. The African and Asian strains of PPR virus may have evolved separately and they have some biological differences.

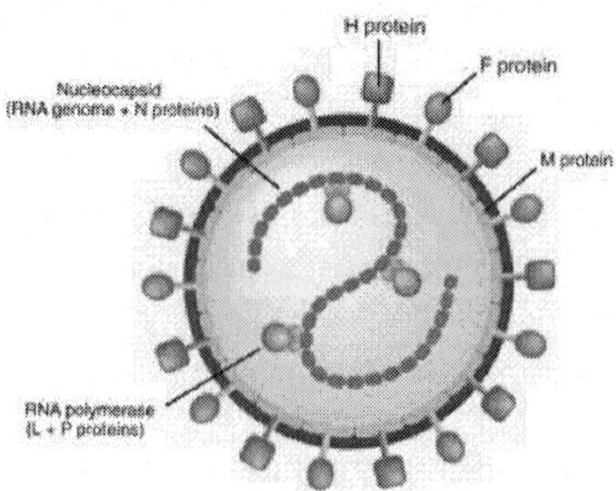

Fig. 1: Morbillivirus structure

Epidemiology

Pigs and cattle do not show any disease symptoms but develop Neutralizing antibodies following experimental infection. Wild sheep, deers and gazelle are prone to the disease but they do not act as "reservoirs" for disease in domestic small ruminants. Sahelian goats and sheep are having innate resistance to the disease virus which they harbour without symptoms and when they co-mingle with dwarf sheep in humid climatic areas, the later develop the disease symptoms. Market goats harbour infection and transmit the same to the Arabian sheep. The disease spreads by close contact of susceptible animals with diseased animals or contaminated fomites. The virus is present in diarrhoeal faeces and other body excretions and infection occurs mainly through inhalation or injection of contaminated feed or through conjunctiva.

Pathogenesis

The virus contaminates "naive" animals through their oral and nasal passages. After entering into the organism, it multiplies first in the oropharynx and local lymphoid tissues. All of the immune cells (lymphocytes, macrophages, and reticular cells) can be a target for virus multiplication. The newly formed virions spread throughout the host's organs and tissues with a preference for digestive, pulmonary, and respiratory mucosa and the immune system.

Lesions

On the macroscopic scale

The resulting tissue damage, which can be observed post-mortem, is responsible for the clinical manifestations of the disease: discharge, lacrimation, diarrhoea.

On the microscopic scale

Biochemical and enzyme analyses show changes in kidney function (high urea and creatinine) through the multiplication of the virus in its cells and low blood parameter values (erythrocytes and haematocrit) linked to internal intestinal and renal haemorrhaging. In parallel, the PPRV infection induces cell death through apoptosis in immune cells, leading to severe immunosuppression. This weakening of the animal's natural defences through leukopenia opens the door to secondary bacterial and viral infections which interfere with the normal progression of the disease and complicate its diagnosis. These opportunistic infections significantly increase the mortality rate associated with PPR..

Clinical Symptoms

The disease is acute more so in goats than in sheep. The disease simulates Rinderpest in cattle as far as diarrhoea is concerned but respiratory involvement especially pneumonia is also present in case of PPR as against its absence in R.P. in cattle, which is a point for differentiation in PPR against R.P.

Incubation period is about 3-6 days after affected animal comes in contact of the susceptible one. In goats, pyrexia above 40^{0}C sets in after anoerexia sneezing, serious discharge from nose and eyes followed by necrosis and minute ulcerative lesions covered with wheat barnlike deposits set in mouth a day or two later. Diptheretic plaques can also appear on oral mucosa. Swollen lips and sore mouth and eye discharge is a common feature of the disease. Profuse diarrhoea with mucoid faeces which may be blood tinged sets in last. Vulvar erosions/ prepucial erosions may be also evident death may occur within one week. Sheep may show less acute picture than goats. Most of sheep may recover after disease. Postmortem picture is almost similar to that in Rinder pest, including typical "Zebra stripings" in last part of intestines. Interstitial pneumonia is a common feature in PPR in contrast with R.P. (Brown, *et al.*, 1991).

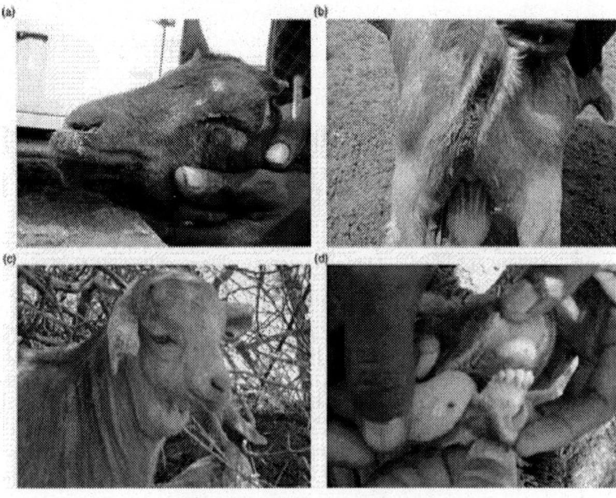

Fig. 2: PPR symptoms

Intra cytoplasmic eosiniphitic inclusion bodies in interstitial crypst epithelial cells in intestine and intracytoplasmic and intranuclear eosinophilic inclusions in respiratory tract mucosa are quite common. The proliferative rhino-tracheitis, bronchitis, bronchiolitis, proliferation of Type II pneumocytes and formation of huge syncytial gians cells are quite characteristics of PPR infection.

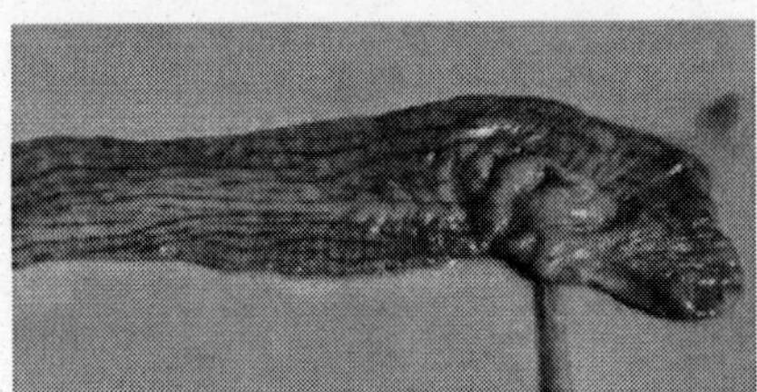

Fig. 3: Characteristic postmortem signs of zebra marking in intestine

Treatment

Use of Rinderpest hyperimmune serum from cattle can be of great help in treating the PPR affected animals along with supportive fluid therapy for dehydration and use of antibiotics for checking secondary bacterial infection is also helpful.

Control

Avoiding bringing unknown sheep or goat stocks from abroad should be followed by quarrantining before mixing in the flocks.

All the newly arrived stock and farm stock in their contact should be vaccinated using tissue culture based kebete "O" strain freez, dried Rinderpest vaccine for getting effective protection against PPR, as this vaccine provides good cross immunity. Vaccination of kids and lambs should be carried out at 3-4 months age i.e. after waning of maternal immunity.

Newly developed vaccines developed as Recombinent vaccines with either vaccinia (Jones *et al.* 1993) or capripox (Romero, *et al.* 1995) as carrier viruses expressing fusion (F) and haemagglutinin (H) genes of R.P. are reported to be very effective.

Homologous PPR tissue cultured vaccine produced in vero cell line by attenuation of PPR Nigerian isolate is also reported to have protection against virulent virus challenge (Jones *et al.*, 1993).

Suggested Reading

Abu-Elzein, E.M.E., Hassanien, M.M., AL-afaleq.A.I.,. Abdlhadi, F. M. and Housawi F. M.T. (1990): Isolation Detection and of peste des petits ruminant from goats in Saudi Arabia.Vet. Rec. 127: 309-310.

Brown, C.C., Mariner, J.C. and Olander, H.J. (1991). An immunohistochemical study of pneumonia caused by peste des petits ruminants virus. Veterinary Pathology 28: 166-170.

Jones, L., Giavedoni, L., Saliki, J.T., Brown, C., Mebus, C. & Yilma, T. (1993). 'Protection of goats against peste des petits ruminants with a vaccinial virus double recombinant expressing the F and H genes of rinderpest virus', Vaccine 11: 961–964.

Romero, C.H., Barrett, T., Kitching, R.P., Bostock, C., Black, D.N. (1995) Protection of goats against peste des petits ruminants with a recmbinant capripox viruses expressing the fusion and haemagglutinin protein genes of rinderpest virus. Vaccine 13: 36-40.

Shaila, MS, Purushothaman, V, Bhavasar, D, Venugopal, K, Venkatesan, RA (1989) Peste des petits ruminants of sheep in India. Vet Rec 125:602

Shaila, M.S., Shamaki, D., Forsyth,M.A., Diallo, A., Goatley, L., Kitching, R.P., Barrett, T. (1996). Geographic distribution and epidemiology of peste des petits Ruminants virus. Virus Res. 43: 149–153.

Taylor, WP (1984) The distribution and epidemiology of peste des petits ruminants. Pre Vet Med. 2: 157–166.

□□□

Chapter 13

Bovine Ephemeral Fever (Three days Sickness)

Bovine ephemeral fever is an arthropod borne virus disease of cattle and buffaloes of the age more than six months characterized by three days of febrile sickness with generally morning remissions. The disease is enzootic in African, continent, most of Asia, Middle East, East Indies and Australia.

Generally morbidity rate is 35% but if environment is favourable for the vector including mosquitoes and the biting midges, the morbidity may reach 100% with no mortality or very negligible mortality, if the host is exotic or highbred.

Probably vectors include mosquitoes belonging to *Aedes* species, *Culex annulirostris, Anopheles bancrofti* and biting midges *Culicoides brevitarsis*.

About the virus

Ephemeral fever is caused by an arthropod-borne *Rhabdo* virus which is a type species of the genus *Ephemerovirus*. Number of strains of *Ephemerovirus* causing the disease varies anigenically. The virus is found closely associated with the leucocyte-platelet fraction of the infected blood, which when inoculated in animal, can transmit the disease. The virus can be easily adapted to adult mice by repeated intracerebral passaging. Lambs, adult rats and guinea pigs are also susceptible.

Method of transmission and epidemiology

Mosquitoes and biting midges mentioned above are the biological vectors and they can transmit the infection within a week of feeding on the infected animal. The reservoir host other than cattle is not yet identified. In Australia, the epidemiological pattern is changed from the disease occurring only once in decade previously to annual occurrence of the disease now-a-days probably due to the establishment of the virus in indigenous vectors (not in any reservoir host). The disease is not spread by physical contact with infected animals or their saliva or ocular discharge or through semen. Spread of the disease occurs in summer months and outbreaks are clustered and relatively short-lived and spread largely depends on the insect vector population and the direction of winds on which vector travel the longer distances.

As almost 100% animal gets infected during the outbreak, immunity develops in whole population and hence, the disease disappears for long periods in the population of animals and re-appears when the resistance of the population is diminished. Recurrence depends on suitable environmental conditions for increase and dissemination of the insect vector.

Pathogenesis

Virus multiplication takes place in Vascular system after the bite from infected vector after incubation period of 2 to 10 days. There is biphasic fever with peaks 12 and 24 hrs apart (Uren *et al.*, 1983). There is generalized inflammation with vasculitis, thrombosis, especially serofibrnous inflammation in serous and synovial cavities and increased endothelial permeability at the same sites (Yong and Spradbrow, 1990). The virus is detected in circulating leucocytes, plasma and serosal/synovial fluids as well as epicardial fluids.

Symptoms and postmortem findings

The disease is acute with sudden onset of fever upto 105^0-106^0F, many times with remissions of 24/12 hours. Off feeding and decreased milk yield also occur stingy nasal and watry ocular discharge with animals shaking their heads and muscular shivering is characteristics. Muscles become stiff with a posture of animal similar to that of laminitis. The febrile reaction reduces by the third day but weakness and lameness persists for 2-3 days. Pulmonary emphysema may develop. Milder cases only show fever. Hypocalcemia and recombancy is found in majority of cases. Postmortem lesions are not dramatic but consistent lesion may be sero fibrinous polyserositis involving with increase in synovial, pleural, pericardial and peritoneal fluid. All lymphnodes are usually enlarged. Pulmonary emphysema with bronchiolitis is generally found.

Treatment

Symptomatic treatment, such as phenylbutazone injection, salisylates by oral route and calcium borogluconate injection by I/V route are useful in treating the symptoms.

Control

Tissue culture based or adult mice brain adapted attenuated vaccines in quil A or frauends adjuvanted vaccines are available in Australia, Japan, Taiwan and South Africa.

Diagnostic tests

Available serological tests include CFT, SNT, FAT and AGID tests (Gard. *et al.*, 1988) or blocking ELISA test is simple and preferred test (Zakrewaski *et al.*, 1992).

Indian Scenario

The disease in enzootic in India, prevailing since ancient times and shows only very mild symptoms in indigenous animals which warrants only symptomatic treatment. Even after starting of cross-breeding programme, there is no much change in the course of the disease and hence, no vaccination is practiced up-to-date.

Suggested Reading

Gard G.P., Shorthose J.E., Weir R.P., Walsh S.J., Melville L.F. (1988). Arboviruses recovered from sentinel livestock in Northern Australia.Vet. Microbiol. 18(2): 109-118.

Uren M.F., St George T.D., Stranger R.S. (1983). Epidemiology of ephemeral fever of cattle in Australia 1975-1981. Aust. J. Biol. Sci. 36: 91–100.

Young P.L., Spradbrow P.B. (1990). Clinical response of cattle to experimental infection with bovine ephemeral fever virus. Vet. Rec. 126: 86–88.

Zakrzewski, H., Cybinski, D.H. & Walker, P.J. (1992). A blocking ELISA for the detection of specific antibodies to bovine ephemeral fever virus. Journal of Immunological Methods 151: 28%297.

□□□

Chapter 14

Blue Tongue in Sheep

Blue tongue is a viral non-contagious disease of sheep and occasionally of cattle, which are transmitted by culicoides or midges, belongs to the species like C. *Varipenis Var. Sonorensis* in U.S.A. or C. *imicola* (pallidipennis in Africa and C. *fulvis, C.inicola,* and *C.orieutalis* in Asia and Middle East while in Australia by C. *wadai,* C. *brevipalpis* and C. *brevitarsis,* etc. The latter two species of culicoides are obligate parasites of cattle (dung breeders) while other species of culicoides can complete their life-cycle without cattle. Hence, blue tongue in cattle is predominantly observed in Australia where C. *brevitarsis* species most extensively dispersed vector (Ward,1994). The distribution and intensity of infection of regions of continents is determined by the climate geography and altitude, as they affect the occurrence and activity of culicoides vectors and by presence of susceptible hosts (sheep & cattle or wild ruminants). Hence, blue tongue activity is continuous in tropics and absence of virus transmission in colder areas.

In endemic areas, the infection of blue tongue (BT) is always present but the clinical BT is seen only in susceptible animals. Generally exotic breeds of sheep like Marinos and Rambuolets, etc. show clinical disease while indigenous breeds' even though show presence of sub-clinical infection do not show clinical disease. Goats generally do not show natural disease but can be experimentally infected.

About the virus

Blue Tongue Virus (BTV) is an arthropod borne *"Orbivirus"* belonging to the family *"Reoviridae"*. There are at least 25 serotypes of BTV worldwide prevailing with the considerable genetic variability within the serogroup. This arises mainly by genetic "drift" of individual gene segments as well as by reassortments of gene segments, when ruminants or the "vectors" are infected with more than one serotype strain at a time. Current view is that whether there is a biological validity of the classification of BTV into strict serotypes (Gorman, 1990; Heidner *et al.,* 1991, Maclachlan *et al.,* 1992).

All serotypes do not exist in anyone infected Area e.g. types 2, 7 and 9 were confined to African continent only while types 10 and 16 did not exist in Africa atleast upto 1970 (as informed by P.G. Howell of Worldwide Reference Laboratory at Veterinary Research Institute, Onderstepoort, South Africa to us at Disease Investigation Section, M.S. Poona vide his report on Blue Tongue material Investigation in 1970 dt. 14.5.1970).

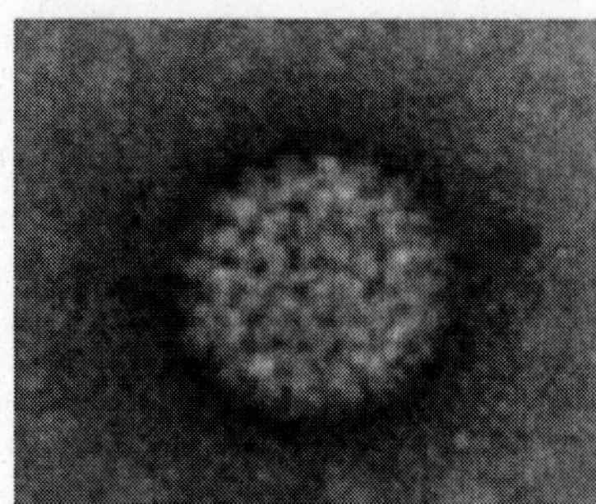

Fig. 1: Blue tongue virus

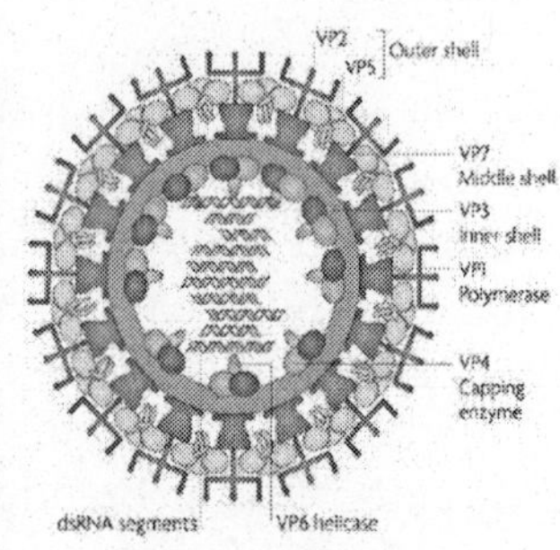

Fig. 2: Schematic representation of BTV

BTV is resistant to decomposition and some standard virucidal agent like Sodium carbonate but are sensitive to acid pH 6.0 and 3% Sodium hydroxide and Idophore compounds.

Epidemiology and disease transmission

Female culicoides feed on cattle sheep, goats and deer and require at least one blood meal for completion of the ovarian cycle. This feeding of blood is nocturnal (night feeding) in open pens and fields and this activity occurs optimally between 13^{0}C and 35^{0}C temperature.

Virus in ingested blood infects cells of the midgut of culicoides by receptor mediated process (XU *et al.*, 1997), where it replicates and then it is released in salivary gland of culicoides which when remain infected for lifetime i.e. period of several weeks (Mellor, 1990). The culicoides may feed two or more times on different hosts and thus, virus transmission is achieved after feeding on viremic animal. BTV is thus maintained in nature by alternating cycles of infection between midge and ruminant species. As the cubicoides are killed by frost, the disease is only seasonal in endemic subtropical high altitude/colder areas. Culicoides breed only in damp wet areas with stream and ponds and hence, disease shows its appearance in sheep and ruminants living in such areas.

Culicoides species show difference in their susceptibility to different sero types of BTV while explains regional differences in serotype occurance (Ward, 1994). Some ticks (*Ornithodoros coriacus*) sheep ked (*Malophagus ovinus*) and mosquites (*Ades lineatopennis* and *Anopheles vagus*) can transmit the disease virus mechanically. Different culicoides species have different host preference some prefer cattle distinctly and not sheep and hence, only cattle get infected in such case without showing infection in sheep in those areas where they exist. This is observed in Australia (Ward, 1994).

Serotype occurrence

In USA, serotypes 10, 11, 13 and 17 were existing for a long time while recently serotype 2 is recorded, serotype 13 was probably derived by re-assortment of vaccine virus (Osburn *et al.*, 1996). In Caribbean Region, and South and Central America serotypes 1 to 4, 6,8,12 and 17 are reported (Gibbs and Greiner,1994; Tanya *et al*, 1992). In Australia, 8 serotypes are recorded, namely 3,9,15,16,20,21 and 23 since 1984 while in Africa, serotype 1,16,18,19 and 24 are major ones isolated and in Asia serotypes 1,4,7,9,10,12,16,17,20,21 and 23 are reported. (Gibbs and Greiner, 1994).

Breed susceptibility

Merinos and British sheep breeds are more susceptible for clinical disease as compared with indigenous breeds which show only infection. In Australia, sheep above 3 years of age only show clinical disease and solar radiation can increase the susceptibility of the solar exposed sheep.

Morbidity and mortality rate

When the disease occurs for the 1st time in susceptible breeds in new areas, morbidity can be as high as 50 to 70% with mortality of 20 to 50%. In Cyprus and Spain, mortality reached upto 70% in affected flocks as unusual case. In South Africa mortality of 2-30% was observed in usual field conditions. Immunity to BTV is strain specific and in epizootics, mortality can continue after introduction of heterogenous serotype strains of BTV one after the other by quick succession in a sheep population. The serotype strain isolated from very severe disease in the field may or may not show very high severity in experimentally inoculated susceptible animal. Mild reproduction of the disease is very common in such cases (Parsonson, 1990; Davies *et al.*, 1992).

Pathogenesis

The bite of culicoides insects carrying BTV in their saliva results into infection of draining lymph-nodes and dissemination of virus in mononuclear cells to secondary sites of replication in lymphoid tissue and lung. Viremia occurs by day 3 which peaks by day 6 to 7 after infection (Stott and Osburn, 1990). This results into localization of virus in vescular endothelium leading to endothelial cell degeneration of necrosis. This causes thromboris haemorrhages and intravascular coagulation of blood (Maclachlan *et al.*, 1994). In cattle, endothelial cell infection is minimal but viremia is highly cell associated especially with erythrocytes and platelets (However, virus is only shielded by them and no replication in erythrocytes (Stott J.L. *et al.*, 1990) but virus in protected from neutralising antibody in circulation.

About the clinical disease

Severe febrile reaction with 105^0-106^{0}F temperature is usual which continues for 5-6 days. After 48 hours of fever, nasal discharge and salivation follows with hyperemia of buccal and nasal mucosa. Nasal discharge is muco-purulent. Swelling of lips, gums dental pad and tongue is evident with offensive odour. Necratic ulcers on lateral aspects of tongue with occasional "purpling" may be evident but not usual. Ulceration of commeasures of lips, buccal papillae and around anus and vulva may be present. Diarrhoea and dysentery can also be observed.

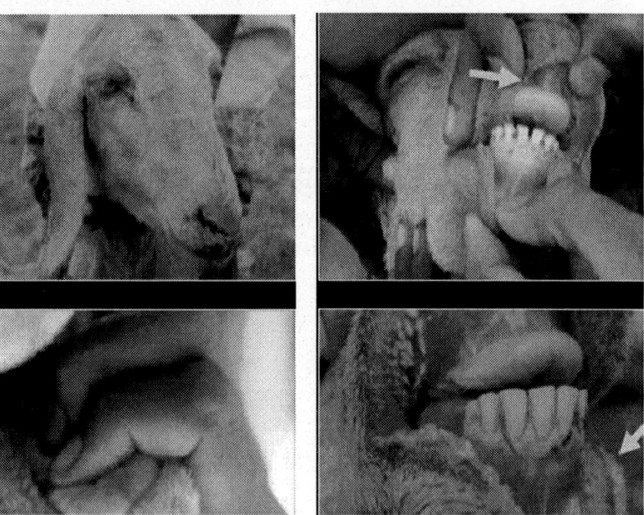

Fig. 3: Blue tongue symptoms in sheep

Coronitis and laminits of one, two or more liombs with lamness is quite often be evident. Dark red to purple coloured band on skin above the carronet is one of the diagnostic symptom of BT in sheep. Twisting of neck (Wryneck) occurs occasionally Hyperemia of non-wooled skin and facial swelling with severe conjunctivitis and lacrimation can be observed in number of affected sheep. Vomiting with subsequent aspiration pneumonia is seen in some cases. Partial or complete loss of fleece is common, causing substantial loss for farmer financially. Cracking of hooves during convalescence is also seen. Pregnant sheep usually get aborted. In sheep in enzootic areas, the disease is much less severe or may be often in apparent.

Post mortem findings

Coronitis skin and facial lesions described above along with pneumonia (Aspiration type), buccal and tongue lesions are evident during the postmortem. Haemorrhagic longitudinal steaks are observed on intestinal mucosa with swollen mesenteric lymph-nodes liver surface may show necrotic lesions of difuse nature. Spleen may be slightly swollen and hyperemic.

Clinical pathology

Packed cell volume (PCV) may fall significantly. Initial leucopenia may be followed by leucocytosis. In severe disease, leucopenia due to lymphopenia may continue upto death.

Diagnosis

Specific diagnosis is either by isolation of virus or detection of viral antigen or nucleic acid or by demonstration of rising C.F. anti-bodies/nuetralising antibodies in acute stage and recovery stage (paired) sera samples from affected sheep. Characteristic haemorrhagic embryo after intra venous inoculation of embryonated chicken egg by suspected blood sample is indicative of presence of BT virus.

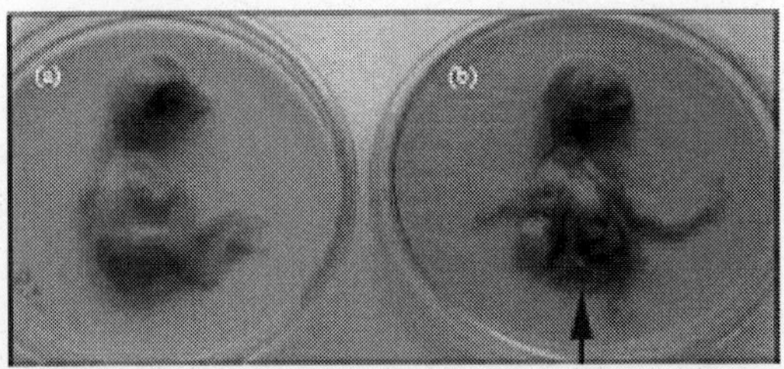

Fig. 4: (a) Normal embryo (b) BT infected haemorrhagic embryo

Virus isolation from febrile viremic stage in affected animal by collection of blood samples in OCG solution and inoculation of the same in embryonated eggs by yolk sac route. The dead embryo can be used for C.F. test or demonstration of viral nucleic acid for confirmation of BTV more reliably. The original host species, namely susceptible sheep (exotic breed) can also be inoculated for virus isolation, confirmed by detection of characteristic symptoms of BT in inoculated sheep and its subsequent challenge by known BT virus isolate of homologous serotype. It should be noted that the compliment fixation test is not type specific but detects only BT virus while the challenge tests or Neutralisation tests are "type specific" used for detection of homologous type.

The commonly available tests for detection of BT group specific antibodies are AGPT and ELISA tests as well as CF test. Klontz *et al.* (1963) described AGPT using baby brain adapted strain of BT virus as positive antigen. This technique could not give satisfactory results at our hands, when we used the same in 1967-68 at Disease Investigation Section, M.S. Poona (under MDC-BT scheme).

Control

Reducing the risk of exposure to infected culicoides vector by using vector repellents and insecticides and housing sheep in insect proof houses (doors and windows provided with meshed doors) during night time may be useful to avoid mosquito and culicoides bites. But this has only limited value due to practical difficulties. Vaccination is the only satisfactory control measure. Vaccination will not eliminate infection but it is successful in keeping losses to a very low level provided immunity to all local strains of the virus is attained.

Currently in counties in which BT virus infections are endemic, such as in Africa and Israel, Polyvalent attenuated vaccines are used while they are available for use in other countries for use, whenever the disease occurs occasionally.

Mason *et al.* (1940) prepared egg adapted BT vaccine consisting of the embryo (infected with BT virus) in buffered saline solution treated with crystal violet. This vaccine was in use for protecting sheep against BT which was then prevalent in Middle East and Africa. However, this vaccine is no more in use as immunity is transient. The live attenuated vaccines are produced in cell cultures and are quite effective. However, they have mild reactions in the vaccinated animals.

These vaccines should not be used in ewes within 3 weeks after mating as anoestrus often results. Annually re-vaccination is recommended one month before the expected occurrence of the disease in particular season of the disease. Immunity is conferred by the vaccine 10 days post vaccination. The live attenuated vaccines should not be used in ewes during pregnancy as vaccine virus can create risk of deformity in lambs or embryonic death danger period being between 4th and 8th week of pregnancy.

There is also a risk of vaccine strain being transmitted sheep to sheep through culicoides vector and getting "exalted" due to serial passaging in nature as evident from emergence of reassortment strain from vaccine virus in United States (Osburn, *et al.*, 1996).

Disease Scenario in India

Blue tongue was recorded in Pakistan in Indian sub continent in 1960 for the first time. Spare (1964) reported number of outbreaks in sheep for the first time in India, showing symptoms of lameness with initial febrile reaction followed by ulcerative lesions on buccal mucosa and lateral aspects of tongue in Ahmednagar and Satara district during the period from 1962 to 1963 which they suspected for Blue Tongue Disease. However, S.N. Sapre, the then Dy. Director of Disease Investigation Section could get confirmation of Blue Tongue Disease in sheep, in India in 1963-64 from "Onderstepoort" world reference laboratory for B.T.V. in South Africa, when his colleagues (Research Assistants), namely S.V. Pandit and V.H. Apte collected paired sera samples and infective spleen and lymph-node material from suspected sheep outbreak of Blue Tongue Disease in Pathardi Taluka of Ahmednagar district and sent the same for confirmation to onderstepoort laboratory. Onderstepoort laboratory also recovered BT "type 10" virus from the material collected by them from outbreak of suspected Blue tongue from Pathardi Taluka. However, refrained to confirm it as "Virus isolation" as sera samples from that particular postmortem animal was not available for detection of homologous antibodies and re-isolation from the material was not possible due to bacterial contamination.

Meanwhile some clinical cases of Blue Tongue were reported from exoitie Russian Merino and Rambullet sheep at Govt. Sheep Breeding farm at Tathawade near Pune (Maharashtra) during 1964-65. Simultaneously local Bannur Breed sheep also were found affected with this disease but they were showing very mild mouth and tongue lesions but lameness of one, two or more legs also evident with mild coronitis. S.V. Pandit and V.H. Apte tried to develop virus isolation technique in egg embryos by yolk sac route and complement fixation technique to diagnose BT at Virus Research Centre of ICMR during their deputation at that institute in 1964 to 1966.

As some evidence of the disease was thus established, further work on problem of Blue Tongue Disease was carried out and persued under scheme on Mucosal Disease and Blue Tongue which was operated at D.I. section, Poona jointly by ICAR and State Govt. The work done under this scheme from 1967 to 1969 threw further light on this incidence of BT in Maharashtra and the occurrence of this disease can be now considered to have been established in Maharashtra State and in India.

30 tissue samples and 46 paired sera samples from 3 outbreaks of suspected Blue Tongue were collected by us (Moghe, R.G., Pandit, S.V. and Apte, V.H.) from sheep breeding farm, Tathawade near Pune during the period 1967 to 1970. All these 3 outbreaks were encountered in exotic sheep (Russian Merino and crossbred sheep) and indigenous stocks of sheep were free from the clinical disease. However, paired sera samples collected from 2 Bannur sheep (local breed) experimentally inoculated with infective blood and spleen/mescentric lymph-node material collected from Russian merino lamb affected with B.T. showed rising C.F. antibody titres, indicating that, indigenous breed like bannur gets only infected but do not get clinical disease from BT virus.

Onderstepoort laboratory (Howell, P.G.) in their official report dated 22nd May, 1970 confirmed existence of Blue Tongue Disease in India on the basis of the tests conducted on exhaustive material sent by us, as mentioned above and stated that they could isolate serotype 16 from infective material sent by us from one sheep, the paired sera from the same sheep showed rising titre against homologous virus, namely type 16 B.T.V. which proved existence of this serotype 16 in India (Maharashtra, Pune) beyond any doubt. This serotype is of African origin and it might have been picked up by exotic Russian merinos during their transit to India via. Pakistan which showed its existence in 1960 in that country as reported by FAO. One particular serum sample was reported to be positive for the antibodies to serotypes 7,9,10 and 11 of BTV, suggesting more than one source of infection which must have entered this sheep at different times. They also communicated serological evidence against BT serotypes 1, 2, 7,9,10 in addition to type 16 from some of the sera out of 46 paired sera samples sent by us. They also stated that 4 out of these sera were positive by C.F. test but they were not showing neutralizing (NT) antibodies against any of the existing 1 to 16 serotype BT viruses, indicating possibility of existence of yet heather unknown types of BTV because these sera were collected 6 weeks after infection, when both CF and Neutralizing antibodies are bound to be present. (C.F. antobidies are only BT specific while neutralizing antibodies are BT as well as homologous type specific). (See final progress Report on ICARs MDC-BT Scheme 1967-70).

After termination of MDC-BT scheme in 1970, very typical clinical Blue Tongue outbreak was detected in Raymonds Exotic sheep Breeding Farm, at Lalling near Dhulia, where characteristics B.T. disease symptoms were seen in a flock of pure exotic Australian sheep imported 6 months before from Australia where there is no Blue Tongue (Australia was declared free from BT during that period) which means that this disease outbreak must have a source of BT virus from indigenous local breeds through culicoides species (Indigenous breeds must be a symptomatic carriers of the virus in their viremic blood.

Attempts for Control of Blue Tongue in India

Inactivated chick embryo based crystal violet treated vaccine with BT-8 embryo adapted strain was made available by Decruz Corporation during mid-1960s (during 1963-65) for field use but data on its efficacy is not available.

Some isolated efforts were made for undertaking serological survey of BTV serotypes existence. Pandit, S.V. and Apte, V.H. tried to develop complement fixation test at VRC, Pune (ICMR) using BT-8 virus strain obtained from California in 1966 (This was originally at 34th passage level in baby mice brain). This was further passaged at VRC, Pune for 10 more serial passages in baby mice brain to get desired titre of 10^{-6} in baby mice brain before using for production of C.F. antigen (Acetone – ether extracted purified antigen as per clerk and cassal method). Known positive hyper immune serum was prepared in adult mice by serial intrapertionial inoculation of the baby mice brain adapted virus BT 8 type CFT was developed as per the standard C.F. technique used for serological survey of Arthropod borne viruses at VRC, Pune (Rock feller Institute Technique).

This test along with BT-8 baby mice brain adapted virus for antigen preparation and hyper immune serum preparation was again established at Disease Investigation Section, Pune under ICAR State Govt. MDC-BT scheme by getting the said virus from VRC, Pune during 1967-70 for conducting serological survey but actual survey could not be undertaken as the said scheme was terminated in 1970.

There is evidence for circulation of at least 22 serotypes in India. BT is endemic in India. Till date, at least 13 different serotypes (BTV-1-4, 6, 9, 10, 12 16-18, 21 and 23) have been isolated under All-India Network Program on Blue tongue (AINP-BT) and by other research laboratories in the country. Diagnosis of BT requires isolation of virus, standard serological methods and several other antigen and nucleic acid detection as says. BTV serotypes are identified by virus neutralization test and sequencing of VP2 gene. Because of a large number of susceptible hosts, BTV serotypes and Culicoides vector, control of BT is not an easy task. Recently, in India, an inactivated pentavalent vaccine (BTV-1, 2, 10, 16 and 23) is developed and commercialized.

Suggested Reading

Davies, F.G., Mungai, J.N., Pini A.(1992). A new blue tongue virus serotype isolated in Kenya. Vet Microbiol. 31: 25–32.

Gibbs, E.P.J.and Greiner, EC (1994): The epidemiology of blue tongue. Comparative Immunology and Microbiology and Infectious Diseases 17: 207–220.

Gorman, B.M. (1990). The blue tongue viruses. Curr. Top. Microbiol. Immunol. 162: 1–19.

Heidner, H.W., Iezzi, L.G., Osburn, B.I. & Maclachlan, N.J. (1991). Genetic variation and evolutionary relationships amongst blue tongue viruses endemic in the United States. Virus Research 21: 91-109.

Maclachlan, N.J., Rossitto, P.V., Heidner, H.W., Iezzi, L.G., Yilma, T., Demaula, C.D. & Osburn, B.I. (1992). Variation amongst the neutralizing epitopes of blue tongue viruses isolated in the United States in 1979-1981. Veterinary Microbiology. 31: 303.

Mason, J.H., Coles, J.D.W.A., Alexander, R.A. (1940). Cultivation of blue tongue virus in fertile eggs produced in vitamin-deficient diet. Nature 145: 1022.

Mellor, P.S. (1990). The replication of blue tongue virus in *Culicoides* vectors. Curr. Topics Microbiol. Immunol. 162: 143–161.

Osburn, B.I., de Mattos, C.A., de Mattos C.C. MacLachlan, N.J. (1996). Blue tongue disease and the molecular epidemiology of viruses from the Western United States. Comp. Immunol. Microbiol. Infect. Dis. 19: 181.

Parsonson, I.M. (1990). Pathology and pathogenesis of blue tongue infections. Curr. Top. Microbiol. Immunol. 162: 119-141.

Sapre, S.N. (1964). An outbreak of blue tongue in goats and sheep. Vet. Rev., 15: 78-80.

Stott, J.L. and Osburn, B.I. (1990). Immune response to Blue tongue virus infection. Curr. Top. Microbiol Immunol 162: 163-78.

Tanya, V.N., Greiner, E.C., Gibbs, E.P. (1992): Evaluation of Culicoides insignis (Diptera: Ceratopogonidae) as a vector of blue tongue virus. Veterinary Microbiology 32: 1–14.

Ward, M.P. (1994). Climatic factors associated with the prevalence of blue tongue virus infection of cattle herds in Queensland, Australia. Vet Rec. 134: 407.

Xu, G., Wilson, W., Mecham, J., Murphy, K., Zhou, E.M., Tabachnick, W. (1997). VP7: 1121 an attachment protein of blue tongue virus for cellular receptors in Culicoides 1122 variipennis. J. Gen. Virol. 78: 1617-1623.

□□□

Chapter 15

Virus Diarrhoea in Calves, Lambs, Kids, Piglets and Foals

Virus diarrhoea other than bovine virus diarrhoea (BVD) is a common diarrhoeal disease of neonatal calves, lambs, kids, piglets and foals caused by several viral families including reoviridae, corona viridae, toroviridae and parvoviridae but the major cause being "*Rotaviruses*" belonging to family *Reoviridae*.

About the viruses causing virus Diarrhoea

Rotaviruses

There are 7 serogroups of Rotaviruses sharing distinctive group specific antigens, namely A to G. Each serogroup is further classified into serotypes based on specific outer capsid proteins VP 7 (G types) and VP4 (P types), there being 14 G and 12 P serotypes of group A rotaviruses which are most frequently detected in farm animals and humans (Saif, 1994). Group B rotaviruses have been isolated from adult cows with diarrhoea (Parwani, *et al.*, 1996).

Corona viruses

Corna viruses produce diarrhoea in calves and piglets.

Toroviruses

They include the Berne virus of horses (foals) and Breda virus of cattle (Scott *et al.*, 1996).

Parvoviruses

They are associated with diarrhoea in calves but not in adult cattle (Sandals, *et al.* 1995). There are Para Rotaviruses from calves, pigs, and lambs which are a typical rotaviruses which do not share common antigens during serological ELISA and immune fluoroscence tests used for Rotavirus detection.

There are many other viruses causing diarrhoea in calves, kids, lambs, piglets and foals but are not described here for want of space.

Epidemiology and disease transmission

The epidemiology of Rotaviruses, coronoviruses, toroviruses and Parvoviruses is similar and hence, Rotavirus epidemiology is described here as "model" for all these viruses. Rotaviruses are ubiquitous in environment and 50 to 100% of adults of bovines, equines, ovines and caprines and swines are seropositive. These infections spread by faeces contamination of feed; water as well as spread is possible by aerosol, when relative humidity of the environment is higher. The adult animal is the primary source of virus to the neonate through faecal contamination.

The rotaviruses of one species can infect only some other species and experimental infection of pigs, calves and lambs with human Rotavirus is possible. The calf rotavirus can infect pigs and foals. Infection of Rotaviruses from one species to the others is not significant in natural infection.

Colostrum antibody and protection of neonatal infection

It is important to note that the protective effect of colostral antibodies depends on its titre, the amount ingested and amount available in the lumen of the intestine. The daily oral dose administration of colostrums containing specific antibodies or hyper immune serum to lambs will protect them against experimental entertitis. The protection is against the disease and is not from infection nor is the excretion of organisms inhibited by colostrual antibodies. Protection lasts only as long as colostral antibodies are present in lumen of intestine and hence, infections generally occur after 5-7 days of age when colostrums feeding is stopped.

Pathogenesis

Lactase (b-Galactosidase) is the "receptor" and "uncoating enzyme" for the rotavirus during its "infection cycle" in the enterocytes on the villi in the small intestines of host calves and in large intestines to a lesser extent. Hence, during rotavirus infections in enterocytes, "Lactase" is "exhausted" from intestine, thus reducing the utilization of "lactose" sugar present in the milk consumed by the calves, thus resulting into "maladorption" of milk sugar and its accumillation in intestine lumen which leads to diarrhoea, dehydration, loss of electrolytes and acidosis. If milk is withdrawn from such diarrhoeic calves and it is replaced with glucose and water, the diarrhoea can be checked. The villous epithelial cell distruction and atrophy of villi is the most important pathological lesion occurs in about 24 hours of rotavirus infection and regeneration of the villi need about 4-6 days after rotavirus infection.

A combined infection of rotavirus with enderotoxigenic *E. coli* infection is more severe which generally occurs in calves during neonatal period.

Clinical symptoms and lesions

Natural disease occurs after 4 days of birth of a calf with profuse diarrhoea with sudden onset. Pale yellow faeces with mucous and flakes of blood are observed. More severe dehydration occurs, when Rotavirus is accompanied by enterotoxigenic *E. coli,* Cornavirus or cryptosporidium infections.

Diagnosis

Samples of intestinal mucosa from several sections of small and large intestines in chilled state should be sent to laboratory for virus detection and isolation.

Electron microscopy is the standard diagnostic technique for rotavirus detection in faeces and intestinal mucosa electron microscopy using specific antiserum can be undertaken on samples collected upto 6-10 days after infection. Protein A-gold immune electron microscopy is valuable test to detect Bovine coronavirus in faeces. Immunofluorescent staining of faecal smcars/cell culture of faecal material is used for diagnosis. Electron microscopy is not possible (Luchelli *et al.* 1992). The ELISA is also equally reliable.

Treatment

Anti-microbial therapy for checking secondary bact infection along with with holding of milk consumption and replaced with oral and parenteral fluid therapy (electrolyte therapy) including a glucose glycine electrolyte formulation is effective.

Control

Principals like: 1) Reduce infection pressure, 2) Insure adequate colostral intake, 3) Vaccinate the dam to induce specific immunity in the colostrums (passive immunization).

Vaccination

1. Stimulation of active immunity by vaccinating the newborn calf with an oral vaccine containing the modified live viruses (MLVS).
2. Enhancement of lactogenic immunity by vaccinating the dam during pregnancy (passive immunity). These 2 approaches can be thought of for protection of newborns.

Oral vaccines

Presence of passive antibodies in the calves given oral vaccines was the hindrence for development of active immunity through MLVS and hence, these were not successful. Vaccination of pregnant dams (Passive immunization) was also unsuccessful due to effect of the colostrums from vaccinated dams is only available as long as colostrums antibodies are present in lumen of intestines of calves only for 5 to 7 days after birth and as soon as feeding colostrum is stopped the effect of antibodies is lost.

Passive Immunization

Feeding of stored colostrums in smaller quantum for 2 to 4 weeks after birth to the calves orally will provide sufficient protection against viral diarrhoea.

Systemic Colostral Antibodies

For many years, it was uncertain if circulating colostral antibodies in calves was transferred back into the intestinal tract. Recent evidence shows that passive immunity to calf rotavirus diarrhoea can be achieved by adequate calf serum colostral antibody titre (Besser *et al.* 1988 a). Calves fed colostrums on the 1st day of life had significant rota virus neutralizing antibody titres IG-4 in their small intestinal lumina for 5 days and 10 days later. Colostral immunoglobulinis administered by parenteral injection can protect the calves against rota virus challenge experimentally (decreased morbidity and case fatality due to diarrhoea in calves) with high concentration of passive serum immunoglobulins (Besser, *et al.*, 1988 b).

Virus Diarrhoea in calves: Indian scenario

No much work on viral aspect of calf mortality (diarrhoeal mortality) is done but field observations indicate that it is difficult to believe that such incidences are not occurring. Only viral isolation work is lacking inspite of high diarrhoeal mortality occurring in the field and baceterial isolations are only done in the diagnosis laboratories from such incidences.

After going through above paragraphs on colostral and serum gamma-globulinas usage for calf diarrhoeal treatment/prophylaxis the author likes to bring to the notice of the readers that this authors work on use of serum gamma globulins from adult animals for control of calf mortality deserves appreciation by readers.

Suggested Reading

Besser, T.E., T.C. McGuire, C.C. Gay, and L.C. Pritchett. (1988a). Transfer of functional immunoglobulin G (IgG) antibody into the gastrointestinal tract accounts for IgG clearance in calves. J. Virology. 62: 2234-2237.

Besser, T.E., C.C. Gay, T.C. McGuire, and J.F. Evermann. (1988b). Passive immunity to rotavirus infection associated with transfer of serum antibody into the intestinal lumen. J. Virology. 62: 2238-2242.

Lucchelli A., Lance S.E., Bartlett P.B. (1992). Prevalence of bovine group A rotavirus shedding among dairy calves in Ohio. Am J Vet Res 53: 169-174.

Parwani, A.V., Lucchelli, A. & Saif, L.J. (1996). Identification of group B rotaviruses with short genome electropherotypes from adult cows with diarrhoea. J Clin Microbiol 34: 1303–1305.

Saif L.J. (1994). In Ed. Kapikian A.Z. Viral infections of the gastro intestinal tract, New York : Marcel Dekker, pp. 289-314.

Sandals, W. C., Povey, R. C., & Meek, A. H. (1995). Prevalence of bovine parvovirus infection in Ontario dairy cattle. Canadian Journal of Veterinary Research, 59(2): 81–86.

Scott, F.M., A. Holliman, G.W. Jones, E.W. Gray, J. Fitton. (1996). Evidence of torovirus infection in diarrhoeic cattle. Vet. Rec. 138: 284-285.

❑❑❑

Chapter 16

Malignant Head Catarrh in Bovines (Malignant Catarrhal Fever)

Malignant Catarrhal Fever (MCF), other wised called as Malignant head catarrh is a highly fatal disease of cattle/buffaloes and farmed deer which is associated with contact with sheep and goats (often lambing ewes) in USA, Canada, Australia, New Zeland, Europe, Scandinavia, Asia and East India and occurs in outbreak form or sporadically. In most instances there are isolated cases and the disease is characterized by Erosive stomatitis, gastro-enteritis, erosions in upper respiratory tract, keratoconjunctivitis with unilateral or bilateral capacity and it is caused by MCF virus either herpes -2 ovine virus or Alcelaphine herpes-1 virus if wild beasts, the later Malignant Fever Virus (MCF) is found in most African countries and the former MCF is a causative agent in other areas of the globe.

About the causative virus

The disease with both herps-2 Alcelaphine herpes-1 virus (AHV-1) and ovine herpes-2 virus (OHV-2) is fatal and both the viruses belong to the genus *Rhadinovirus* of the subfamily *Gammaherpesvirinae,* the former virus is wild beast associated MCF virus transmitted from blue wild beast (*Cannochaetes taurinus*) and the later virus is the sheep Associated MCF virus transmitted from sheep. Neither agent appears to transmit from one bovine to another and neither of the viruses cause any disease in their principal host, i.e. wild beast and the sheep.

Sheep Associated Divine herpest-2 virus does not replicate in tissue culture. It has a close "Association" with lymphoblastoid cells particularly large granular lymphocytes which can be grown in tissue culture and induce MCF, when injected. MCF can also be transmitted to cattle by transfusion of large volumes of blood, if given within 24 hours after collection.

With beast-associated MCF virus can be readily transmitted by several routes. It can be adapted to grow on egg yolk sac and tissue culture and transmission to rabbits of yolk sac to cattle has been achieved. The primary structure of the its genome is described (Ensser *et al.*, 1997).

Epidemiology and transmission of causative agent

Wild beasts are main source of infection for AHV-1 and domestic ewes are source for ovine HV-2 virus in cattle. The recovered cattle show persistant viremia for may months which make them carriers (and O'Toole D. *et al.*, 1997, Vet. Rec. 140:519). The virus is shown to be present in "latent" form (It being herpes virus, viral DNA gets attach to cellular DNA during latency) in cattle by PCR technique, without evidence of clinical signs of MCF. It is possible that "Stress" could activate a latent infection in animals with no sheep contact. The mode of transmission in sheep associated MCF is unknown but it can be probably by injestion. Wild beast MCF is transmitted by aerosol or by injestion of contaminated pasture by wild beasts. Occasional spread by insect bite vector is also suggested. Spread of infection in cattle by ingestion of pasture contaminated with sero positive infected aborted ewes virus containing uterine discharge is also possible (Vanselow B.A. 1980, Vet Rec. 107:15).

Pathogenesis

MCF is multisystemic disease characteristics by lymphoid hyperplasia and widespread "Vascular" epithelial and mesothelial lesions, morphologically associated with lymphoid cells. Development of the epithelial erosions and kerato conjunctivitis is due to the involvement of "Vascular adventitia" (Reid H.W. *et al.*, 1986, Res. Vet. Sci. 41:76). Atypical Proliferation of sinusoidal cells is responsible for lymph-node enlargement and cerebromenigal changes are in fact a form of lymphoid vasculitis in brain.

Clinical symptoms and Postmortem lesions

There are 4 forms of the disease:

1. Peracute disease runs for 1 to 3 days with high fever, dysponea and acute gastroenteritis.

2. In alimentary form, there is a marked diarrhoea and minor eye changes.

3. "Head and Eye" form of the disease is characterized by sudden onset with anorexia, agalactia, high fever (106^0-107^0F), rapid pulse rate, profuse muco-purulent nasal discharge, severe dyspnoea due to nasal obstruction as a result of mucopurulent nasal discharge. Occular discharge with oedema of eyelids, blepharospasm and congestion of sclera versels, superficial necrosis of nasal mucosa and buccal mucosa proceeded by diffuse reddening of mucosa. Necrotic areas appearing on hard palate, gums and gingivitis with painful movement of jaws with smacking sound. Erosive mouth and tongue lesions are evident along with involvement of lips and commissures of the mouth. Cheek papillae are haemorrhagic with eroded tips. Muzzle and nostrils show patches of necrosis, slonghing of skin at the teat tips, vulva and scrotum and covering of the same with tenacious scabs is also evident. Head pushing and dashing, muscle tremours, weekness in one leg followed by paralysis and convulsions may occur in final stages. Enlargement of superficial lymph-nodes and opacity of cornea is present invariably which can be unilateral or bilateral. Exematous weeping and crust formation especially on perineum, around the prepuce, in the ascillae and inside the thigh are prominent skin lesions with shedding of hooves in extreme cases. The death may follow in 7 to 10 days.
4. Mild form of the disease with lesions and symptoms described in "Head and Eye" form in very mild degree also occur rarely with lingering of the disease for long time. A distinctive clinical feature in this form is persistant bilateral ocular leukomata (O'Toole *et al.*, 1997).

Postmortem lesions are described during disease course and also include erosive lesions in abomasums, catarrhal enteritis with swelling and ulceration of peyers patches, erosive lesions in trachiae bronchii and pharynx, swelling and oedema in messenteric and thoracic lymph-nodes and petechial haemorrhages and congestion in brain and menengies, are some other lesios present during postmortem examination.

Diagnosis

Virus isolation is not practical because of instability in harpes and non-replication of virus in case of hepes-2 viruses. Detection of viral DNA by "PCR" technique is possible. A competitive inhibition ELISA using monoclonal antibodies is possible. Histologically "pervascular mononuclear cuffing" in most of the organs is characteristic. The pathognonic lesions is a "necrotizing vasculitis" which features infiltration of the tunica media and adventitia by "lymphoblast like cells and macrophages. Acidophilic, intracytoplasmic inclusion bodies in neurons have been described (Hamilton,1990). Cattle with chronic MCF have chronic bilateral central stromal keratitis with or without corneal pigmentation. An "oblitrative aretiriopathy" is characteristic of malignant head catarrhae and this vascular lesions is present in all major organs (O'Toole *et al.*, 1997).

Treatment

Practically no treatment is useful in this disease to Laltar the fatal outcome of the disease.

Control

Separation of cattle and sheep herds is recommended. Introduction of sheep from areas affected with the disease in cattle should be avoided. Auto-vaccine containing inactivated liver tissue from infected animal as well as tissue culture inactivated vaccines did not produced any favourable effect as probably Virus Neutralising (VN) antibodies are not useful in prevention of the clinical signs of the disease.

Malignant head cattarrh: Indian Scenario

The occurance of the disease in cattle is not described in India. However, Kulkarni, S.G. and Pandit, S.V. presented a technical paper on "An incidence of bilateral corneal opacity of undiagnosed etiology in Buffaloes and cattle in Kolhapur district – A preliminary note" presented in technical seminary of veterinarians held at Nasik polyclinic during 1970, wherein they described sporadic incidences of occurance of cases of bilateral corneal opacity in bufflaoes in Kolhapur and Kagal area of Maharashtra, since with symptoms of rise in temperature upto 104^0-105^0F, profuse salivation, nasal discharge, which is watery initially followed by mucopurulent consistency, characteristic superficial mouth erosions covered with diptheratic membrane with foul odour acute vaginitis with congested vaginal mucosa, semi-liquid faecal diarrhoea containing mucous shreds and costant feature of kerato conjunctivitis (blood red conjunctivitis) followed by bilateral corneal opacity which was a constant feature and death within 14 to 20 days after illness.

The treatment of cases with antibiotics and corticosteroids (locally as ophthalmic ointment) was of no consequence incurring the cases. However, treatment with antimucosal disease (Ajanta disease) serum could cure few cases as per the experience of Dr. Kulkarni, S.G. (serum supplied by mucosal disease controlling scheme unit at Disease Investigation Section, Pune. This serum produced by hyperimmunisation of buffaloes by injecting serial doses of inactivated spleen and lymph-node material from suspected cases of so-called mucosal disease of bufflaloes showing symptoms of erosive intestinal tract lesions as well as "Skin form" of the disease, some of those cases may be the case of possible malignant Head catarrhae (Empirical similarity which is unproved). This mention is made here only to suggest that more scientific investigation of the disease with bilateral corneal opacity is needed which needs complete virological isolation and diagnostic test facilities like ELISA, PCR, FAT and other sophisticated technique facilities including disease containment facilities at Regional level in India for future. The technical article is reproduced as below for details.

An Incidence of Bilateral Corneal Opacity of Undiagnosed

Etiology in Buffaloes & Cattle in Kolhapur District – A Preliminary note

by S.G. Kulkarni, M.V.Sc. & S.V. Pandit, M.V.Sc.

Since 1960, Dr. Pandit came across a peculiar disease condition occurring in bovines particularly in Buffaloes in Kolhapur district, characterized mainly by bilateral corneal opacity. The cases were recorded mostly in sporadic form in the buffalo herds in various villages round about Kolhapur proper and also in Kagal and other talukas of Kolhapur district rarely, more than one cases were also found affected in individual herds.

Symptoms – The typical cases show rise in temperature upto 104^{0}F, to 105^{0}F, off-feed, dullness, followed by bloodred conjunctivitis with mucopurulent eye discharge. Profuse salivation is also observed in many cases. The nasal discharge, watery in the beginning becomes mucopurulent afterwards. The most characteristics and constant symptom is the bilateral corneal opacity which follows the blood-red conjunctivitis and is of difuse nature. The animals loose partial or complete eyesight depending upon the density of corneal opacity in many of the cases. The mouth lesions are also present which are characterized by superficial erosions covered with diptheritic membrane. Few cases show semi-liquid faeces containing mucous shreds with foul odour. But this is not a constant feature of the disease and majority of the cases do not show this symptom. Acute vaginitis and congestion of vaginal mucosa is also observed in many cases.

Sporadic individual cases are occurring in the village herds and the affected cases invariably die after the illness of about 14 to 20 days, if not given proper treatment. Unfortunately the authors could not get chance of carrying out postmortem examination of the suspected carcasses due to the sporadic nature of the disease and due to the fact that the cases were observed in interior villages.

It is observed that Antibiotics, such as Penicillin, Streptomycin, Tetracyclines and Chloramphenicol, etc. by parenteral administration and use of Subamycin, Hycin and other cortisone containing eye ointment are of no value in curing the disease. However, the use of glucose saline helps in prolonging the life of affected animals. The experience of the principal author points out that few cases treated with hyper immune Mucosal Disease Antiserum supplied by M.D.C. unit, cattle market Goregaon, Bombay recovered satisfactorily during the period from 1964 to 1965. Symptomatic treatment, such as Milk-iodine injections and autohaemotherapy, etc. failed to cure the disease.

The authors also tried the use of Anti-Rinderpest serum in two of the affected cases during 7th to 9th post infection days in the doses of 150 cc, 80cc, 40cc, respectively but without any effect and the cases died even after this treatment.

Etiological investigation

Attempts were made recently by the authors to investigate the aetiological agent responsible for the disease. The blood smears of the affected animals collected at the height of temperature were stained with Gram's Giemsa or leishmans staining procedures and were found to be negative for presence of any bacterial or protozoon parasitic infection, including trypanosomes.

The smears collected from the eye discharge were stained with Giemsa and Grams stain and were exmined microscopically for the presence of Rickertsial infection or for presence of Morallxella bovis (haemophilus) or Toxoplasma infection and were found to be negetive for these possible infections.

However, very recently conjunctival discharge smear of one such affected case revealed presence of minutre pink staining bodies found in aggregates scattered intracellularly in the epithelial cells and also in extracellular matrix of the smear when stained with quick Giema staining metod. We could not definitely distinguish these bodies from Rickettsial bodies as well as Eosinophilic granules of cytoplasm of Eosinophilis. This needs further work on possibility of Rickettsial infection (primary or secondary) should not be overlooked.

The absence of bacterial or protozoon parasitic infection in early cases lead us to suspect the other possibilities including Vitamin-mineral deficiencies which can be ruled out by the fact that the disease occurs in area, where there is not sacricity of fodder and greens and the rise in temperature is always associated with the affected animals which indicates the infectious nature of the disease. The clinical symptoms resemble with the following viral disease partially or wholly. These are: 1) Foot and Mouth, 2) Mild Rinderpest, 3) Mucosal Disease Virus Diarrhoea Group, 4) Malignant Head Catarrhae and attempts are made to eliminate the possibilities of these viral disease conditions.

As regards Foot & Mouth Disease, it can be stated that the nature of irregular irrosions with diptheretic membrane observed by the authors has no clinical resemblance with ruptured vesicles of Foot & Mouth disease showing rough reddened erosions. However, the mouth lesions scrapings preserved in Glycerinsaline were submitted for elimination of the possibility of Foot & Mouth disease to the Head of the division Bact & Virology, I.V.R.I. Mukteshwar and surprisingly enough we have received the results stating that, "the residual Foot * Mouth disease virus type O" is recovered from this material and is typed by the C.F. test. From this it can be said that F & M virus type "O" may be one of the causative factor of the said condition. But whether it is the sole responsible factor or just a cocurent factor is just a matter of guess. At this juncture perusal of the literature did not reveal the corneal opacity as one of the symptoms of Foot & Mouth disease to our knowledge.

As regards mild Rinderpest, the clinical feature of the disease and nature of mouth lesions did not indicate the possibility of Rinderpest but the serum sample was submitted to I.V.R.I. for indirect or gel test or N.T. against Rinderpest. It was found negative on biological and serologicl test for Rinderpest Moreover, treatment of affected cases with Rinderpest antiserum did not show any sign of improvement in these affected cases which indicates that the disease is probably not related to Rinderpest. Bilateral Corneal Opacity is described in literature as the feature associated in outbreaks of Malignant Head Catarrhae and other symptoms including nasal and eye discharge, rise in temperature and mouth lesions, etc. are also described under Malignant Head Catarrhae vide Blood & Handerson (1963) and Hagan & Brunner (1957). Similarly the bilateral corneal capacity is also described in few cases in outbreak of mucosal disease/virus diarrhoea group (Merk's Veterinary Mannual). Kerato conjunctivitis is also associated with Infectious Bovine Rhynotrachitis (Huges, J.P. 1964). The vaginitis and vaginal mucous membrane congestion which was present in some of our cases also indicates the possibility of the involvement of viruses of infectious pusturlar vulovaginisis.

The differential leucocytic count of blood smears collected from two cases on 7th and 8th post infection day showed increased in Polymorphs. It may probably be due to secondary bacterial infection or possibility is that it may be indicative of Malignant Head Catarrhae, the viral disease condition in which 'leucocytosis" is possible instead of "Leucopenia" usually accompanying viral disease.s (Blood & Handerson, 1963).

Summary

The progress of investigation is detailed above. It seems from this that positive confirmation of isolation of F & M from one of above cases, needs similar isolation from more cases, if F & M is to be regarded as the etiological factor of bilateral cornel opacity cases described in this paper. The Rickettsial agent as possible cause of the condition as indicated by conjunctival smear examination should also be screened further for confirmation. The possibility of Malignant Head Catarrhae and allied viral disease conditions mentioned above as causative agent need very much specialised type of screening facilities or submission of material to some reference laboratory outside India, which may be undertaken under guidance of state level authorities.

This preliminary note is put forth before this seminar in order to discuss the various possibilities involved in this undiagnosed disease condition and get guidance from the experts and coleagues in this matter, if possible.

Suggested Reading

Ensser, A., Pflanz, R., Fleckenstein, B. (1997). Primary structure of the alcelaphine herpesvirus 1 genome. J Virol. 71: 6517–6525.

Hamilton, A.F. (1990). Account of three outbreaks of malignant catarrhal fever in cattle in the Republic of Ireland. Vet. Rec. 127: 231-232.

O'Toole D., Li H., Miller, D, Williams, W.R., Crawford, T.B. (1997). Chronic and recovered cases of sheep-associated malignant catarrhal fever in cattle. Vet Rec. 140: 519–524.

□□□

Chapter 17

Infectious Bovine Rhinotracheitis

Infectious Bovine Rhinotracheitis (IBR) virus infection produces a disease complex characterized by respiratory, encephalitic and genital syndrome with abortion and conjunctivitis and is caused by an alphaherpes virus (Bovine Herpes Virus-1, i.e. BHV-1).

About the causative virus

Genetic analysis of various clinical isolates of BHV-1 virus revealed at least 3 distinct sub-types, namely respiratory sub-type BHV-1. 1, genital sub-type BHV-1, 2 and encephalitic sub-type BHV=1, 3 respectively (Gibbs *et al.*, 1977). BHV-1.3 sub-type has been renamed as BHV-5 (Jones *et al.*, 1982). The antigenic differences between these isolates of the virus are responsible for the diverse epidemiological and pathological behaviour of the virus.

Epidemiology and virus transmission

The disease complex occurs in most of the cattle raising countries in the world including Europe, Asia, North America, Africa, Australia and New Zealand. Even though clinical incidence of the disease is very low, seroprevalnece of infection is very high in most of the countries. This is because of the fact that the latent infection in breeding animals is very characteristic which causes international trade problems and problems of entry into breeding units.

In Australia, upto 96% of bulls, 52% of cows are sero positive, most of which may be venereal because respiratory disease is uncommon in cattle in extensive range conditions. The genital carrier status is important in maintaining venereal IBR virus and in occurance of sporadaic infectious Pustular vulvo-vaginitis (IPV) and Infectious Pustular balano posthitis (IPB) in these herds. In great Briton, IBV and IPB were quite common during 1960's and 1970's. However, they were reduced in 1980's due to stricter control measures in artificial in semination centres. In 1997, outbreak of IBV/IPV occurred in Dairy herds in great Briton with signs of Respiratory as well as genital form and the isolate from this outbreak was typed as BHV-2b (Pritchard, *et al.*, 1997). The virus (BHV-1) was isolated from wildbeasts in Africa, from wild and pronghorned antelopes in Western Canada and from game animals in Tanzania. The nasal exudates and coughed up droplets is the major source of infection of respiratory form of the disease which spreads by Aerosol route while genital secretions, semen and foetal fluids are the source of genital infection which spreads by venereal transmission. The virus can survive in frozen semen for 1 year at -196^{0}C.

An unvaccinated herd of breeding or a group of feed lot animals is highly susceptible to epidemics of respiratory disease or abortion. Newborn calves are highly susceptible to the systemic form of infection, if the level of specific antibody to the virus in the colostrums is inadequate or if there is failure of passive transfer. BHV-1-1 sub-type produces respiratory disease while sub-type BhV-2.1 causes IPV (Pustular vaginitis) while BHV-2.2 causes abortion. Sub-type BHV-1-3 and BHV-1-5 causes encephalitis while currently available modified live virus (MLV) BHV-1 vaccine strain can cause infertility. Nutritional deficiencies like Vit. B, Pantothenic acid, Vit. B-12 and ascorbic acid status of stressed calves may affect susceptibility to BHV-1, infection. Similar thing occurs due to zinc/copper.

Pathogenesis

BHV-1 affects nasal cavities and upper respiratory tract, resulting into rhinitis, laryngitis and trachetis. Denudation of tracheal columnar epithelium and extensive loss of cillia due to the invasion by the virus is responsible for adverse effects on defence mechanism of the respiratory tract.

Spread of virus from nasal cavity to the occular tissue causes conjunctivitis, peripheral corneal oedema, conjunctival oedema and vascularisation. BhV-1-1 sub-type viral spread from nasal mucosa via the trigeminal preferal nerve to the trigeminal ganglion results in non-suppurative encephalitis of milder type but BHV-1-3 encephalitis sub-type of virus produces severe encephalitis through viremia in colostrums deprived calves (Belknap, *et al.*, 1994). Systemic invasion by virus is followed by localization of the same in different tissues; the virus is transmitted by peripheral leukocytes to the placenta and transferred to foetus causing abortion. When infection occurs in last trimaster of gestation results into Munification of the foetus, abortion, still birth or week calves. The systemic infection of newborn calves results into necrotic lesions in respiratory and alimentary tracts, lymph-nodes, liver, nephiritis and encephalitis.

BHV-1 virus can become latent after a primary infection of field virus or vaccine virus (after vaccination) attenuated virus which may remain latent in definitely.The recrudescence reactivation and shedding of the virus can occur following the use of large doses of corticosteroids which mimic the effects of stress. In nature, transportation of cattle with latent infection can re-activate the virus resulting into re-excretion of the virus which is responsible as a source of infection to the herd in which transported animals are introduced as new entrants.

Aerosal exposure of calves with BHV-1 infection impairs the function of alveolar macrophages which allows pasturella haemolytica to persist and proliferate in the lungs and produce the characteristic lesions. BHV-1 virus can interfere with the function of effector cells, such as macro phages, neutrophils and lymphocytes and can affect the composition of alveolar phospholipids after the function of lung surfactant and compromise pulmonary defense mechanism. This mechanism is responsible for precipitation of pasturella anemolytica/ multocda lung infection which causes so-called "shipping fever" (Lung pasturellosis) in cattle after transporation.

Symptoms and postmortem lesions

Sudden onset of anorexia, loud coughing, fever upto 108^{0}F, severe hyperemia of nasal mucosa, serious discharge from eyes and nose, salivation, slight hyper exitability, marked fall in milk yild, increased respiratory rate, severe tracheitis with dyspnoea, short explosive cough followed by sudden death is present in respiratory form of the disease.

Several animals may show cornial form of the disease with corneal oedema, conjunctivitis and profuse occular discharge. Outbreak of respiratory disease for 10-14 days may follow abortions several days upto 90 days after initial beginning of outbreak. Disease can occur as major occular form with one or both eyes affected. It differs from "Malignant head catarrh" by the fact that no involvement of the alimentry tract/mouth lesions and differs from morexella "infection by absence of corneal affection except slight oedema of cornea and lesions of IBR are limited to conjunctival affection. Calves less that 6 months of age may show encephalitis, marked by inco-ordination, excitement and high mortality rate. Systemic disease in newborn calves is characterized by fatality, sudden anorexia, fever, excessive salivation, rhinitis, uni or bilateral conjuctivitis, erosive lesions of soft palate, acute pharyngitis, laryngitis, respiratory distress with broncho-pneumonia and loud breathing.

Abortion is common sequal after the clinical illnss or parenteral vaccination of non-immune pregnant cows with modified live virus vaccine of bovine tissue culture origin. Abortion may occur upto 90 days following vaccination, if the virus becomes latent in the placenta and infects foetus much later than usual. This happens, if natural infection proceeds safer vaccination. Retention of placenta, endometritis and residual infertility can occur.

In infectious pustular valvo vaginitis form (IPV) frequent micturition, small papules shallow erosions on valval mucosa can occur. In Balano-posthitis form of males, similar lesions occur on preputial mucosa, Rhinotracheitis, bronchopneumonia.

Diagnosis

Isolation of IBR virus from nasal swabs using Bovine kidney tissue culture and identification of the same using ELISA or direct / indirect immune fluoroscence or immuno peroxidase technique or by electron microscopy revealing herpes like virus particles, adjuncted with showing 4-fold rise in antibody titres in paired sera samples from acute and recovered phases of the disease at the interval of 14 to 21 days. The virus can be detected in nasal swabs by use of ELISA technique.

The PCR is more sensitive alternartive for virus isolation for rapid virus detection and is used for detection of virus in semen (Xia *et al.*, 1995). Using restriction endonuclease analysis of viral DNA, it is now possible to distinguish field isolates from vaccine strains which may be useful in investigation of outbreak of IBR originated by vaccine induction. Non-suppurative encephalitis, alimentary tract necrosis in calves with systemic disease aborted foetus autolysed, etc. are the common lesions found in P.M. examination.

Treatment

Use of broadspectrum antibiotics are indicated, if secondary bacterial tracheitis and pneumonia is present but no treatment of primary BHV infection is available.

Control

The virus is ubiquitous and the occarance of the disease is unpredictable with high economic losses from abortion, neonatal disease and respiratory disease. Colostral immunity in calves wanes by 4-6 months of age. The vaccine with prevent abortions due to virus and provide protection against respiratory disease, if vaccination is carried out 10 days prior to natural exposure.

Vaccine development

Two types of vaccines are available:

1. Modified Live Virus (MLV) vaccines.
2. Inactivated adjuvanted vaccines. MLV'S offer 3 advantages over the inactivated vaccines, namely:
   a) Induction of rapid immune response
   b) Relatively long duration of immunity
   c) The induction of local immunity.

Protection from infection and disease both, is observed following intra-nasal or intra-muscular vaccination with MLV vaccines, with in 40 to 96 hours post vaccination, due to rapid development of 'interferon' induced locally. Intranasal vaccination also develops secretary Ig A antibody and cell mediated immunity (Van Drunen *et al.*, 1993). Both parental and intra-nasal vaccines stimulate circulating humoral antibodies also.

In Europe, "Temperature-sensitive" intra-nasal mutant containing BHV-1, MLV Vaccine which grows only in the upper respiratory tract has been developed using 'chemical' for temperature sensitive character development.This makes this modified live vaccine virus to stop replication at body temperature of the animal, thus restricting its multiplication only in upper respiratory tract and not allowing the multiplication beyond that. Prebreeding vaccination of replacement heifers with this vaccine provides total protection and it is efficacious as well as safe for use in pregnant cows. It develops immune antibodies within 2 months post vaccination and is protective in 91% cows even after 30 months (Van der Poel *et al.*, 1995). Extensive use of MLV vaccines has reduced incidence of clinical disease but there are certain disadvantages of these, namely:

a) Parenteral administration of MLV vaccine is potentially "abortigenic" and hence, can not be used in non-immune pregnant cows:

b) The MLV vaccine virus can become "latent" after vaccination.

c) Fatal generalized BHV-1 infection has been reported in calves under 3 days of age and in HF calves vaccinated at 1 and 3 weeks age intranasally in commercial combined MLV/PI3/BRSV vaccine MLV (Furuoka *et al.*, 1995).

d) MLV vaccinated non-immune calves were shown to be shedding vaccine virus 9 hours after vaccination (Baker *et al.*, 1989).

e) Calves vaccinated with temp. Sensitive mutant of BHV-1 were protected against clinical disease but they were found to be excreting the virus after treatment with corticosteroids (Nettleton *et al.*, 1984).

f) MLV vaccines sometimes produce immune suppressive effect by multiplying in macrophages of lung alveoli and reduce body defence mechanism of lung macrophages and thus, precipitate past multoceda infection similar way as done by field IBR virus (BHV-1-1) infection.

Inactivated vaccines

As against MLV vaccines, inactivated vaccines do not cause abortions, immune suppression or latency. However, inactivated vaccine can not stop development of latency by field challenge after inactivated vaccination. Inactivated vaccines do not cause shedding and hence, are safe for use in and around pregnant animals.

Inactivated vaccines are, however, may not be as efficacious as MLV vaccines because of potential destruction of some of the protective epitope on viral antigens during inactivation process. Moreover, both MLV vaccines and inactivated vaccines are unable to allow differentiation of vaccine virus and field virus after vaccination in the endemic areas and hence, they are disadvantageous for use of eradication programme.

Sub-unit vaccines / genetically engineered vaccines

These vaccines have advantages over conventional vaccines in respect of possibility of allowing differentiation of field and vaccine virus incidence in the field during eradication programme.

Infectious Bovine Rhinotracheitis Incidences and Prevalence of BHV-1 virus infection: Indian scenario

Scanty literature on actual incidence of IBR in India is available BHV-1; virus responsible for IBR was first isolated from a case of Kerato conjuctivitis in calf by Mehrotra (1977). The mention of occurance of cases of IBR in India by S.N. Singh of BAIF, Wagholi (1994) in his article on "Bio-technology in Animal health strategy for Livestock development read in XIV Annual Conference and National Symposium on Recent Advances in Production and Testing of Vet. Biological conducted by IAVMI at Pune 29-31st Jan, 1994 pp.90. In the same conference Shukla D.C. of IVRI, Izatnagar stressed the need for development of inactivated BHV-1 vaccine or subunit/Bio-engineered vaccine for protection against IBR to avoid shedding of BHV-1 virus which brings about threat to frozen semen banks, taking into consideration of global incidences of contamination of semen in frozen semen banks abroad by BHV-1 virus (pp 50 of the above mentioned report of conference).

It seems necessary that the Vet. Scientists (Virologists/ Vaccinologists) should give priority to the development of proper diagnostic facilities using modern Bio-technological skills to survey the extent of IBR infection in the country and develop proper vaccines for effective control of the same in India according to them. Khillari, S. and Singh, S.N. *et al.* (2000) reported production of IBR oil adjuvanted vaccine and its extensive field trials resulting into long lasting immunity.

Suggested Reading

Baker, J.C., Steven, R.R., Walter, D.R. (1989). Transmission of a vaccinal strain of infectious bovine rhinotracheitis virus from intra-nasally vaccinated steers commingled with on vaccinated steers. Am J Vet Res. 50: 814-816.

Belknap, E.B., Collins, J.K., Ayers, V.K. & Schultheiss, P.C. (1994). Experimental-Infection of Neonatal Calves with Neurovirulent Bovine Herpesvirus Type-1.3. Vet. Pathol. 31: 358-365.

Furuoka H., Izumida N., Horiuchi M., Osame S., & Matsui T. (1995). Bovine herpesvirus meningoencephalitis association with infectious bovine rhinotracheitis (IBR) vaccine. Acta Neuropathol. 90: 565-571.

Gibbs E.P.J., Rweyemamu M.M. (1977). Bovine herpesviruses. Part I. Bovine herpesvirus 1. Vet Bull. 47: 317–343.

Jones G.E., Field A.C., Gilmour J.S., (1982).Effects of experimental chronic pneumonia on body weight, feed intake and carcass composition of lambs. Vet Rec., 110: 168-173.

Mehrotra, M.L., (1977). Isolation of respiratory viruses from cattle and their possible role in genital disorders. Ph. D. Thesis. Agra. Univ., Agra.

Nettleton, P.F. (1984), In : Latent Herpes virus infection in Vet Medicine Eds. Witman G. *et al.*, Boston : Martinus Nijhoff pp. 211-228.

Pritchard, G.N. Cook and M. Banks (1997). Infectious pustular vulvovaginitis/infectious pustular balanoposthitis in cattle. Vet. Rec., 140: 587-587.

Van Drunen Littel-van den Hurk, S., Tikoo, S.K., Liang, X. & Babiuk, L.A. (1993). Bovine herpesvirus vaccines. Immunology and Cell Biology 71, 405–420. Van der Poel W H M, Kramps J A, Quak J, Brand A, van Oirschot J T. (1995). Persistence of bovine herpesvirus 1-specific antibodies in cattle after intra-nasal vaccination with a live virus vaccine. Vet Rec., 137: 347–348.

Xia J.Q., Yason C.V., Kibenge F.S.B. (1995) Comparison of dot blot hybridization, polymerase chain reaction, and virus isolation for detection of bovine herpesvirus-1 (BHV-1) in artificially infected bovine semen. Can J Vet Res., 59: 102–109.

❑❑❑

Chapter 18

Vesicular Exanthema in Swines and Vesicular Stomatitis in Cattle, Horses and Swines and Swine Vesicular Disease

Vesicular exanthema of swines is an acute febrile, infectious disease of swine, in distinguishable clinically from foot and mouth disease (FMD) in swine, vesicular stomatitis in swine and swine vesicular disease, caused by calicivius and is characterized by vesicular lesions in oral cavity and feet. Vesicular stomatis is a disease of cattle, horses and occasionally pigs caused by vesiculovirus in the family *Rhabdoviridae* characterized by vesicular lesions or healing ulcers on oral mucosa, teats and prepuce. Swine vesicular disease is restricted to pigs only and is caused by an entero virus (family *Picornaviridae*) related to human coxackie B5 virus.

Epidemiology of vesicular diseases

The vesicular stomatitis virus can be biologically transmitted by black flies (*Stimulus vittatum*) and mechanically by *Culicoides* species. Ingestion of contaminated materials through contaminated feed and water troughs and contaminated pasture. Vesicular exanthema is transmitted through excreted saliva and faeces of affected animals. Raw garbage containing infected pork scraps are the source of virus. Similar way swine vesicular disease is also tramitted.

Pathogenesis

In vesicular stomatitis, there is primary viremia with subsequent localization in mucous membrane of mouth and coronets but frequently the classical vesicle formation is absent, only dry necrotic lesions occur. In vesicular exanthema, lesions are limited to non-hairy areas including snout, coronary band and tongue. Mild viral encephalitis can occur.

In swine vescicular disease, viremia occurs and localization of virus in snout, tongue, coronary band and myocardium occurs.

Symptoms and lesions

In vesicular stomatitis, vesicular lesions or healing ulcers on oral mucosa, teats and prepuse occurs. In vesicular exanthema, fever, vescicles on mouth, snout, teats and udder and in between claws occur. In swine vesicular disease, fever, lameness, vesicles on coronary bands occur, disease runs for 2-3 days.

Differential diagnosis

Virus isolation, polymerase chain reaction (PCR) and serology with rising titres can be done in case be vesicular stomatitis. FAT is also possible. In case of vesicular exanthema, lab identification of virus and differentiation from other vescicular disease is required. CFT is diagnostic. In case of swine vesicular disease demonstration of antigen in tissues and virus in cell culture. ELISA is diagnostic.

Suggested Reading

Brocchi, E., G. Zhang, N.J. Knowles, G. Wilsden, J.W. McCauley, O. Marquardt, V.F. Ohlinger, and F. De Simone (1997). Molecular epidemiology of recent outbreaks of swine vesicular disease: two genetically and antigenetically distinct variants in Europe, 1987-94. Epidemiol. Infect. 118: 51-61.

Dekker, A., P. Moonen, E. A. de Boer-Luijtze, and C. Terpstra (1995). Pathogenesis of swine vesicular disease after exposure of pigs to an infected environment. Vet. Microbiol. 45: 243-250.

Vescicular Stomatitis : Knight A.P. et al. (1983). Vesicular stomatitis comp. cont educ., 5: 5117-5522.

❑❑❑

Chapter 19

Equine Infectious Anaemia (Pink Eye Disease or Swamp Fever)

Equine Infectious Anaemia is an emerging viral disease of equines caused by a *Retrovirus* belonging of the subfamily *Lentivirinae* and is characterized by persistant anaemia, relapsing type of fever and chronic disease with intermittent relapses in some horses. The major clinical signs and lesions of equine infectious anaemia (EIA) are attributable to the host immune response to the virus rather than direct viral damage to tissues.

About the virus

EIA virus (EIVA) is non-oncogenic retrovirus with presence of an enzyme reverse transcriptase. It has RNA directed DNA Polymerase (RDDP) enzyme in peptide and oligomucleotide map of glycoprotein. This enzyme is similar to those from a number of RNA tumour viruses. It catalyzes the production of a DNA provirus that is integrated into the genome of persistently infected cells of equines. The family *Retroviridae* (Animal Retroviruses) is classified in 3 sub-families (namely O*nchornavirinae, Spuma virinae* and *Lentivirinae*). EIAV is classified under*Lentivirinae* belonging to animal Lentivirus group while HIV (Human Immunodeficiency virus) a primate Lentivirus. Both EIAV and HIV are closely related phylalogically (HIV is more complex virus with 7 genes while EIAV and other animal lentiviruses have 3-4 genes). The virus has one major group specific antigen "P 26" which is basis for AGID and ELISA dagnostic tests. Two surface glycoprotein antigens are present on the virus, namely gp-45 and gp-90 which show frequent antigenic drift, when the animal infected with EIAV chronically (but stopped showing symptoms), suddenly starts showing symptoms i.e. relapse again due to some stress conditions, due to the random mutations of the virus frequently, which are related to the lack of a "proof reading capacity" of the viral "reverse transcriptase" enzyme.

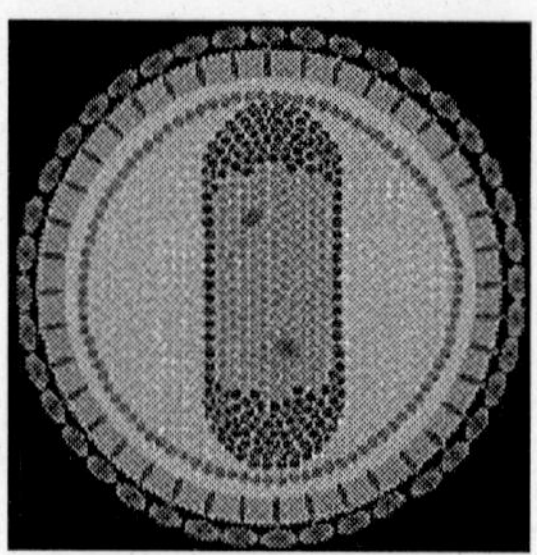

Fg. 1: EIA virus structure

Epidemiology and methods of virus transmission

An infected horse is a source of all new infections of EIAV. Horses, donkeys or mules are "persistently infected" and clinically normal infected animals are a source of virus (Coggins, 1984). Transfer of contaminated blood or blood products is responsible exclusively for transmission of EIAV either through biting insects like horse flies (*Tabanus* species) or *Stomoxys calcitrans* (stable fly) or even through blood transmission from infected to non-infected horse. The insect transmission is purely "mechanical" while feeding from infected animal body to non-infected one and especially when the feeding of fly is "interrupted", as it infects while feeding on other animal just in close viscinity. Use of biological preparation of equine orgin or use of contaminated surgical equipment or semen from infected stallion is some other source of transmission of infection.

Pathogenesis

After infections, virus multiplies in organs with aboundant macrophages like liver, spleen, lymph-nodes, lungs and kidneys, as mature tissue macrophages are the target cells of virus multiplication and not the circulating monocytes. After multiplication in tissue macrophages, virus concentrates in blood (viremia), which is responsible for fever and other clinical signs, within 2-7 days of infection. Viremia attained in few days and then persistant viremia of low level remains throughout the life. There is considerable distracrtion of macrophages during virus multiplication.

There is high and strong immune response to the virus infection and development of antibodies detectable in 7 to 10 days post infection especially antibody response is against "P-26 antigen (coreprotein)" which can be detected by AGID test in 45 days post infection and by

60 days post infection antibodies against gp-45 and gp-90 antigens are developed which leads to production of "Hyper gamma globinemia" which is due to neutralising antibodies and CF antibodies. There is rise of cytotoxic T-lymphocyte population also. This high immune response brings about termination of viremia. Antibodies against gp-45 & gp-60 glycoproteins do not neutralise virus completely and hence, most virus in persistant viremic horses is "virus-antibody complex" which is readily phagocytosed by cells of reticulo endothelial system which is responsible for fever, depression, thrombocytopenia, anaemia and glomerulo-nephitis characteristics of the disease.

Red Blood Cells (RBCs) in circulation which are normally destroyed in 138 days (normal life span) get destroyed within 38 days. This happens due to the fact that RBCs of infected animal get coated with virus antigen-antibody complex on the surface and combination of complement with this complex on surface of RBCs make them either "lyse" (haemolysis) or agglutinate with subsequent "intravascular" removal of lysed RBCs from Reticulo-endothelial system. This brings about "Anaemia" characteristics of this disease. Similar "Phenomenon" occur in case of Thrombocytes (platelets) and "Thrymbocytopenia" develops.

The ability of retrviruses to splice a DNA copy of their genome into the genome of the host cells is important in persistence of virals infection, although viral DNA is not detectable in "clinically normal but persistently infected" horses (Rice, N.R. *et al.*, 1989, J. Viral 63:5194). This viral strategy allows the virus to escape immune surveillance of the host and remain "latent" in the host for remaining period of life of host. The 'latency" of virus make the infected animals appear "normal" for the time until "replase" of the clinical disease occurs due to "causes" or "stresses" which are not yet defined, when "antigenic drift" occurs in gp-45 and gp-90 surface glycoprotein epitopes which allows the "mutated virus" to show clinical symptoms again.

After less frequent "reccurance / relapse" of these clinical episodes, the host (horse) becomes "permanently asymptomatic" due to achievement of appropriate level of immune response sufficient to protect it from antigenic epitopes that are common to all "EIA virus variant strains".

Symptoms and postmortem findings

On 1st exposure to infection, after 2-4 weeks of incubation period, Anorexia, depression, profound weekness and loss of condition Ataxia followed by intermittent fever upto 105^{0}F, jaundice, oedema of ventral abdomens, prepuce and legs and petechial haemorrhages especially under the tongue and on conjunctional mucosa occurs which gives the name "pink eye" to this acute stage of the disease. Characteristic rise in rate and intensity of heart sounds and serosanguineous nasal discharge occurs. Abortion of pregnant mares is usual. After this acute/subacute phase of 3 days to 3 weeks, "temporary recovery" may occur or some may become progressively weak and die. "Relapse of disease" can occur in temporary recovered animals at the intervals of 2 weeks but relapses cease to occur after a year's period. Apetite is not affected in such horses. Survivers can persist as "symptomless carriers" of the disease.

Diagnostic conformation

Haematalogical exam shows "Thrombocytopenia and "normocytic and Normocromic" anaemia. Thrombocytopenia is marked during relapse period. The presence of sideroleucocytes (Leukocytes containing haemosiderin) in high numbers is highly suggestive of "EIA" infection. Increase in serum bilirubin concentration and decrease in serum iron levels is detected. Coggins AGID test which detects "p-26 core antigens" and competitive ELISA (CELISA) which also detects the same antigens, is diagnostic of EIA Infection, both have equal sensitivity and specificity.

Postmortem findings

In acute disease, subcutaneous oedema juaundice and petechae or echymotic subserosal haemarrhages, enlargement of liver, spleen and local lymph-nodes are common. Bone marrow is reddened due to the increase in haemopoietic tissue with focal infarcts. Chronic cases show ematiation and pallor of tissues. Histopath examination reveals haemosidersis, perivaseular infiltration of round cells and extensive proliferation of the mononuclear phagocytic cells through out the body.

Treatment

Only supportive treatment including blood transfusion and haematinic drugs may be useful in clinical recovery but the recovered horses remain persistently infected and carriers of the disease.

Control

The control of the disease is still based on eradication of the disease by identifying the infected, clinically normal "carrier" animals with serological tests, such as "ELISA" or AGID. The disease was eradicated from Hong Kong by such test and destroying the "positive" animals. This control programme has come under despute elsewhere due to the opinion of horse-owners that the "asymptomatic animals" with very low infectivity are being destroyed un necessarily.

Restriction of introduction of infected horses into new clean herds by carrying out strict "quarantine" for during "testing" and not allowing "positive" carriers to enter the clean herd is a wise policy "Retest" after 1-2 months is also better idea. Surveillance after every 6 months for segregation of "positive" reactors is also useful. In countries where the incidence is high, it is usual to control horse movement by system of permits and certificates of freedom from the disease and to insist on skin branding or lip-tattoing of all horses (Issel and Cook, 1993). Draining of marshy area for control of bitings insects as well as use of insect repellents and staling horses in "screen meshed" stables is useful for controlling spread of infection through insect bite. Vaccines (killed vaccines) (whole virus) are safe and are available in certain countries only. "Subunit" vaccines may actually enhance the occurance of the disease (Issel *et al.*, 1992).

Equine Infectious Anaemia (EIA), Indian Scenario

Uppal and Yadav (1987) from India reported 11 cases in horses with clinical symptoms simulating EIA and their sera were found "positive" with conggins AGID test.

It was learnt that Uppal, P.K. undertook regular serological survey programme later on by using Coggins test in race horses in stables round about Pune city under diagnostic lab facilities of Royal Turf club and established presence of this disease in the country and implemented control measures.

Suggested Reading

Coggins, L. (1984). Carriers of equine infections anaemia virus. J.Am. Vet. Med. Assoc. 184: 279-281.

Issel, C.J., D.W. Horohov, D.F. Lea, W.V. Adams, Jr., S.D. Hagius, J.M. McManus, C. Allison, and R.C. Montelaro, (1992). Efficiency of inactivated whole-virus and subunit vaccines in preventing infection and disease caused by equine infectious anaemia virus. J. Virol. 66: 3398–3408.

Issel, C. J., and R. F. Cook (1993). A review of techniques for the serologic diagnosis of equine infectious anaemia. J. Vet. Diagn. Invest. 5: 137–141.

Uppal, P.K. and Yadav, M.P. (1987). Outbreak of equine influenza in India. Vet. Record., 121: 569-570.

□□□

Chapter 20

Maedi-Visna and other Retroviral Infections including Caprine Arthritis - Encephalitis Virus Infections of Sheep and Goats

Maedi - Visna - Caprine Arthritis - Encephalitis disease complex can be described as a multisystemic disease complex caused by closely related non-oncogenic *Retrovirus* belonging to the animal Lentivirinae group, characterised by infiltration of mononuclear cells in the affected tissues and producing slow incidious, chronic disease.

Visna is a chronic progressive paralytic disease of sheep characterised by inflammatory menigo encephalitis and demyelinating entity of central Nervous system and Maedi is a progressive dyspnoeanic condition of sheep characterized by chronic interstitial pneumonitis with mononuclear cell infiltration and lymphoid hyperplasia, carpal/tarsal non-suppurative arthritis and indurative mastitis with mononuclear cell infiltration in interstitial mammary glandular tissue. While caprine arthritis-encephalitis (CAE) infection is characterized by Arthritic and encephalitic lesions in goats similar to those of Maedi-Visna disease complex of sheep. Antigenic relatedness between virions of CAEA, Visna (VV) and Maedi viruses due to nucleotide homology and serological properties was found (Pyper *et al.*, 1984).

Maedi (Ovine progressive pneumonia) was earlier reported in South Arica and United States (De Boer, 1975) but this was 1st reported in 1933, in Iceland from where it was eradicated by 1965. Maedi-Visna was also first recorded in Iceland but was not seen in that country after 1951 due to eradication. Caprine Arthritis Encephalitis (CAE) virus infection was 1st reported by Cork *et al.* (1974).

About the viruses of maedi-visna and CAE

Maedi-visna virus and ovine progressive pneumonia virus are ovine lentiviruses which are non-oncogenic ovine retroviruses which constitutes a species of the lentivirus genus. There is a high degree of relatedness with the lentivirus associated with caprine arthritis encephalitis (CAEV) virus. The deduced genetic organized visna virus resembles most closely that of AIDS virus (HIV) which also belongs to lenti group of retro viruses. Although maedi-visna CAEV belong to a single virus species, isolates obtained from naturally infected sheep/ goats are genetically heterogenous. "Antigenic drift" is common and antigenic variation of the surface protein facilitates the persistence of the virus in the host. There is evidence for variation in pathogenic potential between isolates. There is evidence that the North American strains of ovine lentivirus may have originated from cross species transmission of caprine arthritis encephalitis (CAEV) virus than from maedi-visna lentivirus (Karr *et al.*, 1996).

Persistance of visna virus is being explained by its immunologically silent nature. Most infected cells harbor the virus in the latent state (Provirus form) in which viral antigens are not produced in sufficient quantities for detection and destruction of the infected cells by immune surveillance mechanism of the body. The genetic information of the infective RNA virus transcribed into viral DNA, which in turn is transcribed into RNA of mature newly synthesized virions. It has been found that the replication of visna virus proceeds by way of DNA intermediate and this DNA (intermediate) "provirus" is integrated into the host cell DNA and viral "provirus" genome forms a stable association of even the "antibodies".

Virus is "Cell Associated" and hence, isolation of virus requires 2-3 passages in cell culture using infective "cell explants". Virus is readily propogated in fibroblastic cell cultures from choriodi plexus, with CPE characteristic of multinucleated giant cell formation.

Etiology and virus transmission

The virus is transmitted from the infected animal to the susceptible animal in the herd by aerosol route or from infected Ewe to the neonate lambs or kids through colostrums or milk. The Icelandic breed of sheep is more readily and severaly infected in this way as compared with British sheep breeds. The infected sheep with "persistant latent infection is able to excrete free virus particles only in few numbers through terminally differentiated macrophages from Lungs and udder as the virus replication is markedly "restricted" in most of the infected cells of matured monocytic cells in circulation.

Pathogenesis

The whatever free virus particles enter the newly infected sheep through nasal portal or through oral route with colostrums/milk in neonate are able to infect monocytes in which they multiply in cytoplasmic vacuoles and then get spliced into genomic DNA of these cells by mechanism of "reverse transcription" and persistently remain latent in the form of "Provirus" in these cells (Haase *et al.*, 1977).

Owing to the latent viral genome in most of infected host cells, viral proteins will not be present and so are not likely to be detected by the hosts immune surveillnce mechanism which enables Visna virus (VV) to escape host defence by assuming the proviral form, without becoming target for antibodies form, without becoming a target for antibodies or cellular defence mechanism. This explains the "persistence of infection" for lifetime.

The nature of lesions in visna is of inflammatory type and they are immunologically mediated. There is consistency in the cellular reaction irrespective of the site lesions eg. There is interstitial type of inflammatory reaction with uniform monocytic cellular infiltration observed in lungs and udder tissue (interstitial pneumonia and interstitial mastitis with induration in both tissues). In the central nervous system, virus replication is observed in oligodendrocytes and astrocytes in the foci of demyelination. These cells get access to the virus through contact with monocytes. It is stated that visna is caused by a virus infection in which some cells carry virus in provirus form. Gradually more and more provirus carrying cells undergo "activation" with the expression of virus specific antigens that provide the target for cell mediated immune responses (CMI) of host. This CMI response causes lesions of visna with subsequent functional disturbances.

Symptoms and postmortem lesions

In maedi-visna, there is a long clinical course and disease is incidious. Even though the neonate gets infected with colostrums/ milk, the clinical signs develop only after 1-3 or 3 years. The disease is characterized by Dyspnoea (increase in respiratory rate) and interstitial pneumonia with coughing and nasal discharge. Clinical signs last for

3 to 10 months with total consequences. Disease also is characterized by wasting condition. Involvement of udder with induration of glandular tissue and secondary mastitis can be present ("Hard bag" condition). Arthritis can be seen occasionally. In visna, involvement of nervous system with encephalitis and demylination of spinal cord can occur. CAE infection also shows similar symptoms.

Lung lesions are characterized by interstitial pneumonia with infiltration of monocytes and macropheges in interstitial tissue which makes collapse/atrophy of the alvioli responsible for dyspnoea. The weigh of lung tissue is increased considerably. The lung tissue and udder tissue shows characteristic bluish discolouration.

Diagnosis

Agar get immune diffusion test (AGID) tests and Elisa tests are used in most of the countries for diagnosis. AGID detects antibodies directed against the major surface glycoprotein, namely gp-135. It is highly specific but lacks sensitivity especially because of slow development of antibody following infection which gives negative result.

Treatment

There is no satisfactory treatment of these infections.

Control

Two methods are used, one is test and segregation policy which is effective in control of the disease. But there is a danger of renewed infection, as the negative herd is fully susceptible and segregated positive reactors are required to be maintained inspite of being non-productive. Second method is test and cull policy but it is costly to cull the positive reactors by slaughter. Currently there is no effective vaccine available for protection.

Visna maedi – CAEV infection of sheep and goats: Indian scenario

Spontaneous cases of Maedi in India were identified for the 1st time by Rajya and Singh (1964). Chauhan and Singh (1970) recorded a significant increase in erythrocyte sedimentation rate (ESR) in sheep affected with maedi along with other clinico-pathological studies. Subsequently its epizootology, clinical pathology and pathomorpholgy were reported by number of workers and were reviewed by Sharma (1982)). Later on, studies on experimental transmission of the disease and isolation of etiological agent were carried out at Veterinary College, Mathura and IVRI, Izatnagar, U.P. (Sharma *et al.*, 1975) C.M. Singh (1985) diagnosed and attempted control of caprine Arthritis - Encephalitis (CAE) syndrome in Imported Sanen goats in Thailand (FAO consultancy Report FAO/RAPA, Bankok).

Suggested Reading

Cork, L.C., W.J. Hadlow, T.B. Crawford, J.R. Gorham, and R.C. Piper. (1974). Infectious leukoencephalomyelitis of young goats. J. Infect. Dis. 129: 13.

De boer, G. (1975). Zwoegerziekte virus the causative agent for progressive interstitial pneumonia (maedi) and meningoleucoencephalitis (visna) in sheep. Res.vet. Sci. 18: 15-25.

Haase, A.T., L. Stowring, O. Narayan, D. Griffin, and D. Price. (1977). Slow persistent infection caused by visna virus: role of host restriction. Science 195: 175-177.

Karr, B.M., Chebloune, Y., Leung, K. & Narayan, O. (1996). Genetic characterization of two phenotypically distinct North American ovine lentiviruses and their possible origin from caprine arthritis-encephalitis virus. Virology 225: 1–10.

Pyper, J.M., J.E. Clements, S. Molineaux, and O. Narayan. (1984). Genetic variation among lentiviruses: homology between visna virus and caprine arthritis-encephalitis virus is confined to the 5' gag-pol region and a small portion of the env gene. J. Virol. 51: 713-721.

Thormar, H. (1961). An electron microscope study of tissue cultures infected with visna virus. Virology, 14: 463-475.

□□□

Chapter 21

Enzootic Bovine Leukosis

Enzootic Bovine Leukosis is an infectious disease of cattle which exists in the form of leukosis alone or leukosis with persistant lymphocytosis or leukosis with tumours and is caused by Bovine Leukemia Virus (BLV) which is an exogenous C-type onchovirus belonging to the family *Retroviridae.*

The disease was originally described in Germany in 1871 (Johnson and Kaneene, 1992). The disease became common after World War II in most of the countries in the world which raise cattle. Now it occurs in U.S.A., most of the Europe and South America and Canada. The spread of the disease is very high in infected herds as shown by AGID test (even upto 80%) but herd to herd spread is slow. The occurance of clinical lymphosarcoma in affected countries is only about 1 per 1000 animals per annum. Dairy cattle are much more commonly infected as compared with beef cattle, even though all breeds are susceptible to BLV infection.

About the virus

BLV is an oncogenic exogenous C-type RNA virus which belongs to the family *Retroviridae*. The virus exists in the form of "Cell Associated Virus" in lymphocytes and is cultured in lymphocytic cultures through infected lymphocytes and "not as cell free" virus.

The virus causes a chronic B-cell proliferative disease in cattle and is an important model for human T-cell leukemia virus type-1 (HTLV-1) infection because of many shared molecular and biological features. However, it is not a zoonosis. It has a leukemogenic activity, can be grown in tissue culture and produces specific antibodies in calves and sheep (Johnson and Kaneene, 1992). Bovine Leukemia Virus (BLV) belongs the family *Oncornavirinae* which is further divided into mammalian and other oncornaviruses. As mentioned previously, structure of BLV'S pro-viral genome is similar to that of HTLV-1

Kuman virus and Magnesium) is required for its maximum activity. The identification of the immunological cross-reaction between BLV and HTLV internal proteins P-24 nd P-12 are most remarkable (Burny *et al.* 1984). BLV being an oncogenic retrovirus, it differs from other viruses by presence of reverse transcriptase enzyme which brings about "reverse transcription" of its original RNA genome and catalyzes the production of a DNA provirus that gets integrated into the genome of persistently infected lymphocytes of the host animal.

Epidemiology and disease transmission

The virus is present in lymphocytes in blood, milk and tumour masses. Most susceptible cattle become infected by exposure to the infected lymphocytes and not by cell free virus. Minimum 10 microlitres of lymphocytes (240 lymphocytes) or 1 microlitre of whole blood (with 4524 lymphocytes) from a BLV seropositive cow when injected into calves, results into infection and sero-conversion. Probably 100 BLV infected cells are minimally required for establishing infection in cows. Natural transmission occurs by insectbite or batsbite between in contact animals mechanically through transmission of infected lymphocytes from blood of infected animal (Klintevall *et al.*, 1995).

The vaginal secretions and placentas from cows infected with BLV as well as contaminated calving instruments may serve as sources of infection through infected blood cells. The semen and artificial insemination is neither a method of spread of BLV, nor does embryo transfer spread the same. However, semen collected by massage of donors urethra/accessory glands per rectum can contaminate semen collected by this method through bleeding containing infected lymphocytes and hence, it can become a source of infection. The infection can be transmitted by vaccines containing blood from infected animals and by surgical instruments contaminated with blood from infected animals as well as through blood transmission from infected animal source. Mechanical transmission of infected animal blood through insect bites is also a source of infection.

Pathogenesis

The virus establishes a "Persistant infection" in lymphocytes by integration of "Proviral DNA" into the hosts cellular DNA after exposure of cattle to BLV virus as above in 4 possible ways of the final outcome :

1. If animal is genetically resistant, it fails to become infected.
2. Animal become permanently infected and develops detectable levels of antibodies (These animals become "latent carriers" of the infection).
3. Animal becomes permanently infected and becomes sero positive as well as it develops persistant lymphocytosis which is a benign lympho proliferative process but not preclinical stage of lymphosarcoma.
4. Animal becomes permanently infected sero positive and develop neoplastic malignant tumours - lymphosarcoma.

The outcome of the infection developing into anyone out of above 4 forms depends on the "genetic make up" of the animal. The outcome also depends on animal's immune status and size of infective dose of virus. In calves, visceral lymph-nodes, spleen and liver are the commonest sites of development of lesions while the abomasums, heart; visceral and peripheral lymph-nodes are commonly affected organs. The symptoms developed depend on the site of lesions development.

The tumours consist of aggregation of neoplastic lymphocytes or reticulo-sarcomas. They are highly malignant and metastasize widely. Large number of immature lymphocytes in the blood smear is a reliable indicator of the disease presence.

Disease symptoms and postmortem lesions

The disease is characterized by occurance of multiple cases of adult multi centric lymphosarcomas with tumours developing rapidly in many sites with great variation in clinical signs depending on sites of the lesions. Incubation period is 4 to 5 years and hence, the malignant form (Form No. 4 above) is present only in adults. Persistant lymphocytosis form (Form No.3 above) is present in calves above 2 years of age. Form No.2 and 1 are present without clinical signs in calves below 2 years of age.

In acute cases with lymphsarcoma, the sudden death with rupture of abomasal malignant ulcers or spleen tumour with severe haemorrhage occur with or without showing prior wasting of animal body. Most of the cases show subacute form of clinical disese 75-90% cases show skin lesions with enlarged haemolymph nodes. Enlargement of visceral lymph-nodes, palpable by rectal examination, deep inguinal and iliac lymph-node enlargement with local oedema may be observed.

Involvement of abomasal wall results in reduced appetite, persistant diarrhoea with melanin (dark coloured blood from abomasal ulcers) and chronic moderate bloating due to tumours of mediastinal lymph-nodes.

Right side congestive cardiac failure due to tumours in heart (right side) with hydropericardium may occur. Oedema of brisket, inter-mandibular space can occur due to heart lesions. Malignant lesions of nervous system can cause posterior paralysis and other paralytic symptoms.

Diagnosis of the BLV infection

AGID test can be used for diagnosis of herd or individual animal infection. Radio Immune Assay (RIA) is suitable for individual case diagnosis which is most sensitive, which uses virion GP antigen as well as serum ELISA on pooled serum for herd diagnosis. (Johnson and Kaneene, 1992).

Milk ELISA for individual milk sample or pooled milk sample is more sensitive than AGID test. PCR is a sensitive and specific for direct diagnosis of BLV infection in perferal blood lymphocytes.

Persistant lymphocytosis for more than 3 periods was used for diagnosis of BLV infection until the other serological tests were not developed. The lymphocytes in such cases are mostly normal in morphology microscopically when form No. 3 without malignancy occurs. However, when few lymphocytes show "mitotic figures" in such persistant lymphocytosis, the form No.4 (malignant tumour form) can be diagnosed.

Treatment

There is no known treatment for this infection.

Control programme

The disease can be controlled/eradicated from the country or the herd depending upon prevalence of the disease, value of the animals in the herd and whether Govt. is offering indemnity for sero positive animals. The herd slaughter policy was continued in Denmark until 1982, after which "AGID" test was made available for slaughter of individual infected animal. "Voluntary eradication programme" was applied by European member countries of European community. In

Britain, BLV disease was made in reportable disease in 1992. Sweden introduced national eradication programe in 1990. In Canada and USA, all control programs of this disease are voluntary and herd based as disease is having high sero positive cases prevalence.

Infection in calves can be prevented by feeding colostrums from sero negative cows and avoiding exposure to maternal blood at the time of parturition and management of calf housing (Thurmond, 1991). No vaccine is available for prevention of the disease, as it should be non-infectious, non-onchogenic and should not interfere with sero-diagnosis.

Indian Scenario

Studies on Bovine lympho sarcoma particularly in Indian buffaloes have been carried out since mid-1960's at IVRI, Izatnagar under the leadership of Singh, C.M.The unique features of involvement of respiratory tract, mainly lungs of buffaloes in this syndrome was described by Singh, C.M. *et al.* (1973) at the 5th International symposium on comparative Leukemia Research held at Padova, Italy. Involvement of most of the parenchymatous organs and lymph-nodes, including reproductive and endocrine organs of buffaloes by gross and histopathological lesions of lymphosarcoma has been illustrated amply by Singh, C.M. 1975, Singh, C.M. *et al.*, 1979, Singh, C.M. *et al.*, 1980 and Singh, C.M. 1981 elsewhere as referred to by Singh, C.M. 1988 at the 75th Indian Science Congress, Pune (Platinum Jubilee year lecture on "Retro-viruses as Biological Threat to Man and Animals). He informed the gathering of the said congress (1988) that "Besides the observation of "C" type virus particles under electron-microscopy, studies on immune-diffusion, radio immune assary (RIA) Enzyme Linked Immuno sorbent Assay (ELISA) and radioimmune precipitation tests conducted at Ecole National Veternaire, maision Alfort, France. Free university of Brussels, Belgium Hospital, Cochin, Paris and Central Vet. Institute, Roterdam have revealed that replicating fifterable agent is associated with lymphosarcoma in buffaloes and further investigation elucidated that it may have different antigenic configuration than those of other known leukemogenic viruses. Further studies for characterization of the viral agent, its role in causation of the disease, molecular integration of cellular DNA, etc. may provide the answer. For further studies on these aspects, it is necessary to make available appropriate facilities for molecular level studies with virus containment facilities in India.

Suggested Reading

Burny, A., Bruck, C., Chantrenne, H., Cleuter, Y., Dekegel, D., Ghysdael, J., Kettman, Rr., Leclerque, M.J., Jeunen, J., Mammerickx, M. & Prtetelle, D. (1980). Bovine leukemia virus: molecular biology and immunology. In Viral Oncology, pp. 231-289. Edited by G. Klein. New York: Raven Press.Johnson R, Kaneene, J.B. (1992). Bovine leukemia virus and enzootic bovine leukosis. Vet Bull 62: 287–106.

Klintevall, K., Berg A., Svedlund G. (1993) Differentiation between enzootic and sporadic bovine leukosis by the use of serological and virological methods. Vet Rec., 133: 272.

Thurmond, M.C. (1991). Calf management to control 6: 285-290. Bovine leukemia virus infection. Cornell. Vet., 81: 227-231.

□□□

Chapter 22

Enzootic Pneumonia of Calves

Enzootic Pneumonia of calves is the single important cause of calf mortality in India as well as in the world between the age group of 2 to 20 weeks of age after enteritis. Enzootic Pneumonia is a complex entity caused by multifactorial etiology including viruses like Bovine Respiratory Syncytial Virus (BRSV) and Para influenza-3 (PI-3) paramyxo-virus mycoplasma speices like *M. bovis, M. bovigenitalium, M. bovirhinis and M. dispar,* etc. and bacterial infections including *Pasturella multoceda, Pasturella haemolytica* may act synergistically to cause more severe and fatal pneumonia. Other bacterial species like *Streptococci* and *Staphylococci, Fusobacterium* species and *Haemophilus* species can also act as secondary invaders in calf pneumonia cases. Most of the routine disease diagnostic and investigation laboratories in India recorded bacterial isolations only as the causative agents of calf pneumonias in the past probably due to lack of virological isolation facilities.

Enzootic pneumonia occurs most commonly in housed dairy claves with 30% of all deaths of calves from birth to 16 weeks of age (Sivula, *et al.,* 1996).

About the causative agents in enzootic calf pneumonia

Bovine Respiratory Syncytial Virus (BRSV) appears to be a major important causative agent of Enzootic pneumonia in housed dairy calves, weaned beef calves and even adult cows (Uttenthal, *et al.,* 1996). Serological surveys in Canada indicated 60 to 80% prevalence of this virus infection in cattle population; even though clinical incidence of this virus is much lower (Lynch and Derbyshire, 1986).

The Para Influenza -3 (PI-3) virus has been isolated most commonly from affected pneumonic calves which when inoculated in colostrums deprived calves resulted into a pneumonia resembling naturally occurring disease (Kiorpes, *et al.,* 1988).

The mycoplasma is considered as primary pathogens and probably the most important and most common etiological agents of calf pneumonia. M. bovis has been isolated from severe epidemics of pneumonia in calves imported into our country from the other and it produces clinical pneumonia experimentally in calves (Doherty, *et al.*, 1994, Reilly, *et al.*, 1993). Morbidity rate may reach 100% with mortality usually less than 5%, however, on an average morbidity rate of 25.6% with 2.25% mortality is recorded in dairy hards.One estimate reports that the disease accounts for 50% of all calf mortality and a reduction of 7.2% in live weight gain.

Epidemiology and mode of transmission

Aerosol infection and direct contact are the methods of transmission and both are accenturated in crowded, inadequately ventilated conditions. Most of the pathogens described under etiology are found in the respiratory tract of normal claves as "commensals". It is generally presumed that environmental risk factors like changes in ambient temperatures during winter or rainy seasons, increase in relative humidity, bad air quality, population density are all responsible for precipitation of the disease.

The onset of calf pneumonia occurs between 2 and 4 weeks of age, when concentration of serum Ig G_1, IgG_2 and IG A in the nasal secretions are lowest. The incidence of the disease begins to decline, when the concentration of Ig G_2 begins increasing at about 2-4 months of age. The spectrum of colostral antibodies present in home raised adult cows. Hence, feeding of colostrums to newborn calves is very important for preventing incidences of enzootic calf pneumonia. The practice of not feeding colostrums to the calves due to using the same for commercial sale or not feeding the male calves with colostrums for economic reasons, is responsible for precipitation of the disease in young calves.

As the disease is of multifactorial etiology, the immunological status of the calves of various age groups in the herd against the possible infectious agents responsible for calf pneumonia is important in precipitation of particular causative agent. The calf pneumonia of early age groups of calves (2 to 8 weeks) occurs due to "previously non-existant" etiological agents on the herd, as these calves are prevented from the disease due to "previously existent" infections in the herd due to getting immunoglobulins against the same from colostrums of their mothers which have suffered from pneumonia due to those infections in their calfhood. General feeding practices, quality of perinatal care provided by the personnel age of weaning of calves, use of prophylactic antimicrobials and health management of the dams are all the management risk factors that can influence the incidence rate and mortality of calves due to enzootic pneumonia (Brunning Fann, *et al.*, 1992). Feeding of coccidiostats to pre-weaned calves and incidence of "Twin births" has an influence on precipitation of calf pneumonia (Sivula, *et al.*, 1996).

The infectious agents like mycoplasma disper and pasturella multoceda have been cultured from respiratory tracts of calves 1-2 months old which show "colonization" for periods upto 2 years in dairy herds. Following natural infection of young calves, the presence of PI-3 virus may persist for several weeks in the herd in respiratory tract of calves and may predispose respiratory disease by interfering with normal pulmonary clearance mechanism and allowing secondary invasion by bacteria or mycoplasms. BRSV (Bovine Resp. Syncytial Virus) may be present in older cows as persistant sub-clinical infection from previous outbreaks and become a source of infection to young calves which are colostrums deprived, which results into enzootic calf pneumonia.

Pathogenesis

To understand the complex mechanism of pathogenesis of enzootic pneumonia of calves in natural outbreaks, the following observations on individual etiological agents out of the multifactorial causative complex of this disease entity may be useful. The experimental data on each etiological agent has the following highlights:

1. Calves experimentally inoculated with mycoplasma species including *M. bovis, M. disper* and other mycoplasma species produce characteristic peri-bronchiolar and Peri-vascular cuffing of (mononuclear cell infiltration surrounding the branches) catarrhal bronchioli and blood vessels) and at electasis. Thus mycoplasma species are synergistic with each other, viruses and bacteria in producing the lesions of enzootic pneumonia (Reilly, *et al.*, 1993).
2. In experimental intra-nasal inoculation of the PI-3 virus into colostrums deprived calves, there is bronchitis, bronchiolitis and

cellular exudates in bronchiolar lumina. Alviolar cell thickening and hyperplasia also occur. PI3 virus affects alviolar macrophages which may impair the lung clearance mechanisms and allow pasturella haemolytica to produce a secondary bacterial broncho-pneumonia.

3. Bovine Respiratory Syncytial Virus (BRSV) in calves causes rhinitis, trancheitis, bronchitis and proliferative and exudative bronchiolitis with accompanying alveolar collapse with the formation of multinucleated syncytial giant cell formation in the epithetial lining and in their lumen of the bronchioli and alvioli (Bryson, 1993). The changes in lung tissues caused by BRSV may affect lung clearance mechanism and predispose to secondary bacterial infection.

It is suggested that hypersensitivity caused by BRSV may be important pathogenic mechanism causing lung injury after the initial mild attack of the virus, resulting into the fatal consequence during second phase of the disease after initial partial recovery.

Symptoms and postmortem findings

The disease in calves starts with mucopurulent nasal discharge. The breath sounds are loud, harsh due to consolidated lung. There is high fever more that 106°-07° F, with harsh hazing cough, stimulated after pinching of trachea. Intensity of the heart sounds is increased. The usual course of the disease ranges from 4 to 7 days. There can be immediate death within a day due to viral pneumonia. PI-3 virus generally causes mild respiratory disease with coughing and nasal discharge and recovery in few days. BRSV pneumonia is generally severe, polypnoea and dyspnoea, becomes worse with mouth breathing and on expiratory grunt and death may follow in 2-4 days. Mycoplasma pneumonia causes sudden onset with severe dysponoea, fever and death inspite of treatment. When secondary bacterial broncho pneumonia occurs, fever toxaemia and dyspnoea is more severe especially when pasturella species are involved.

Diagnosis

Nasopharyngeal swabs and lung lavage samples may be used for isolation of viruses of BRSV/PI-3 using cell culture techniques. The immunofluoroscent antibody test for antigen detection is most rapid, reliable and sensitive test for BRSV from tracheal aspirates, nasal swabs and lung samples. Isolation of mycoplasma species and special media. The other bacteria can be isolated using usual media specific for specific organisms. The standard serological test is a Virus Neutralisation (VN) test using microtitre plates. Other tests include FAT, indirect haemagglutination and ELISA test, the last one is more sensitive and specific and given rapid results in several hours. VN test requires 5-6 days. CFT is less sensitive and less specific than ELISA for BRSV.

Treatment

There is no specific treatment for viral (PI-3 and BRSV) enzoolic pneumonia but bacterial complications can be dealt with by using broad spectrum antibiotics like long acting oxytetracyclins, trimethoprim potentiated sulphonamides. Danofloxacillin has excellent in-vitro activity against mycoplasma species involved in enzootic pneumonia and can be used with success in-vivo.

Control

Control depends on management of environmental and housing factors responsible for the precipitation of enzootic pneumonia, such as inadequate space, overcrowding and ventilation of houses, etc. Recently purchased calves should be isolated from the housed calves. Management of hygiene of calving sheds is also very much important to avoid infections. Feeding of colostrums immediately after birth and proper weaning practices followed during rearing of calves play a very important role in avoiding calf pneumonia. Feeding of calves with nutritious diet containing adequate Vit. A, E & D is very important and the formulation of milk replacers in this respect play a significant role in avoiding precipitation of Enzootic pneumonia.

Vaccines and Immunisation

The instra-nasal inoculation of calves with modified strain of PI-3 virus vaccine stimulates the development of both serum antibody and nasal secretion antibody which is dose dependent. Challenge exposure of these calves provided protection against the clinical disease. These factors should be considered in the development and administration of PI-3 viral vaccines. The inactivated PI-3 virus oil adjuvanted vaccine will induce high levels of serium antibodies and prevent pneumonic pasturellosis if PI-3 precedes the bacterial infection (Stott, *et al.*, 1987).

The vaccine containing inactivated past haemolytica bacterial extract and Haemophilus somnus along with a modified live BRSV vaccine has been used to aid in the control of Enzootic pneumonia in beef calves vaccinated at 3-5 weeks of age (Van Donkersgoed, *et al.*, 1992).

Viral pneumonia in older calves, yearlings and Adult Cattle (Bovine Respiratory Syncytiel Viral Pneumonia)

The Bovine Repiratory Syncytiel Virus (BRSV) is capable of producing "BRSV Pneumonia" as a "separate entity in calves under 6 months of age as well as in yearlings" and adult cattle. BRSV is a "Pneumovirus" in the family paramyxoviridae and is already described under the etiology of enzootic pneumonia of calves caused by multi-factorial etiology in the beginning of this chapter. Herd epidemics of clinical disease occur during fall and winter months usually but clinical disease can occur in nursing beef calves during summer months.

BRSV causes rhinitis, tracheitis, bronchitis and bronchiolitis and mild interstitial pneumonia with widespread emphysema and oedema through out the lungs. The acute faetal disease proceeded by a mild respiratory disease several days previously which suggested that hypersensitivity may be a pathogenic mechanism causing lung injury, the virus specific IgE antibody may be playing the important role of pathogenesis of hypersensitivity and this brings about injury to bronchiolar epithelium including hypertrophy, hyperplasia and formation of "syncytia".

The diagnosis of BRSV is already described under the diagnosis of enzootic pneumonia in this chapter earlier. Several modified live virus and inactivated virus vaccines are available for the control of BRSV infection, as described under enzootic pneumonia but the inactivation of vaccine virus functionally after important epitopes of BRSV and hence, live modified vaccines are preferred to inactivated vaccines (Ellis, *et al.* 1995). Ag negative BHV-1 vector vaccine carrying a gene coding for G protein of BRSV induced the same high degree of protection in calves against BRSV infection and BHV-1 infection as multivalent commercial vaccine.

India scenario

Even though, problem of calf mortality due to respiratory disease complex including calf pneumonia in India especially (in various Pinjrapols in Maharashtra) in calves as well as at Arrey Milk Colony and Goregaon (in buffalo calves) is quite rampant and simulates the clinical picture described under enzootic pneumonia, no much virological work including virus isolation is carried out probably due to the lack of virus isolation facilities and only bacteriological isolations are made by most of the workers from disease investigation section. It is now high time to undertake virus isolations which should be aimed at getting BRSV, PI-3 virus isolates; mycoplasma isolates in order to develop effected vaccine (multivalent viral/bacterial combined vaccine).

Attempts should also be made to design an "immunoglobulin product" derived from slaughter house adult cattle serum, containing antibodies against all possible agents involved in "enzootic calf pneumonia complex". The author struggled to develop similar product while working at BAIF, Wagholi during early eighties but could not get opportunity to complete his aimed objective.

Suggested Reading

Bruning-Fann, C. and J.B. Kaneena. (1992). Perinatal diseases. Vet. Bull. 62, 399. Quoted by Blood D.C. 1994. Vet. Medicine, Eighth Ed., ELBS, London. pp. 107-112.

Bryson, D.G. (1993). Necropsy findings associated with BRSV pneumonia. Vet. Med. 88: 894–899.

Doherty, M.L., Mcelroy, M.C., Markey, B.K., Carter, M.E. & Ball, H.J. (1994). Isolation of Mycoplasma bovis from a calf imported into the Republic of Ireland. Veterinary Record 135: 259-260.

Ellis, J.A., Hassard, L.E., Morley, P. (1995). Bovine respiratory syncytial virus-specific immune responses in calves after inoculation with commercially available vaccines. J Am Vet Med Assoc. 206: 354–361.

Kiorpes, A.L., Dubielzig, R.R. & Beck, K.A. (1988). Enzootic pneumonia in calves: clinical and morphological features. Compendium on Continuing Education for Practicing Veterinarians 10: 248–261.

Lynch, J.A., Derbyshire, J.B. (1986). Application of a modified indirect fluoroscent antibody test to the detection of antibodies to bovine respiratory syncytial virus in Ontario cattle. Can J Vet Res; 50: 384-389.

Reilly, G.A., Ball, H.J., Cassidy, J.P. and Bryson, T.D. (1993). First reported isolation of Mycoplasma bovis from pneumonic calves in Northern Ireland. The Veterinary Record, 133: 550 551.

Sivula, N.J., Ames, T.R., Marsh, W.E. (1996). Descriptive epidemiology of morbidity and mortality in Minnesota dairy heifer calves. *Prev Vet Med.*; 27: 155.

Stott, E.J., Thomas, L.H., Howard, C.J. and Gourlay, R.N. (1987). Field trials of a quadrivalent vaccine against respiratory disease. Vet. Rec., 121: 342-347.

Uttenthal, A, Jensen N.P., Blom, J.Y. (1996). Viral aetiology of enzootic pneumonia in Danish dairy herds: diagnostic tools and epidemiology. Vet Rec 139: 114–117.

Van Donkersgoed J. (1992). Meta-analysis of field trials of antimicrobial mass medication for prophylaxis of bovine respiratory disease in feedlot cattle. *Can Vet J.* Dec; 33(12): 786–795.

❑❑❑

Chapter 23

Haemorrhagic Septicaemia of Cattle and Pasteurella Infections of Cattle, Sheep, Goats, Horses and Pigs

Haemorrhagic Septicaemia (H.S.) is an acute bacterial highly foetal septicaemic disease of cattle caused by *Pasteurella multocida var boviseptica* organisms and is characterized by multiple petechieal haemorrhagic lesions in visceral organs.

About the Causative Organisms

Pasteurella multocida var boviseptia is a gram negative coco-bacillary rod shaped capsular organism with bipolar staining characteristic in tissue and blood smears. There are a number of immunologically distinct types of pasteurella multoceda which have been classified as type 1 (or B), 2 (or A), 3 (or C) and 4 (or D) and there is a loose relationship between serotypes and host species as well as some relation between the serotype and the disease produced.

Septicaemic Pasteurellosis is caused only by type 1 (B) and occasionally type 4 (D) and type E. (Francis, *et al.*, 1980). It is the classical form of the disease of southern Asia including India. The electrophoretic profile of *P. multocida* isolates from animals with haemorrhagic septicaemia (H.S.) can be placed in two distinct groups on the basis of their country of origin. The differences can be co-related with the serotypic properties of individual isolates; those of Asian and North American Origin (Carter B group) and those of African Origin (Carter E. group), each can be distinguished on the basis of their electrophoretic patterns (Johnson, *et al.*, 1991).

Occurrence

Septicaemic Pasteurellosis (Haemorrhagic septicaemia) occurs in cattle, yalks, camels and water buffaloes and to lesser extent in pigs and horses.

It is observed in southern and south-east Asia including Indonesia, Malaysia, Thailand, Phillipines, India, Africa, Europe (Southern), Russia and Near East. It is also observed in bisons and cattle in United States.

Animals of all age groups are susceptible but mostly it occurs between 6 months to 2 years of age. There is no breed susceptibility all breeds are equally susceptible. Morbidity and mortality is between 50 to 100%. Buffaloes are more prone to the disease as compared to cattle.

Epidemiology and Pathogenesis

The outbreaks occur in wet humid weather and rainy season. The organisms remain as commensals during intervening periods and persist on the tonsillar and nasopharyngeal region of the carrier animals on mucosal surface. About 45% of animals in herds which show disease occurrence harbor the organisms on their naso-pharyngeal mucosa as compared to only in 3-5% of cattle unassociated with the disease. (Mustafa, *et al.*, 1978).

The change of weather brings about the stress on the carrier animal and allows the multiplication of the commensel organisms on tonsillar/ nasopharyngeal mucosa and gain virulence which precipitates the septicaemia in this animal. This animal becomes the source of infection to other animals in the herd for starting the outbreak. Spread occurs by the injection of contaminated food/fodder stuffs from clinical cases or carrier animal source and also by biting insects, biting flies and ticks (Mocadam,1962). The epidemiology of haemorrhagic septicaemia in India is described by Dutta, *et al.*, 1990.

The portal of entry of infection is thought to be the tonsils and fulminating septicaemia occurs, which is associated with capsular material of the organism. The effects of septicaemia are most severe in respiratory and gastrointestinal tract and on heart.

Symptoms and Postmortem lesions

The disease is characterized by sudden onset and per acute deaths in the beginning of outbreak. Afterwards, the affected animals exhibit profuse salivation, very high fever upto 106^0-107^0 F, submucosal petechae, severe depression followed by death in 24 hours. Development of warm painful swellings around the throat, dewlap, brisket and perineum is characteristics of the disease in subacute cases.

Severe respiratory obstruction with dyspnea occurs followed by pulmonary and alimentary tract involvement. Pasturellae may be isolated from saliva and blood circulation.

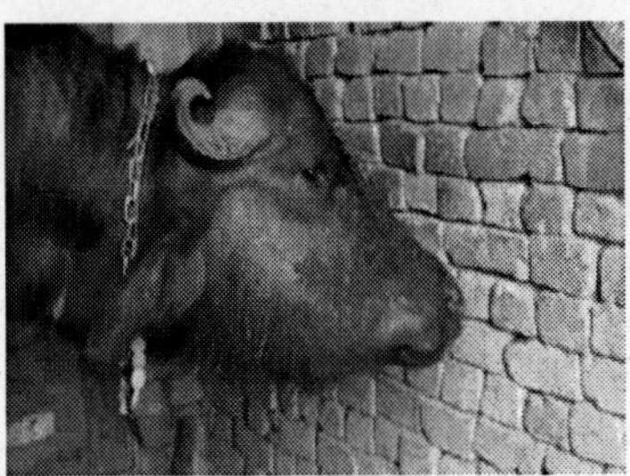

Fig. 1: Haemorrhagic septicaemia symptoms

The gross pathological lesions involved are generally characterized by generalized petechial haemorrhages, particularly on epicardial fat, endocardium and serosal surfaces of alimentry tract, oedema of lymph-nodes and lungs and haemorrhages on tracheal and bronchial sacrosae. Subcutaneous infiltrations of gelatinous fluid may be present. In few animals early pneumonia and severe haemorrhagic gastroenteritis may be present. Thoracic lymph-nodes are enlarged and haemorrhagic.

Diagnosis

Laboratory diagnosis is based on isolation and identification of causative organisms i.e. pasturella multoceda from heart blood from carcass or from blood, from ear vein of affected animal during the septicaemic phase of the disease. Heart blood sample from the suspected carcass or long bones "marrow" is used for culturing on blood agar surface of isolation of pinpoint non-haemolytic colonies, showing typical pasteurella organisms with capsule and bipolar staining characteristics. Heart blood cultures when injected in white mice, will be killed the same within 48 to 72 hours and their heart blood smears will reveal typical bipolar staining capsular organisms when stained with Giemsa stain. A rapid ELISA is now available for identification of the specific serotype of pasturella multiceda responsible for Haemorrhagic Septicaemia.

Treatment

Sulphonamide (Sulpha mezathene or sulpha diazine with trimethoprim or sulphadimidine as well as broad spectrum antibiotics including oxytetracycline or terramycine are all useful for treating the affected animals. Haemorrhagic Septicaemia (H.S.) antiserum is used for therapeutic purposes in 50 to 100 ml quantities by subcutaneous or intravenous route per affected animal along with Penicillin or other antibiotics or sulfa group of drug.

H.S. antiserum was being produced in U.K. and USA by serial inoculation of killed cultures (formalized) of appropriate local typed strain of pasturella multoceda organisms in bulls, in increasing doses at the interval of 1st, 8th, 18th, 28th, 38th and 48th days and bleeding the same on 10th, 20th, 30th, 40th and 50th days at the rate of 8 ml per lb of body wt. of the animal for separation of the serum which is pooled for use.

In India, the said serum was being produced by giving 5 injections of 100 ml of avirulent broth culture of past multocida in buffaloes weekly at the interval and bleeding the same at the rate of 6 ml per lb of body weight of the animal at 8th, 18th, 28th, 38th 48th and 50th days for separation and pooling of serum for use. Other method used was pasturella multocida adjuvanted vaccine used for injection in animal for hyperimmune serum production. These methods were in use in India, in fifties and sixties for H.S. antiserum production which were discontinued later on as the incidences of H.S. outbreaks reduced due to the increasing use of prophylactic vaccinations for prevention of the disease. (For details of H.S. antiserum production, please refer to ICAR publication entitled "Vety Biological Products" by Seetharaman, C. and Sinha, K.C., 1962).

Prevention and Control

Early H.S. vaccines were mere anaecultures, i.e. pasturella mltoceda organisms grown in nutrient broth aerobically for 18 hours (in phase I) for keeping the capsular material in fact on the organisms and inactivating the same (organisms) using 0.5% formaldehyde. However, plain broth anaecultured vaccines were poor antigens which were able to protect the animals only for 2-3 months or less. The precipitation of capsular material with potassium alum treatment improved the antigenicity of the vaccine to some extent but duration of immunity could not be improved only by alum treatment. Early vaccines in UK, USA, Australia and India ageists H.S.were of this type. Dhande, M.R. and Seetharaman, C. at IVRI, Mukteshwar demonstrated the importance of preservation of capsular material of the organism during their classical work on H.S. at IVRI Mukteshwar during late fifties and early sixties of 20th century and they showed that the antigenicity of H.S. vaccine seed cultures deteriorates by serial cultivation of Pasturella multocida on media without presence of blood in the culture medium and even the culturing of seed on blood agar also deteriorates the antigenic capsule which can be improved, if seed culture is passaged through inoculation of the same in the live susceptible calves every six months interval for revival of capsular antigen. This quality control of H.S. seed bank is very important for good H.S. vaccine production. Work of Bain and Dhanda, M.R. on capsular antigen in fifties made good improvements in H.S. vaccine production.

Based on this work, stable H.S. vaccine composed of 18 hours broth culture with good capsular antigen containing P-52 strain past multoceda organisms in an adjuvant base containing paraffin and lanolin was prepared at IVRI, Izatnagar (using solid medium containing Difco peptone, yeast extract and creatnine). This vaccine gives solid immunity against H.S. for 18 months period but has some disadvantages of injectability due to very thick emulsion produced by use of lanolin (emulisifying agent) and liquid paraffin. (Bain, 1954; Iyer *et al.*, 1955; Handa *et al.*, 1956). De Alwin (1994) reported that paraffin and lanolin based H.S. oil adjuvanted vaccines are highly effective especially when used prophylactically, although vaccination in the face of an outbreak may also reduce losses. Only disadvantage is the development of persistant swelling at the site of inoculation. Anaphylactic shock may occur in upto 1% batches of vaccine.

A live streptomycin dependent mutant P. multoceda vaccine provides good protection (De Alwis and Carter, 1980). Similar live vaccine containing P. multoceda, serotype B:3,4 isolated from fallow deer in UK has been developed which provides good protection, avoid anaphylactic shock, and relatively small dose, when vaccine is produced in freeze-dried form, is available as described by Myint and Carter (1990).

Indian Scenario

H.S. is prevailing in India since ancient times. H.S. 0.4% formalin killed whole culture vaccine produced in plain broth with virulent P. multiceda phase I. organism was the most ancient vaccine produced as IVRI before independence (1947) which was further improved by use of some organisms grown in Rouse flask agar cultures and agar wash was used for production brew for further formal inactivation which was adjusted to opacity table No. 10. This being more concentrated as compared to broth vaccine, is considered as more active. However, the oil adjuvanted (Paraffin-lanolin based) vaccine was best which was developed later on by Iyyar's and Dhanda's efforts at IVRI. S.S. Joshi and Gholap, L.D. of IVBP, Pune, 1994 described cultivation of P.multoceda (P.52 strain) in Indigenous made fermentor for production of oil adjuvanted H.S. vaccine on experimental basis.

BAIF, Wagholi started production aluminium hydroxide adjuvanted H.S. formalin inactivated vaccine in 1982 using 300 litre capacity fermenter for cultivation of vaccine brew of P.multoceda on larger commercial scale, as described earlier in this chapter. Presently H.S. outbreaks are certainly minimized due to large scale vaccination programmes undertaken by State Government in India.

Pasteurellosis in other species

Manjrekar, S.L., 1953-54 reported occurence of Pasturellosis caused by strain R_1, R_2 and R_4 in sheep and found oil adjuvant vaccine containing these strains to be useful.The author (S.V. Pandit) while working at disease investigation section M.S., Pune during 1963-1974, happen to investigate number of cases of deaths in sheep and goats at thathawade sheep breeding farm and Govt. sheep farm at Pune 16, where in he could isolate pasteurella cultures, indistinguishable from P. multoceda on the basis of their culture and biochemical characteristics, from sheep of Merino, Ronnimarsh and Ramboilet breed as well as Bannur breed from either their heart blood or their consolidated lungs. These sheep carcasses revealed either pneumonia or pneumonia and enteritis as their cause of deaths. These were the routine sporadic mortality cases of the sheep farms and were not found in outbreak form.

Pavari and Apte (1967) reported a fatal septicaemia in horses and donkeys in India (Pune and round about districts) in which P.multoceda appears to be implicated as a causative agent. Khot *et al.* of Bombay Veterinary College, 1962-63, reported number of Buffalo calves deprived off colostrums dying in Milch buffalo stable round about Goregaon Aarey Milk Colony due to pneumonia and enteritis from which pasteurella like organisms were isolated. Their detailed cultural characteristics by seralogy were not studied and identification was not possible. Hence, it is not possible to comment wheather they were the cases of shipping fever pneumonia (caused by *P. hemorrhagica*).

Suggested Reading

Bain, R.V.S. (1954a). Vaccination against Haemorrhagic septicaemia of bovines. Nature, 173: 583.

De Alwis, M.C.L. and Carter, G.R. (1980). Preliminary field trials with a streptomycin dependent live vaccine against haemorrhagic septicaemia. Vet. Res., 186: 435-37.

De Alwis, M.C.L. (1994). Pasteurellosis in production animals: A review. Proceedings of the international workshop on diagnosis and control of haemorrhagic septicaemia. May 28th-30th, 1996, Natour Kuta Beach Hotel, Bali, Indonesia.

Dhanda, M.R., Das, M.S., Lall, J.M. and Seth, R.N. (1956). Immunological studies on Pasteurella Septica., 26: 273-84.

Dutta, J, Rathore, B.S., Mullick, S.G., Singh, R., Sharma, G.C. (1990). Epidemiological studies on occurrence of haemorrhagic septicaemia in India. Indian Veterinary Journal, 67: 893-899.

Francis, B.K.T., Sehels, H.P. and Carter, O.R. (1980). Type E, Pasteurella multocida associated with haemorrhagic septicaemia in Zambia. Veterinary Record, 107: 135.

Iyer, S.V., Gopalakrishnan, S. and Ramani, K. (1955). Studies on haemorrhagic septicaemia vaccines. The effects of adjuvants upon the immunizing value of formalin killed P. boviseptica organisms. Ind. Vet. J., 31: 379-82.

Johnson, R.B., Dawkins, H.J.S and Spencer, T.L. (1991). Electrophoretic profiles of Pasteurella multocida isolates from animals with haemorrhagic septicaemia. American Journal of Veterinary Research, 52: 1644-1648.

Macadam I. (1962). Tick transmission of bovine pasteurellosis. Vet Rec 74:689-690. Mustafa A.A., Ghalib H.W. & Shigidi M.T. (1978). Carrier rate of Pasteurella multoceda in a cattle herd associated with an outbreak of haemorrhagic septicaemia in the Sudan. Br. Vet. J., 134: 375–378.

Myint, A. and Carter, G.R. (1990) Field us e of live haemorrhagic septicaemia vaccine. Vet Rec 126(26): 648.

□□□

Chapter 24

Anthrax in Domesticated Animals and its Zoonotic Importance

Anthrax is a bacterial disease caused by *Bacillus anthracis*, characterized by peracute or acute foetal septicaemia in cattle, sheep, goats, horses and pigs with zoonotic importance, as it is easily transmitted to human being through animal products to cause foetal human infection and vice versa. Anthrax has worldwide distribution. However, the prevalence varies from sporadic cases to "Anthrax belts" in which it occurs enzootically.

In developed countries, it occurs as "multicentric foci of infection" in which many sudden deaths occur without prior symptoms when appropriate climatic conditions, such as summer followed by heavy rains, arise. These incidences almost always have a history of disease occurrence as long ago as 30 years previously. This happens because the anthrax spores from old buried carcasses from old epidemic come out and sporulate on soil or on fodder, on soil and infect the graizing cattle.

In tropical and subtropical countries with heavy annual rainfalls persistant soil infection brings about frequent serious outbreaks of Anthrax and in some countries, they occur almost every summer. In temperate cool climate, only sporadic outbreaks occur. Accidental ingestion of contaminated bone meal or pasture contaminated by tannery effluent are more frequent causes. In Africa, disease occurs every summer and reaches a peak in years with heavy rainfall. Wild buffaloes, hippos and elephants are the victims with the predators acting as inert carriers of the infections (Webb *et al.*, 1987).

About the causative organism

Anthrax is caused by Gram positive, rod-shaped bacteria which show central or sub-terminal spores. The organisms from affected tissues and septicaemic blood smears under microscope show typical capsule around them which when stained with matured polychrome methyl blue stain show typical pink colouration. This is called as Ascoli's reaction. The septicaemic blood when cultured on blood agar show typical "Modusca head" colonies, surrounded by clear haemolysis.

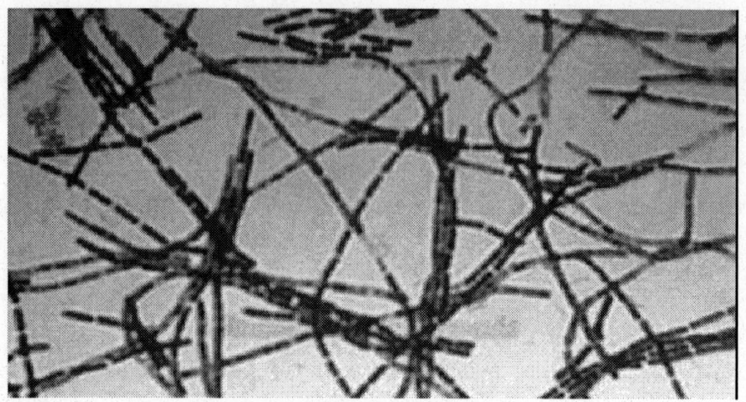

Fig. 1: *Bacillus anthracis*

The infective blood from the carcass, if inoculated in guinea pigs, rabbits or white mice, kill these animals within 24 hours and their heart blood smears stained with polychrome methylene blue stain show typical pink capsulated organisms in singles, pairs or short chains.

Epidemiology and the disease transmission

The disease occurs in 2 phases of the infection cycle. Phase 1 consists of picking up the Anthrax spores by susceptible animal directly from the soil infected by old buried carcass from previous older outbreak or from fodder grown on such infected soil. Spore of Anthrax can be picked up also from contaminated bone meal protein concentrates or from infective excreta, blood meal or other materials of infected animals/carcass origin. Water contaminated by tannery effluent or infected carcasses or by flooding and deposition of anthrax infected soil can also be a source of the 1st phase of infection cycle. Migratory Avian (bird) scavengers like gulls, vultures and ravens can also carry spores to considerable distance.

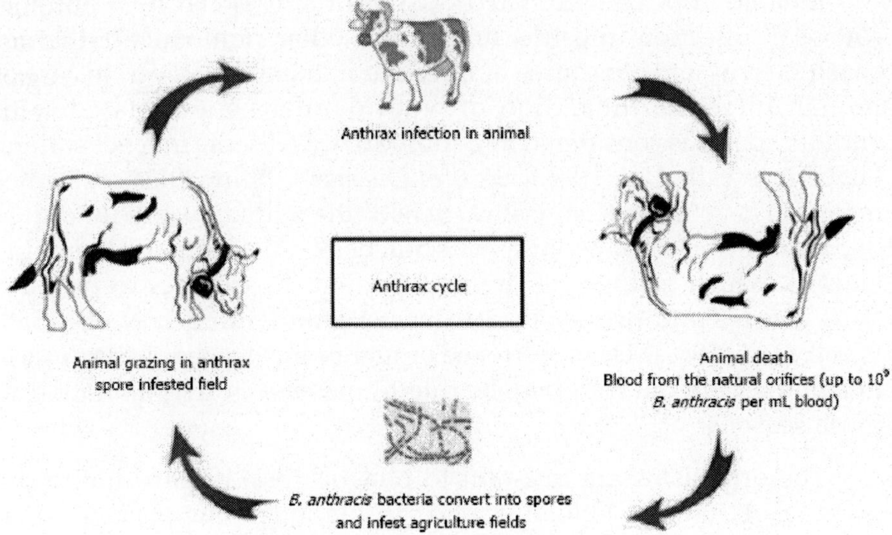

Fig. 2: Anthrax transmission cycle

The single animal infected in the 1st phase of the disease generally has peracute infection with sudden death without showing any symptoms. But this infected animal in 1st phase contaminates the soil surface or fodder grown on the soil which becomes a source of infection to many animals in 2nd phase of the disease which precipitates an outbreak with many cases showing acute clinical symptoms.

Importation of bone meal, hides, hairs, wool and fertilizers of animal origin which are contaminated with Anthrax spores become a source of Anthrax outbreak. In recent years, 50% of consignments of bone meal imported in U.K. have been shown to be contaminated with anthrax spores. There are instances of precipitation of Anthrax outbreaks in cattle vaccinated with Anaplasma vaccine containing blood due to accidental contamination of same with Anthrax spores. There are also reports of Anthrax outbreaks after vaccination inadequately attenuated spores containing Anthrax spore vaccine.

Pathogenesis

After ingestion of spores, infection occurs through intact mucous membrane or through defects in oral mucosa around erupting teeth or through scratches from tough fibrous fodder/feed materials which facilitates invasion of the organisms.

Inhalation of contaminated dust with spores can be a possible source of infection in cattle, horses and other ruminants but is not considered as a major source of infection in them. However, in case of human infection inhalation of wool dander contaminated with anthrax spores is considered as a source of this disease in wool sorters, hence it is called as "Wool Sorters Disease". Biting flies and other insects also act as mechanical carriers of the anthrax spores and they deposit the spores on wounds or scratches on the skin of susceptible animals which further get drained through lymphatics to produce local disease and further lead to bacteremia (Humber, *et al.*, 1988; Webb, *et al.*, 1987). The occurrence of higher incidences of the disease in summer and autumn may be due to increase in fly population in those seasons.

The organisms are resistant to phagocytosis in part due to the presence of the poly D-glutamic acid capsule and proliferate in regional draining lymph-nodes, subsequently passing via lymphatic vessels into blood stream which is followed by septicaemia and massive invasion of body tissues. B. anthraces produces a lethal toxin which causes oedema and tissue necrosis, death resulting from shock and acute renal failure with terminal anorexia.

Disease symptoms and lesions

Sheep & cattle

In peracute form of the disease, which occurs during initial beginning of an outbreak, animals are found dead. Suddenly animal collapse with convulsions within 1 to 2 hours after very short phase of fever and muscular tremors, thus resulting into haemorrhages from natural openings of the body, namely nostrils, mouth, anus and vulva as well as teat canals. The oozed out blood is characteristically tarry in appearance and is not clotted.

In acute form of the disease, which runs for about 2 days, severe depression, listlessness is followed (sometimes preceded by excitement) with high body temperature upto 107^{0}F deep and rapid respiration and congested haemorrhagic mucosae. There is anorexia and ruminal stasis. Reduction in milk yield with blood tinged milk and diarrhoea / or dysentery is evident. Tongue, throat, sternum, perineum and flanks may become oedematus.

Pigs

Fever, dullness anorexia and inflammatory oedema of throat and face are characteristics with obstruction to swallowing and respiration. Skin shows petechial haemorrhages. Baby pigs show respiratory form of the disease with lobar pneumonia and pleurisy.

Horses

Enteritis and septicaemia with colic is observed in infection through oral route and oedematous swellings on throat, lower neck, lower floor of thorax, abdomen, prepuce or mammary gland is a characteristic when infection is through insectbites. Postmortem examination is generally strictly prohibited, as this is a scheduled disease by law in all the countries. However, postmortems when conducted in advertantly due to mis diagnosis during clinical examination, reveal striking absence of "Rigour Mortis" and gaseous decomposition of the carcass is undergoing quickly with tarry unclotted blood oozing out of all natural aurifices. Widespread ecchymotic haemorrhages in all visceral organs and respiratory as well as alimentary tract are observed. Spleenomegally bloodstained serous exudates in thoracic and abdominal cavity are other characteristics features of the postmortem lesions.

Diagnosis

Demonstration of pink coloured capsules surrounding bacterial blue rod-shaped organisms in single pairs or short chains in polychrome methylene blue stained blood smears obtained from ear vein or blood oozing orifices of the anthrax suspected carcass in enough for anthrax diagnosis, as the postmortem examination of the carcass is prohibited by law due to the risk of spread of this "scheduled" disease.

In laboratory, careful handling of blood sample from ear vein of affected animal is needed for inoculation of rabbit, guinea pig or white mice and blood smear examination of heart blood of sacrificed / dead laboratory animal after 4 days P.I. using polychrome methylene blue stain gives confirmatory diagnosis of Anthrax, if pink capsule is demonstrated in rod shaped organisms in blood smear. Further culture on blood agar will show typical "medusa head" colony characteristics with surrounding haemolysis and will reveal final confirmation of Anthrax. PCR and Immunofluoroscence are also presently used for diagnosis.

Treatment

Animals in early febrile stage can be treated with penicillin or streptomycin or higher antibiotics 20000 units per KG body wt. and 8-10 gms per day in 2 doses are the appropriate dosages for pencillin and streptomycin respectively while 5 mg/kg body is the dose for oxytetracycline. Simultaneous treatment with hyper immune anthrax antiserum (100-250 ml daily for 5 days) by subcutaneous or intravenous route can be successfully used for complete recovery of the animal.

Vaccination and control measures

Placing of the farm in quarantine and proper disposal of carcasses (without opening for postmortem) by incineration and disposal of incontact feed/fodder/discharges by burning is the most proper way for arresting the further spread of the disease. Deep burial of carcass (2 metre deep trenches) with lime powder is also useful. Vaccination of the animals in contact of the affected animals on the farm using Avirulent Anthrax spore vaccine will be able to contain the disease within 10-12 days period after vaccination.

No importation of animals without the certification of vaccination and no import of animal products including wool, hair, bone meal, blood meal and meat pork and ham or other meat products should be allowed without certification for absence of Anthrax spores by random sample testing as per procedure laid down by WHO/OIE regulations to avoid occurrence of Anthrax outbreaks in the country.

Vaccines for Anthrax Immunization

Vaccines which consist of living attenuated strains of the organisms with low virulence but capable of forming spores have been most successful. Sporulation character is useful for long viability of vaccines. However, the disadvantage of these vaccines is that same species of animals show varying susceptibility to the vaccines and anthrax may result after vaccination in some situations. This can be avoided by use of saponin or saturated saline in the diluent used for vaccination to delay absorption. This is the basis of the "Cabazoo Anthrax Vaccine" (Shlykhov, *et al.*, 1996).

The stern avirulent spore vaccine has overcome the risk of causing anthrax by vaccination and produces a strong immunity. This vaccine is also safe for human handler of the vaccine. It produces sufficient immunity within 8 days post vaccination. This vaccine is used now in most of the countries including India. Milk of the vaccinated cows is not used for 72 hours after vaccination.

Indian Scenario of Anthrax

Anthrax exists in India since ancient times. Holmes prepared Anti-Anthrax Serum in India, in 1913 by injecting susceptible cattle with graduated doses of *Bacillus anthracis* in culture (based on the knowledge of production of anti-serum against anthrax by scalvo in 1895 using sheep and donkeys for immunization followed by Sobernheim, 1902 who advocated sero-vaccination using attenuated culture along with anti-serum prepared in calves and sheep as coated by Seetharaman, C. and Sinha, K.C. and their monograph of the Veterinary Biological Products and their uses 1962, pp.23) (ICAR Publication). IVRI started producing this Anthrax anti-serum in 1902 for prophylaxis (dose 50 ml) of the disease as well as treatment of the clinical cases in conjunction with Novarsinobilon and strepto-penicillin or tetracycline (dose of anti-serum 100 to 150 ml per animal). Initially, attempts were made to produce anthrax vaccine in India on lines of Pasteur. Bannerji and Cooper were deputed to bring the attenuated seed of Anthrax vaccine from Pasteur Institute, Paris at the beginning of 1st decade of 1900 (Seetharaman, C. & Sinha, K.C. 1962, ICAR publication). Later on stern type Avirulent spore vaccine was being produced at IVRI and some other State Vety. Biological production units including IVBP, Pune for preventive vaccination against Anthrax. It was a practice to undertake Anthrax vaccination for anthrax prevention in June-July every year especially where the disease was occurring in this season.

The author (S.V. Pandit) experienced sporadic incidences of Anthrax in imported sheep (Merino and Romnimarsh breed as well as Afghan breed (Goat and Sheep) at sheep breeding farm, Tathawade (near Pune) during 1962-63. During 1972-73, this farm was converted into composte livestock farm and Jersey and Holstein frezian cows and heifers were installed in some sheds in this farm. One Holstein frezian heifer was reported to have died suddenly in 1973 due to suspected cobra bite which was finally proved to have died due to Anthrax; the source of Anthrax was traced back to the burial of sheep carcass (which was proved as anthrax case) at the site of the shed exactly 10 years back. The preventive vaccination using anthrax spore vaccine (avirulent) in other animals in contact was undertaken urgently to avoid spread of the disease.

Two junior staff members of disease investigation section, M.S., Pune conducted few postmortems of sheep near Shahpur (Thane district). Which they suspected to have died of blue tongue disease and hence, they brought their spleens, lymph-nodes and blood smears for investigation purposes to D.I.S., Pune. The author (S.V. Pandit) before processing the material for virological investigation examined the blood smears from these cases for bacteriological elimination and to his surprise blood smears stained with poly chrome methylene blue showed typical pink coloured capsular organisms in single, pairs and short chains indistinguishable from anthrax organisms. The biological test of P.M. material in guinea pigs confirmed the diagnosis of Anthrax in those sheep. The attendant of those investigation officers complained of having slight swelling on his hand near his palm which was having a wound of postmortem scissors. He did not take any chance for further agriviation of possible "human anthrax incidence" and immediately treated him with strepto-penicillin injection on his arm near his shoulder. This stopped further progress of his local lesion of possible anthrax.

Suggested Reading

Humber, K.A.; Sweeney, R.W.; Saik, J.E.; Hansen, T.O.; Morris, C.F. (1988). Clinical and clinicopathologic findings in two foals infected with Bacillus piliformis. Journal of the American Veterinary Medical Association. 193: 1425–1428.

Webb, D.M., Harrington, D.D., Boehm, P.N. (1987). Bacillus piliformis infection (Tyzzer's disease) in a calf. J Am Vet Med Assoc. 191: 431–434.

□□□

Chapter 25

Black Quarter (Black leg) in Cattle & Sheep and Braxy in Sheep and Lambs

Black Quarter (BQ) is an infectious bacterial disease of cattle and sheep, caused by anerobic organisms, namely *Clostridium chauvoei* and sometimes mixed infection of *Clostridium chauvoai* and *Clostridium septicum* (especially in India).

True Black leg (Black quartors) occurs in the cattle which may be called as infectious myositis and is caused by *Cl. Chauvoei* only occasionally it is seen in sheep also, wherein only legs and quarters are affected. BQ is caused by trauma. Braxy is another disease of sheep in which infection occurs through "wounds" caused by shearing and docking or wounds caused by "fighting" in groups of young ewes and rams and the causative agents involved in Braxy is "Clostridium septicum". Wounds due to castration and dystocia are also other reasons for this clostridial infection.

About the causative organisms

Clostridium chauvoei and *Clostridium septicum* are both gram positive, spore forming rod shaped bacteria. The spores occur sub-terminally. These organisms are fastredious anaerobic organisms without capsule and can be grown on "Cooked meat & liver" particle containing medium or sodium thioglycolate containing liquid medium. In anaerobic solid medium, the organisms produce "lenticular" colonies (boat shaped). The spores are highly resistant to environmental changes and disinfectants and persist in soil for many years.

Epidemiology and transmission

The disease is enzootic in particular areas, especially when they are subjected to flooding. Such areas may vary in size from a group of farms to an individual field.

Black quarter is a soil borne infection especially black cotton soil harbours the spores of the causative organisms. However, the portal of entry of the organisms is still in dispute.

It is presumed that the organism enters the body through the alimentary tract mucosa after consumption of contaminated feed and fodder or is associated with eruption of teeth. The bacterial spores may be found in spleen, liver, alimentary tract or muscles of limbs of normal animals. True black leg develops when spores lodged in normal tissues are caused to proliferate by mechanism, such as trauma due to hit or accidental injury produces "anorexia" in muscles/spleen/liver tissue. This produces the initial first case of "black leg" which may die rapidly and decomposition of this carcass may contaminate fodder and soil with "activated virulent organisms" which may precipitate the disease in cattle/sheep population through injection of contaminated fodder.

In case of Braxy, the sheering, docking, fighting & distocial wounds are presumed to be responsible for local anorexia of skin, vulva or vagina of sheep which brings about proliferation of organisms and triggering and virulence in them which precipitates the discase in farm population.

Pathogenesis

In true black leg, the stimulus which results in growth of the latent bacterial spores is unknown. There is usually no history of trauma observable in every outbreak. However, trauma while passing through an alley is reported as the likely inciting factor in one outbreak. Toxin formed by organisms produces a severe necroting myositis locally in skeletal mucscles and systemic toxemia which is usually fatal. In cattle and sheep, atypical outbreaks of sudden death occur in which lethal lesions is a clostridial cardiac myostis (Glastonbury, *et al.*, 1988).

Disease symptoms and Post mortem lesions

The outbreak may start with per acute case with sudden death. In acute cases, the animal may show anorexia, ruminal stasis and high temperature upto 106^{0}F and pulse rate upto 100-120 per minutes. Pyrexia is not a constant symptom. Cattle may show severe lameness with hot and painful swelling of hind quarters or front shoulder in some cases in the beginning of the disease. But swelling may become colder later on and painless also. Palpation of the swelling will reveal emphysema with cracking sound. The skin at the affected site may be discoloured and will soon become dry and cracked. There may be oozing out of blackish red coloured fluid with frothy bubbles. The lesions being present on black leg in most of the cases is the reason for the name "Black quarters" to the disease. However, sometimes lesions can be seen at other locations, such as the base of the tongue, heart muscle, diaphragm or psoas muscles, the brisket and udder. The lesions can be at multiple places in one animal. Death can occur 12-36 hours after appearance of 1st signs.

In sheep, one or more number of legs can get myositis with stiffgait, which results into lameness. Subcutaneous oedema with gaseous crepitations is not felt during life but is felt only after death only discolouration of the affected part is observed while skin necrosis and gas gangrene do not occur.

In braxy, in sheep occurring through wounds of the skin, valve or vagina, there is extensive local lesions. Local head swelling with oedema and bleeding through nose with high fever, anorexia, depression may be observed in braxy in sheep. Sheep and cattle with cardiac myositis due to Cl.chauvoei infection are usually found dead suddenly.

Postmortem examination of affected carcass reveals typical posture of BQ which is characterized by carcass lying on one side with the affected hind limb stuck out stiffly. Carcass bloats and putrifies quickly with blood stained fourthly exudates from the nostrils and anus but clotting of blood occurs quickly. Incision of the affected muscle reveals dark red to black swollen tissue with rancid odour and oozing out of sanguineas fluid with gas bubbles. The thoracic cavity and pericardial sac may contain blood stained fluid with fibrous clothes. Lungs may be congested and atelectatic due to abdominal tympany.

In sheep lesions of muscle are more localized and deeper while subcutaneous oedema is not much marked except around head. Gas is present in lesser quantum as compared with cattle. Typical lesions are found in the walls of udder and vagina or uterus.

Diagnosis

As the putrifaction of the carcass of animal died of BQ sets in very early, the tissue material and its smears should be collected quickly after death of animal to avoid confusion between causative organisms and putrefactive anaerobe. Formalin fixed sample of suspected muscle tissue from quarter lesions is used for demonstration of myonecrosis, emphysema, neutrophilic cellultis with gram positive typical clostridial rod shaped organisms in tissue sections microscopically. Air dried lesions smears can also be used for demonstration of clostradial organisms. Anaerobic culturing of fresh tissue lesions material reveals typical lenticular colonies of clostridium chauvoei/septicum in deep solid agar cultures. Flourorscent Antibody Technique can also be used for demonstration of specific organisms using known positive fluoroscent dye tagged BQ hyperimmune serum prepared in rabbit or guinea pigs for FAT staining of tissue sections or tissue smears.

Treatment

Large dose of crystalline penicillin by intravenous route (40,000 units/kg body weight) followed by long acting tetracycline is useful.

BQ anti-serum was being prepared in suitable animals by hyperimmunisation with culture of virulent clostridium chauvoei organisms (monovalent) while in India, polyvalent BQ hyperimmune serum using both clostr. Chauvoei as well as closter septicum organisms killed by formalin for inoculation of Buffaloes subcutaneous by (i.e. BQ vaccine) by serial dosing on 1st, 9th, 30th, 42nd, 54th, 66th days respectively. This serum was being used for therapeutic use in dose 100 ml dose in cattle, 30-40 ml dose in cattle as well as for preventive purposes in doses of 15 ml in cattle and 7-10 ml in sheep as quoted by Seetharaman, C. & Sinha, K.C. (1962) in Vet. Bio. Prod. and their uses, ICAR publication. Now the production is discontinued at IVRI.

Control

Annual vaccination of all cattle between 3 and 6 months with 2 vaccinations given 4 weeks apart followed by annual booster vaccination is recommended for preventive purposes. During olden days anaculture (0.5% formaldehyde treated whole bacterial culture of clostridium chouvoei (monovalent) or both *Cl. chauvoei* and *Cl. septicum* (polyvalent) grown anaerodically in suitable medium was being used for production of BQ vaccine.

Indian Scenario

Black quarter disease is existing in cattle, in India since ancient times. There is no mention about the year in which BQ vaccine and BQ anti-serum production was started for the first time at IVRI in India in the book on Vety. Biological Products by Seetharaman, C. and Sinha, K.C. 1962, ICAR publication. However, while describing the standardization of BQ vaccine and BQ antisera; they have mentioned the reference of British Vet. Codex, 1953 for standardization of these products which gives the idea that these 2 products were under production at IVRI since 1953 onwards at least. The Author remembers of BQ Broth Vaccine (Anaeculture) was under production at Lazareto section of Bombay Veterinary College during 1958, where Biological Production Division was located during those days. Biological Production Section, Poona and IVRI Izatnagar, U.P. both were producing BQ vaccine in 1962, as listed out in Seetharaman, C. & Sinha, K.C.s Book on Vet. Biological Products (ICAR publication). This vaccine was being produced using conventional broth cultures containing Sodium thioglycolate for production of anaerobiasis during cultivation of the production brew of clostridium chauvoei or clostridium septicum organisms in production flasks of small capacity and the vaccine was containing the formalized whole culture without any adjuvant and hence, the immunity produced was shortlived (3 to 4 months after vaccination).

In India, there are two monsoon seasons in South (In Tamil Nadu, Kerala and Part of Andhra Pradesh), namely South West monsoon followed by South-East monsoon and hence, 2 season of occurence of Black Quarters every year and hence, 3 to 4 months shortlived immunity for BQ vaccine is not enough to take care by single vaccination against BQ, if the simple unadjuvated BQ broth vaccine is used annually. Hence, author (S.V. Pandit) and his team prepared Aluminium hydroxide gel adjuvanted formalin inactivated BQ vaccine at B.A.I.F., Wagholi during 1982 which proved successful in producing immunity for 18 months for taking care of BQ during both the monsoon seasons every year. (The immunity was proved by challenge experiment in cattle also). The vaccine production on large scale was also achieved by use of 300 litre fermentor for production of anaeculture of BQ organisms.

Suggested Reading

Glastonbury, J.R.W., Searson, J.E., Links, I.J. & Tucket, L.M. (1988). Clostridial myocarditis in lambs. Aust. Vet. J. 65: 208-209.

□□□

Chapter 26

Brucellosis in Cattle, Buffaloes, Sheep, Goats and Pigs

Brucellosis is a bacterial disease of cattle and buffaloes (caused by *Brucella abortus*), sheep (caused by *Brucella ovis*), Goats (caused by *Brucella melitensis* in sheep and goats) and pigs (*Brucella* suis), the principal manifestations of disease are reproductive failures, such as abortions or birth of unthrifty newborns in the female and orchitis or epididymitis with frequent sterility in the male. The disease has universal existence.

Mode of spread of this disease is characterized by direct transmission of the infection from affected animal to susceptible animal by uterine discharges which contaminate feed and fodder and infect the susceptible animals through ingestion. Congenital infection also occurs in case of *Brucella abortus* and *Brucella melitensis* infections. The venereal infection is a characteristics of *Brucella ovis* infection in sheep and *Brucella suis* infection in pigs while true venereal infection does not occur in case of *Brucella abortus* infection in cattle, even though *Brucella abortus* is excreted by affected bull in the semen and hence, it can be transmitted through artificial insemination as the organisms are well preserved in frozen semen.

Persistant (life long) infection is a characteristic of *Brucella* organisms (all species) as they are facultative intracellular organisms with shedding in reproductive and mammary secretions (i.e. milk). It is also an important Zoonosis causing debilitating disease in humans.

About the causative organism

Brucella is a gram negative, rod shaped organism which is micro-aerophilic in nature and needs presence of 5% carbon dioxide tension in atmosphere during its cultivation. *Brucella* species do not ferment most of the sugars during their growth and hence, no gas or acid is produced in these sugar media including glucose, lactose, galactose, inocital. On Methyl Red-Brilliant green agar, *Brucella abortus* reduces Methyl Red while *Brucella melitensis* do not reduce Methyl Red and produce pink colonies while *Brucella suis* reduces the same, thus colonies are not pink in colour. Hence, this medium is used for differentiation of *Brucella* species. *Brucella abortus* exists with 9 Biovars. Biotype-1 is present in about 5% infections of cattle in the world. Biotype-2 was found in Canada in 1986 while Biotypes

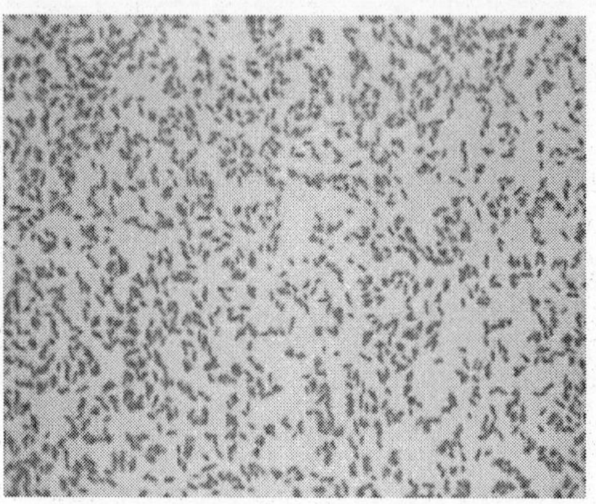

Fig. 1: *Br. abortus* organisms

1-4 are found in USA. Biotype-1 is also isolated from Bison in Canada (Forbes and Tessaro, 1996). Biovar-1 is highly fatal in "mouse" which is the dead end host of the organism. *Brucella suis* has 5 Biovars of which Biovars 1, 2 and 3 are important in swine. Biovar-4 occurs in rangiferines and Biovar-5 is causative organism of Murine Brucellosis. Biovars-1-4 cause a rare disease in cattle. *Brucella melitensis* in sheep and goats has 3 biovars.

Mode of Transmission and Epidemiology

Brucellosis is an important disease of cattle, sheep, goats, pigs and buffaloes. In cattle abortions occur most commonly in outbreaks in unvaccinated heifers after the 5th month of pregnancy. Brucella infection occurs in all age groups of cattle but most commonly in sexually mature animals. Bulls are affected with orchitis, epididymitis and seminal vesicles. The disease also occur in bison, elk, deer, raccons, moose and other wild ruminants but with no evidence that they can be a source of infection to domesticated animals.

Horses show presence of Brucella organisms in fistulous withers, poll evil and bursal enlargements as secondary invadors along with Actinomysis bovis.

Dogs naturally acquire infection of Brucellosis from cattle (cows) on the farms, as they have the habit to eat placental materials which can be a source of brucella organisms, when it is from Brucella aborted cows. Dogs do not show the disease but can act as "Carriers" of the organisms for spread of brucellosis on affected farm and from farm to farm spread. The infection is transmitted by ingestion, penetration of intact skin and conjunctiva. Grazing on infected pasture or consuming other feedstuffs and water supplies contaminated by placental material and discharges from uterus and vagina of infected cows and contact with aborted foetuses and infected newborn calves are the most common sources and methods of infection. Horizontal transmission is usually by the direct contamination.

Congenital infection may occur in calves born from infected dams but its frequency is low. The infection occurs in utero and may remain latent in the calf during its early life, the animal may remain serologically negative until its first parturition, when it then begis to shed the organisms. Frequency of latent infection may range from 2.5 to 9% and such animals can remain a source of infection later on.

Even vaccinated heifers from sero positive dams (about 2.5%) can harbor a latent infection and become a threat to a re-established herd.The organisms can survive for 100 days on grass in temperate climate and for only 30 days in summer. Cow's tail contaminated with uterine discharge can pass on brucella infection, if it comes in contact of intact skin or conjunctiva of susceptible cow. Infected cows shedding Brucella organisms in milk can contaminate other uninfected animals through milk. Bulls do not usually transmit infection from infected to non-infected cows mechanically (through venereal infection) but infected bulls shedding Brucella organisms in their semen can be a source of infection to other cows through artificial insemination. Embryo transfer from infected donor cows may be achieved without transfer of brucella infection, as super ovulation is unlikely to reactivate the release of brucella into the uterus during the period, when embryos are normally collected. Thus, embryo transfer is a safe procedure for salvaging valuable genetic material.

Pathogenesis

Brucella organisms are facultative intracellular parasites capable of multiplication and survival within host phagocytes. The organisms are phagocytosed by PMN leucocytes in which some survive and multiply. They are then transported to lymphoid tissues and foetal placenta as well as to other site, such as the reticulo-endothelial system. The organism is able to survive within macrophages because it has the ability to survive phagolysosome present in them. Thus, survival of brucellue in both neutrophils and macrophages afford them protection from humoral and cellular bactericidal mechanisms during the periods of haematogenous spread (Enright, 1990).

After the entry of brucella infection in animal through ingestion or through intact skin or conjunctiva or through infected semen in vagina, localization of brucellae occurs initially in lymph-nodes draining these areas. The spread further occurs to other lymphoid tissues including the spleen and mammary/itiac lymph-nodes. Congenital infection in newborn calves occurs as a result of in vitro infection and persists in small proportion of calves which are sero-negative until upto their 1st parturition or abortion. In the adult, non-pregnant cow's localization of infection occurs in udder and the uterus, if it becomes gravid, is infected from periodic bacteremic phases originating in the udder. So, infected udders are clinically normal looking but they become source of infection to human being through their milk-secretions and source of re-infection to the uterus and bring about infection to calves drinking the milk.

Erythritol, a substance produced by placenta and foetus is secreted in placental and foetal fluids and is responsible for stimulation of brucella organisms and their localization in these tissues. Thus, the invasion of brucella in the gravid uterus and placental tissue results in a serere ulcerative endometritis of the inter-cotyledonary spaces. In acute infection of pregnant cows, upto 85% of the bacteria are invading and cotyledons, placental membranes and allanotic fluid, leading to the displacement of the foetus from mother cows uterus resulting into abortion. Abortion occurs principally in the last 3 months of pregnancy.

Disease Symptoms and Pathological Menifestations

Brucellsis of cattle

In highly susceptible non-vaccinated pregnant cattle, abortion after the 5th month of pregnancy is the typical feature of the disease. In subsequent pregnancies, generally abortions are absent except in few animals 2nd or 3rd abortion can occur. Retention of the placenta and metritis occur after abortions which sometimes leading to secondary bacterial infections, septicaemia and resultant death occasionally. Storm of abortions may occur in the highly susceptible herds, which may last upto 1 year period. After the period of stormy abortions in the herd, the abortions are largely restricted to first-calf heifers and new additions as the rest of the herd acquire partial resistance.

Occasionally, orchitis and epididymitis occur in bulls and one or both scrotalsacs may be affected with swelling and testing undergoes liquefication necrosis and may eventually destroy. Seminal vesicles may also be affected. The affected bulls, thus become partially or completely sterile. Often, the cattle may show non-suppurative synovitis with hygromatous swellings of joints (Knees). Sometimes, cotton strain 19 vaccination of some calves can also lead to non-suppurative synovitis and arthritis of stifle joints. In horses from Brucella abortus infected cattle farms, the cases of fistulous whethers or enlargement of naval bursac or bursal enlargement of neck occur occasionally.

Brucellosis in sheep and goats

Brucella melitensis infection of the foetus during pregnancy does not nccessarily result in abortion, kids and lambs may be born alive but week. The infection of naïve flock will produce an abortion storm following which most animals are infected but immune and hence, in small flocks, infection becomes self-limiting but in large flocks where new introductions are frequent, the new-comers may get infected, if they are susceptible and problem of abortion continues. Brucella ovis produces disease only in sheep and infertility in rams is due to epididymitis.

Brucellosis in pigs due to *Br. suis*

Many times presence of high positive reactors without clinical signs are observed as manifestation of disease depends on site of localization of organisms. The incidence of abortions is low and abortion occurs only once and occurs in 3rdmonth of pregnancy. Infertility, irregular oestrus, small litters are some other findings in sows. Orchitis with scrotal swelling and necrosis of one or both testicles followed by sterility, lameness, in co-ordination and posterior paralysis occur quite commonly in boars. Arthritis and osteomyelitis of lumbosacral vertebrae can occur. Heavy mortality of piglets may occur during 1st month of life or still births or death within a few hour after birth may occur.

Brucella Diagnosis

Diagnosis of abortion due to brucella organisms on cattle, buffalo, sheep, goats and pigs is attempted by isolation of organisms by culture, from the organs and lymph-nodes of the foetus, the placenta, milk, vaginal mucous or uterine exudate, which provides the direct evidence of Brucellosis and avoids false diagnosis. A nucleic acid probe assay for detection of organism is very sensitive and faster than conventional cultural method for clinical diagnosis is developed (Hopper *et al.*, 1989).

The major objective in the laboratory diagnosis of brucellosis is to identify animals which are infected and potentially shedding the organisms and spreading the disease. This enables the farm management to cull/dispose off the shedder animals in order to eradicate the brucella infection from the farm. Most of the shedder animals are identified by the serological test but few animals are sero negative but still shed the organisms and are "latently infected". On the other hand few animals which are sero positive but no actually "Shedders". These diagnostic problems make the control and eradication programme more difficult.

Serological Testing Programme for detection of infected animals

The following antigens are available for detection of antibodies against brucella infection is animals:

1. Brucella Abortus Quick Plate Test Coloured Antigen

This is a suspension of pure smooth cultures of *Brucella abortus* strain 99 in Phenolized glycerine saline, bacteria being coloured by addition of crystal violet and brilliant green. This is a greenish violet coloured reagent and when mixed with the suspected serum produces specific agglutination on a slide/plate which indicates that the animal from which the said serum collected is a positive reactor which may be a potential shedder of the *Brucella abortus* organisms. However, the specificity of the reaction is not absolute, as it detects specific as well as non-specific antibodies from Br. abortus infection or vaccination. "Powdery" type of agglutination may be a border line case and needs further retesting using "standard tube test" antigen to know the exact titre of agglutination.

2. Brucella Abortus Plain Antigen for Standard Tube Test

It is a suspension of pure smooth culture of *Brucella abortus* strain 99 in Phenol saline which is opalescent liquid containing dead bacteria in suspension. It is used for tube test which requires incubation of tubes containing serial 10 fold dilutions of "test serum" and constant tube test antigen for 24 hours before reading for agglutination. Titre of 1:40 and above is taken as positive for brucellosis in cow and 1:20 and above is positive for brucella for breeding bull. However, Standard Tube Test (STT) detects antibodies in vaccinated animals also and hence, it should be adjunted with heat inactivated serum tube test (HTT) which should give the above mentioned standard titres for declaration of animal positive for brucella infection. HTT is negative or shows titre less than 1:40 in case of vaccination in case of cow and less than 1:20 in case of bull. While in case of infection, HTT is higher i.e.>1:40 in cow and > 1:20 in case of bull respectively. HTT titres are always less than STT titres in case of vaccination and there is no difference in STT and HTT titres in case of infection. This is based on the principle that heat inactivation (HTT) destroys IgM class of immunoglobulin while it has no effect on IgG class of immunoglobulin (In case of Brucella infection due to either field infection or vaccine virus infection, IgM appears first followed by appearance of IgG later on in the serum antibodies. IgM disappears later on in case of vaccination and only IGG persists). In case of Brucella field infection, IgM persists for longer time along with IGg and there is reduction in total titre in case of field infection after HTT while total titre is not reduced in case of vaccination, as it is totally IgG titre and IgM is absent.

3. 2-Mercapto – Ethanol and Reavnol Test

The tube test is carried out on sera samples after treatment with "2-mercapto-ethanol" or "Revanol" after using the untreated sera for STT. There is reduction in total STT litre after mercapto ethanol treated sera testing (MET) or after Revanol treated sera testing (RVT). There is reduction in MET titre as well as RST titre as compared to (STT) titre in case of sera from Brucella abortus positive field infected animals, while there is no titre reduction in MET/RVT tests after STT in case of vaccinated animals. This is based on the same principal in case of HTT, as ME/RV both can destroy IgM.

4. Rose Bengal Antigen for Plate Test

This antigen in prepared in a similar way as Brucella abortus. Crystal violet + Brilliant green coloured antigen is prepared except that rose Bengal dye in specific acid buffer replaces crystal violet and brilliant green dye in the antigen. Acid buffer gives more specific agglutination reaction by avoiding non-specific antigenic fractions precipitation is avoided in acidic environment. The antigen has rosy pink colour.

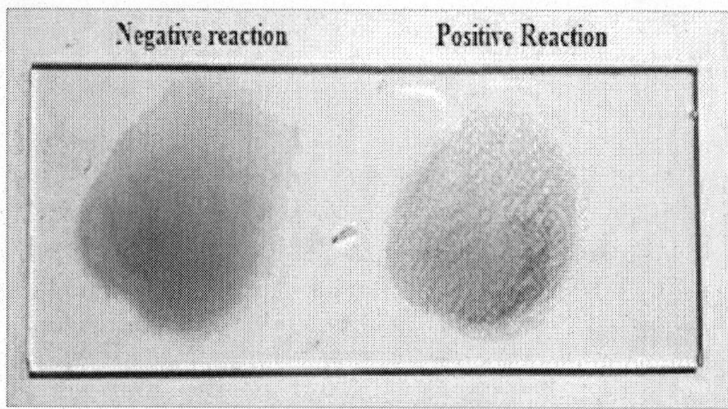

Fig. 2: Rose Bengal plate test

5. Milk Ring Test Antigen

This antigen is reddish in colour and is prepared by using methyl Red colour for dying Brucella abortus strain-99 antigen suspension. This antigen is used for testing a pooled milk sample from a herd of 25 cows each. This test is used for testing milk samples from various small herds at milk collection centre. This antigen is used for pooled milk samples in test tubes which are incubated for 2-3 hours after addition of Milk Ring test antigen which agglutinates the brucella antibodies present in milk samples and agglutinated masses floating along with fat globules come to the surface of creamy layer and produces reddish pink coloured ring which indicates presence of antibrucella antibodies secreted in milk by infected cows which means that the sample is from brucella positive herd of cows. If the test is positive, that particular herd is to be tested for individual cows sera to know specific cow's positive for brucella infection.

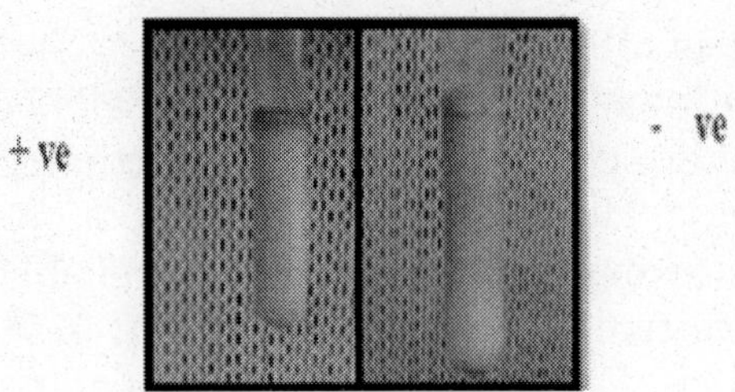

Fig. 3: Milk Ring test

6. Complement Fixation Test

CFT antigen is produced by heat-lysis of Brucella abortus culture organisms and the test used for detection of Brucella abortus infected potential shedder animals more specifically as compared with STT tested positive reactors. CFT antibodies appear earlier than STT antibodies in brucella infected animal and remain for longer period in chronically affected animals.

7. Enzyme Linked Immunosorbent Assay (ELISA)

This test is available in 2 formats, namely indirect ELISA and competitive ELISA. It is used for screening after vaccination programme during eradication programme or as supplementary test to CFT which gives comparative advantage over other serological tests as ELISA detects antibody of all isotopes unlike the other conventional tests mentioned previously (Nielsen K.H. *et al.*, 1995, Vet. Immunol. Immunopathol 46: 285).

Sensitivity and Specificity of Serological Tests

It is recommended that either the Rose Bengal Buffered Plate Antigen Test or indirect ELISA be used as screening test and either CFT or indirect ELISA is appropriate for use as confirmatory test in situation requiring a high specificity (Dohoo, I.R. *et al.*, 1986, Can J. Vet. Res. 50:485). In Brucella Free herds, Rose Bengal Buffer Plate Test (RBPT), STAT, SPAT, 2-MET and CFT correctively classified all sera as "Negetive", thus proving specificity.

On a sample of "culture positive" cattle analysis of relative sensitivity of six agglutination tests give the following ranking from highest to lowest sensitivity : BPAT, RBPAT, SPAT, STAT while 2-MET ranked between BPAT and RBPAT. BPAT is recommended as a screening test followed by CFT. Milk Ring Test (MRT) is generally used as a screening test for detection of Brucella positive herds, which is carried out at least 3 times annually as recommended by regulatory agency in Canada. However, ELISA using potassium chloride extract of Brucella organism is highly specific and reliable test for monitoring Brucellosis Control Programme (Thoen, C.O. *et al.*, 1995, Vet. Microbiol.45 :185). ELISA using polysaccharide, as antigen has 95% sensitivity and 99.95% specificity while comparing milk samples from Brucellosis free and Brucellosis infected herds (Nielsen, *et al.*, 1996). Combined use of ELISA and PCR gives 100% sensitivity (Romero *et al.*, 1995).

False positive reactors due to exposure of animals to *E. coli* O: 116 and O:157 Pseudomonas maltophilia, Vibrio cholera, etc. which share antigencity pose as big problem in eradication programme, as these reactors get unnecessarily slaughtered inspite they are non-specific and they cannot be differentiated easily.

Treatment

As *Brucellae* are intracellular parasites, the treatment with any antibiotic is unsuccessful.

Control and Eradication

Most countries with brucellosis have programme designed to control and ultimately eradicate Brucellosis. All breeding cattle in the herd are tested and positive reactors are culled and then sent to slaughter to remove infected cows from the herd and reduce exposure and transmission within the herd. Particularly, it is important to detect and remove infected cows prior to parturition.

It is necessary to quarantine the negative reactor cows after the 1stbrucella testing and retest them after a period of twenty-one days during which time if any negatively testing animal is in incubation period, it will become sero-positive and will be detected during the second testing. The retesting progrmme should be repeated until 2 consecutive tests are negative and positive reactors are eliminated by segregation and slaugher to avoid cross infection again. Doubtful reactor should also be separated and retested after 3 weeks to confirm the real status of the animal. If more than 33% animals are positive reactors in a herd, it is to be totally destroyed.

The disease can be eradicated by either 1) test and slaughter policy or 2) test and slaughter and vaccinate rest of the negative herd policy, the later policy is not successful as vaccination with cotton strain 19 can stop abortion but cannot eliminate the shedding of organisms in uterine discharge during and after parturition and also in milk from udder of vaccinated but infected cow.

Complete eradication of Brucellosis by test and slaughter policy is achieved by great Briton in 1981, but 3 in 1985, it was found that 99.8% herds were free from brucellosis but small foci of infected herds persisted and outbreaks occurred in West England during 1984-86. The co-operative state federal Brucellosis eradication programme of United States is making progress. In U.S., in 1992, 29 states were classified as "class-free", when no cattle or bison in a state are found infected for 12 months. 19 states maintained "Class A" status with infection rate of less than 0.25% while only 2 states were in "Class B" with infection rate of less than 1.5% (See details of U.S. programme for Brucella eradication on pp.880 of book entitled Vet Medicine disease of cattle, sheep, goats, pigs Otto M. Radostitis et al. W.B. Sounders. 9th edition year, 2000).

Australia, New Zeland and Canada are also other countries in which systematic Brucella Eradication programme are undertaken and progressing (see details in above mentioned reference text book).

Control by Vaccination

Brucella abortus, cotton strain 19 has a low virulence and is incapable of causing abortion except in proportion of cows vaccinated in late pregnancy although it can cause "undulant fever" in human, if it gets accidental entry in human vaccinator through injury/cuts in skin of hand due to negligent handling of vaccine without use of hand gloves during vaccine handling. Strain 19 Br. abortus has 2 other weakness, namely 1) its failure to completely prevent infection of udder and 2) the persistence of vaccinal titres in some animal during adult hood after late calfhood vaccination.

The optimum age for vaccination is between 4 and 8 months. The serum agglutination test returns to negativity by the time the animals are of breeding age, except in some 6% animals, titres upto 1:20 to 1:40 still persist upto 18 months. These titres interfere during the sera testing programme during eradication compaigne. However, infected animal titres and vaccination titres can be differentiated by

CFT, 2-MET, RVT and HTT in adjunction with STT as described in preveius paras of this chapter. In some control programmes, cotton strain 19 vaccination is permissible upto 12 months of age of calves, if adult testing programme includes CFT, MET, RVT, HTT or ELISA which can differentiate the "Vaccination titres" and "Infected titres".

Vaccination of bulls with strain 19 vaccine is not advisible as vaccinal organisms can produce orchitis in some bulls and excretion of organisms in semen (Nicoletti P. 1990, in Animal Brucellosis, pp. 283-299, Boca Raton F.L. CRS press). Cotton strain 19 vaccine markedly reduce number of abortions and reduction of shedding of Brucellae due to increased resistance of vaccinates to infection but total shedding is not stopped.

Economic Importance

Brucellosis has major veterinary and human importance in affected countries, costs include production loss associated with infection in animals preventive programme and human disease. Production loss includes decreased milk production by aborting cows, loss of calves and common sequel of infertility increases the period between lactations, prolonged intercalving period of several months which interfere with breeding programme, heavy culling of valuable cows due to metritis and retained placenta problems.

Zoonotic implications

Drinking of infected milk and handling of abortion cases by veterinarians may bring about accidential zoonotic problems. The human infection is characterized by undulant fever (biphasic fever), arthritis, occasional orchitis. Handling of infected animals including cattle, sheep, goats and pigs during slaughter is also important source of zoonotic importance.

Control of human brucellosis

The major source of human brucellosis infection is milk from brucella infected cows. Generally flash treatment of pasteurisation is effective method for killing brucella organisms in milk. Instant heating of milk to 80^{0}C for few seconds followed by instant cooling is undertaken at milk processing plant for pasteurisation of milk for this purpose which makes the milk completely safe for drinking.

Boiling of milk and milk products as well as cooking of pork and ham -products and cooking of meat and beef makes the products safe for human consumption and avoiding zoonosis. Smoking and injection of potassium nitrate in ham and pork as well as freezing of pork, ham, beef and meat is of no use in killing brucella organisms in meat and pork industry. Veterinarians handling distokia cases, parturition and abortion cases should use protection clothings, aprons and hand gloves with proper disinfectant measures to avoid professional hazard of zoonosis.

Brucellosis in domesticated Animals Indian Scenario

Brucellosis Incidence in India is present since ancient times. Seroprevalence of Brucellosis in Bovines was reported by many workers (Mohan, 1954; Mukharjee, 1960; Chaudhari & Chatterjee, 1975; Mathus, 1966). While working at Disease investigation section, M.S. Poona from 1962 to 1974 the author (S.V. Pandit) came across brucella "positive reactor" animals in significant number during Brucella testing at various cattle and buffalo breeding farms as well as during testing of "breeding bulls" during working as a member of bull selection committee at cattle/buffalo fairs/bazaars for selection of breeding bulls for use of artificial insemination centres State Govt. STT and HTT were standardized using Brucella crystal violet brilliant green stained plate test antigen, Brucella plain antigen for standard tube agglutination test and Heat inactivation tube agglutination test (HTT). While testing we came across fast positive "No Visible Lesion (NVL)" reactor bulls which when destroyed and their number of lymph-node samples from each bull were subjected for cultural examination proved negative for presence of Brucella organisms as well as their semen samples also proved negative for isolation of Brucella organisms, inspite of these bulls showing more than 1:20 STT and HTT titres for which no definite explaination could be obtained.

Even though we were able to destroy positive reactors bulls as well as Cows/buffaloes, after confirmation of Brucella tests using STT, HTT and Cultural examination from State Govt. Farms we worked only in advisory capacity to advice elimination of positive reactors from private herds for want of specific legal provisions for brucellosis control programme from Govt. of India/State Govt. we came across incidence of brucella reactors from 1 to 33% from various farms including Govt. buffalo dry farm and Govt. pure bred jersy and Holstein frezian farm both at Palghar (Distt. Thane).

When the author (S.V. Pandit) was working at BAIF'S vaccine project, Wagholi, he participated in development of Rose Bengal plate test antigen STT plain antigen, Milk Ring Test (MRT) antigen production and Brucella strain 19 vaccine in liquid as well as in freeze dried form. We at BAIF, undertook calfhood Brucella strain 19 vaccination programme on some Pinjrapol's crossbred young stocks (at age between 4-8 months) and studied STT & HIT control programme monitoring during early 1980's. We could find that both STT and HTT antibodies were present in titres > 1:40 (upto 1:120) after 14 to 21 days after vaccination and titres were completely "negative" by 12 months (By STT & HTT). We used MRT for detection of Brucella positive farms by testing pooled milk samples at milk collection centres of some sugar factories in Maharashtra State successfully.

Author (S.V. Pandit) participated in 1972-73 in investigation of an outbreak of Brucellosis in pigs and piglets at Regional Pig Breeding Farm, Aarey Milk Colony, Goregaon, Bombay suburban Distt. Maharashtra, where in symptoms of abortion, delayed heat, repeat breeding among breeder sows and gilts and late reactor boars were noticed. The postmortem of the sows at "Bacon Factory" plant of the state Govt. to which this farm was attached, revealed severe endometritis and multiple abscesses along the walls of uterine horns and fallopean tubes which were very prominent lesions.

The author (Pandit, S.V.) alongwith and under the guidance of Dr. G.P.Sen of IVRI, Mukteshwar undertook serological examination of 70 sera samples using SAT, HTT and MET and Allergic test with brucella lysate (Brucella suis) brought by Dr. G.P. Sen from IVRI, Mukteshwar by Interdermal inoculation in pigs. 25 animals out of 70 were positive for brucella infection by Allergic test while 35 animals +ve by HTT as the most confirmative test (Sen *et al.*, 1976). Barbuddhe *et al.*, 1994 of IVRI, Izatnagar, Div. of Vet. Public health demonstrated that dot ELISA using 599 strain brucella abortus autocalve extracted antigen detected more number of positive samples as compared to Rose Bengal Plate Test (RBPT), STAT and CFT used for diagnosis of Brucellosis in sheep, goats and human (Report on XIV Annual Conference and National Symposium on Recent advances in production and testing of Vet. Biologicals, conducted by Indian Association of Vet. Microbiologists immunologists and specialists in infections disease pp.26 (BM-10) (IAVMI) at Pune, 1994).

In the above mentioned symposium report, Gupta, P.K., Takale, M.N. and Singh, S.N. (pp 26, BM-11) 1994, demonstrated that plate ELISA, using enzyme digested extract of Brucella abortus S99 as antigen and bovine serum dil of 1:400 could detect 67% positive samples out of 170 bovine sera tested while Rose Bengal Plate Test (RBPT) could detect only 47% samples.

Suggested Reading

Enright, F.M. (1990). The pathogenesis and pathobiology of Brucella infection in domestic animals. In Animal brucellosis (K. Nielsen & R. Duncan, eds). CRC Press, Boca Raton, Florida, 301–320.

Forbes, L.B., Tessaro, S.V (1996). Infection of cattle with Brucella abortus biovar 1 isolated from a bison in Wood Buffalo National Park. Can. Vet. J. 37: 415-419.

Hopper, B.R., Sanbom, M.R., Bantle, J.A. (1989). Detection of *Brucella abortus* in mammalian tissue using biotinylated, whole genomic DNA as a molecular probe. J Am Vet Med Assoc 50: 2064-2070.

Nielsen, K.H., Kelly, L., Gall, D., Nicoletti, P., Kelly, W. (1995). Improved competitive enzyme immunoassay for the diagnosis of bovine brucellosis. Vet Immunol Immunopathol. 46: 285–91.

Romero, C, Gamazo, C, Pardo, M, Lopez-Goni I (1995). Specific detection of *Brucella* DNA by PCR. J Clin Microbiol 33: 615-617.

❑❑❑

Chapter 27

Enterotoxaemia of Domesticated Animals caused by *Clostridium Perfringens* Types A,B,C, D and E

Enterotoxaemia is an acute disease of domesticated animals including sheep, goats and cattle and sometimes horses and pigs, caused by blood circulation of toxin produced in enteric tract by clostridium perfringens organisms belonging to either one of the types A,B,C,D and E. *Clostridium perfringens* (types A,B,C,D and E) organisms are toxin producing spore bearing bacteria of soil origin, contaminating pasture and other feedstuffs and foodgrains of farm origin, capable of producing enterotoxins, such as alpha, beta, and epsilon toxins under suitable anaerobic conditions in enteric tract of animals under the specific local stress.

About the organisms

Clostridium perfringens which was previously known as *Clostridium welchii* is a gram positive rod shaped non-capsulated bacterium (with central or subterminal spore) in single, pairs or short chains. It is a facultative anaerobe and produces spore under unfavourable conditions which can survive for long periods in soil or in intestines of animals.

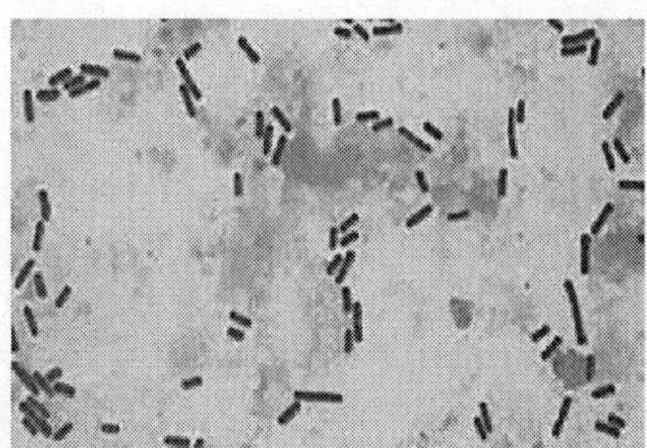

Fig. 1: *Clost. perfringens* organisms

Clostridium perfringens exists in various serotypes, namely *Clostridium perfringens* types A,B,C,D and E, each serotype produces specific exotoxins in intestinal tract of animals as follows:

1. *Clostridium perfringens* type A produces alpha toxin, which possesses phospholipase C. and Sphigomyelinase activity with haemolytic.
2. Clostridium perfringens, types B and C, both produce alpha and beta toxins. "Alpha toxin is a "lethal toxin" which is a "phospholypase" which brings about hydrolysis of membrane phospholipids in erythrocytes (RBG), platelets, leukocytes and endothelial cells results in cell lysis and other forms of cytotoxicity. The Beta toxin is a "necrotizing" toxin and initially produces damage to the microvilli with degeneration of mitochondria with eventual destruction and desquamation of the intestinal epithelial cells and the production of a haemorrhagic enteritis and ulceration of intestinal mucosa. Beta toxin also increases permeability and may facilitate its own "uptake" from the intestine (Rood and Cole, 1991; Songer, 1996). Age incidence of the enterotoxemia disease can be explained partially by the observation that "Betatoxin" is highly sensitive to inactivation of "Trypsin" which is a component of normal "pancreatic proteases". Colostrum contains a "trypsin inhibitor" and trypsin is decreased or absent in affected pigs. Experimentally administered soyabean floor used as a protease inhibitor converts experimentally induced "clostridial enteritis" from a "non-fatal" to a "fatal" disease.
3. *Clostridium perfringens* type D produces number of toxins of which the "Epsilon toxin" is the most important and results into "Vascular damage"as well as damage to "nervous system". Epsilon toxin also increases the "permeability" of the intestinal mucosa and facilitates its own absorption. "Epsilon toxin" is responsible for the rapid autolytic and liquifactive changes in the kidney and brain tissues. This is responsible for severe neural symptoms and "pulpy" kidney lesion observed in postmortem examination of sheep died of pulpy kidney disease caused by Clostridium perfringens, type D. A receptor for epsilon toxin has been identified on vascular endothelial cells which are responsible for strong affinity of epsilon toxin to vascular endothelium and damage caused it by "epsilon toxin" and its increased permeability (Finnie *et al.*, 1992; Sakuri, 1995).

Occurrence of the diseases

A. *Clostridium perfringens*, type A causes equine Intestinal clostridiosis in adult horses.This is characterized by profuse watery diarrhoea with high mortality in adult horses. Haemorrhagic caecaitis and colitis and death following exercising (Wierup, 1981). This organism also produces diarrhoea in pigs, with watery yellow diarrhoea in piglets under 5 days of age with high morbidity and low mortality (Songer,1996).*Clostridium perfringens* type A is also associated with haemolytic disease in sheep and cattle in Australia and Haemorrhagic enteritis in calf and adult cattle in U.K. and Australia, and Haemorrhagic Enterotoxemia in foals in Australia and Japan.

B. Clostridium perfringens, type B, C and E produce enterotoxemic disease conditions with haemorrhagic enteritis and ulceration of intestinal mucosa resulting in diarrhoea and dysentery in young lambs, goats, claves, piglets and foals in different parts of the world and are given specific names in those countries as follows:

   i) Lamb dysentery occurs in Great Britain Europe and South Africa and Australia. This disease is predominantly caused by type C organisms.

   ii) Necrotic Enteritis of piglets is most common in United States, Europe and Britain and occurs in sporadic form and sometimes become endemic in swine units.

   iii) Enterotoxaemia of foals due to type B and C predominates in reports from North America (Pearson, E.G. *et al.*, 1986, J. Am. Vet. Med. Assoc. 188: 1309).

   iv) "Enterotoxaemia" in calves occurs due to types B and C and is characterized by outbreaks with severe dysentery and deaths in 7-10 day old calves.

   v) "Struck" in sheep is manifested only by sudden death without symptoms, but rarely with abdominal pain and convulsions before death and it occurs only in Britain.

C. Clostridium perfringens, type D causes typical enterotoxaemia in sheep, goats and in calves and it especially occurs during the beginning in rainy season, when newly grown lush green pasture is available for graizing on the fields which is eaten up by the sheep and goats voraciously and hence, it is also known as "Over eating disease". Primarily, lambs and young calves are affected with clostridium perfringens type D worldwide. In North America, it is a main cause of due to enterotoxaemia in feed lot lambs.

Epidemiology and Disease transmission

Clostridium perfringens which is primarily an organism from soil is of universal presence and normal grazing animal's pickup small numbers of such soil clostridia through pasture grazing in routine course. Small numbers of clostridial organisms are always present in normal intestinal containts of sheep, goats and calves without any disease problem.

However, when young lambs, kids, calves, piglets and foals are weaned from their mothers and are introduced to the "feed lots" for the first time suddenly in the grazing fields with lush green pastures they get "stressed" due to "overeating" and "intestinal stasis" increases the number of clostridial spores concentration in intestine. The intestinal stasis also favours accumulation of trypsin from duodenal pancreatic secretion which favours desolution of clostridial spores chitinous walls and vegetative phase of the clostridial organisms brings about multiplication of the same in "anaerobiasis" created by intestinal stasis. This brings about production of entero-toxins including alpha, beta, iota, epsilon and other toxins by clostridial organisms. The variety of toxins produced depends on serotypes of these organisms and the special pathogenic effects produced by the toxins will depend on their specific toxogenic effects which ultimately determine the nature of the enterotoxic disease produced by them.

Pathogenesis

Nature of pathogenesis depends on the serotype of the clostridium perfringens according to the specific toxin(s), they produce as follows:

A. *Clostridium perfringens* serotype "A" produces only Alpha toxin which has "haemolytic" effect as described in details under the heading "About the organism" in the beginning of this chapter. This toxin produces haemolytic enterotoxaemia in sheep, cattle and foals.

B. *Clostridium perfringens* serotype B; C & E produce Alpha and Beta toxins. Alpha toxin is responsible for "heamolytic" effects as well as lysis of platelets and entothelial cells which produce haemorrhages which B toxins produce necrotizing effects and increase permeability of endothelial cells, thus these organisms produce an enterotoxaemia with "haemorrhagic" and "Necrotic" enteritis, including bloody dysentery and abdominal pain.

C. *Clostridium perfringens* serotype D produces protoxin of "epsilon" which is converted into active "epsilon" toxin by the action of pancreatic juice containing trypsin" enzyme which has a proteolytic action. Epsilon is a powerful toxin which brings about severe vascular damage as well as damage to the nervous system, thus these organisms produce severe lethal enterotoxcemia with sudden death or produce liquefication of brain tissue with acute nervous symptoms prior to death.

Clinical symptoms and Postmortem lesions

a) Enterotoxemia caused by "Type A" organisms: In equines and in pigs' symptoms include acute profuse watery diarrhoea with high mortality in adult horses. Acute colic is observed before death. Mucosal pallor, Jaundice, haemoglobururia and severe abdominal pain is characteristic. P.M. lesions include swollen liver, hydropericardium and pulmonary oedema.

b) Enterotoxemia due to serotypes B & C and E produce lamb dysentery in hill breeds with small litter size but with high milk production (serotype B & C) Necrotic enteritis in piglets, enterotoxemia in foals under 7 days of age and in calves 7 to 10 days old as well as "struck" in sheep. The symptoms in all these diseases are characterized by acute disease with absence of "sucking drive" in affected young ones, severe abdominal pain with bloating, stretching and looking at abdomen, passing of brown fluid faeces containing blood and defecation with painful straining, passing, necrotic debris some times. In very acute cases, death occurs in few hours. "Struck" in sheep is characterized by sudden death.

Type C enterotoxemia is common in "single born" lambs of 1 to 4 days of age and especially in lambs and kids of ewes in "Cold weather" and which are kept confined to small yards or fields for lambing or kidding as the gross contamination of such places is bound to occur in these circumstances. Incidence of 15-20% and mortality upto 100% is found in such outbreaks of type C enterotoxemia.

P.M. lesions in all above mentioned young ones of different species of animals with type B infections show common lesion, namely localized areas of necrosis most evident in ileum. The intestinal mucosa is dark red with large ulcerations about 2.5 c.m. in diameter. Intestinal contents are blood stained with fibrin clots in them. In type C infections, the necrotic areas are more widespread throughout the intestine.

Histopathological features of type B,C and E type enterotoxemia include mucosal haemorrhages, necrosis, fibrin exudations and neutrophilic infiltrations in enteric tract and large number of gram positive clostridial rods lining the luminal surface of these lesions.

c) Enterotoxemia due to type D occurs mainly in lambs of sheep, age 3 to 10 weeks and in goat kids aged same as in case of sheep. Most common age group of 1 to 4 months is affected in calves with type D enterotoxemia. The disease occurs due to overeating of lush green pastures as explained previously, within 5 to 14 days after introduction in feeder lot. Horses are rarely affected. Adult sheep and goats also can get affected after overgrazing in pastures after starting rainy season.

Lambs & Kids are found dead without showing any previous symptoms especially at the start of outbreak (peracute form). In acute cases, dullness, depression, yawning, smacking and facial movement with lack of interest in feed followed by convulsions with frothing at the mouth and rapid death may occur. Some show cases may show severe clonic convulsions, green pasty diarrhoea, staggering, recombancy, opisthotonos, calves also show similar symptoms in addition to bellowing mania and convulsions.

Postmortem lesions are characterized by presence of clear straw coloured pericardial and thoracic fluid which clots on exposure due to fibrin contents. Hydro pericardium and hydro thorax, epicardial and endocardial haemorrhages are predominant with pulmonary oedema. Patchy congestion of the abomasal and intestinal mucosae is usual. Contents of large intestine may be dark green and watery.

Kidneys are "Pulpy" in consistency which is "characteristics" lesions of type D enterotoxemia only if observed within few hours after death otherwise putrefaction may mislead. In sheep died of enterotoxemia of milder type and taken longer time for death, symmetrical areas of haemorrhage, oedema and liquefication of brain especially in area of basal ganglia is observed.

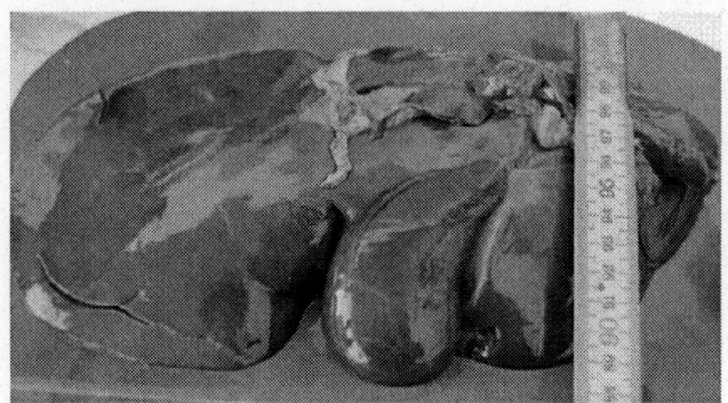

Fig. 2: Pulpy kidney in Enterotoxaemia

Diagnosis of Enterotoxaemia

Gram stained smears of ingesta and intestinal mucosa taken from various levels of intestine if show uniform presence of gram positive short, fat rods typical of clostredial morphology with almost absence of any other contaminant organisms, during postmortem examination of fresh carcass of sheep/goat kid/calf strongly indicates the diagnosis of enterotoxemia.

Bowel filtrates from "intestinal loop" collected during postmortem examination of fresh carcass, if injected intravenously into white swiss mice via tail vein will produce circling movements in mice within few seconds of injection and kill the mice instantaneously will confirm the case of enterotoxemia and if the filtrate is treated with suitable dilution of specific antiserum against l, b and epsilon toxin separately and then injected by intravenous route in mice after incubation at 37^{0}C for one hour and if mice survive without showing "toxic" symptom, the presence of specific "toxin" symptoms, the presence of specific "toxin" can be identified and clostridium perfringens type can be determined which is responsible for the outbreak of enterotoxemia. Passive Latex Agglutination (RPLA test) test using Alpha/Beta anti-toxins adsorbed on latex particles, as antibody for detection of toxins (Alpha/Beta) in intestinal contents is also useful for diagnosis.

PCR technique detects genes encoding the major toxins and are promoted for replacing in vivo test for toxins and can detect and differentiate toxogenic clostridia in pathological material from non-toxogenic clostridia from normal animals. An ELISA test shows good specificity and sensitivity for epsilon toxin.

Addition of one drop of chloroform to the loopful of enteric material collected for toxin diagnosis is useful for preservation of those contents for period upto one month. Intestinal contents absorbed on filter paper and transported at ambient temperatures can be used for immune-Assay for 74 days.

Treatment

Hyperimmune serum produced against l, b and epsilon toxins is unable to save the peracute cases of enterotoxemia due to sudden deaths. However, the less acute cases can be saved with the use of hyperimmune serum parenterily and sulpha diamidine administered orally.

Control measures

Reduction of the food intake, administration of antitoxin and vaccination are the 3 principal control measures, out of these 3 reduction of the food intake is not of much use. Antitoxin can be administered to all sheep/goats/other animals as soon as outbreak commences. Administration of epsilon antitoxin 200 unit/kg body wt. will provide protective level passive antibody for 21-29 days and immediate losses are prevented. Toxoid is cheapter but takes longer time for development of antibodies and hence, will allow some toll to take place before development of immunity.

Vaccination

Vaccines available are toxoids. They are improved by addition of adjuvants. Activated alum precipitated toxoid is the common vaccine in use, two vaccine doses at the interval of atleast one month with the last vaccine about 4 weeks prior to lambing/kidding/calving of the mother, calve/cow will result in good passive immunity may last upto 8 weeks of age in 97% young ones and upto 12-16 weeks with moderate protection level. Thus, their highest risk period is covered for protection. Older animals previously vaccinated should receive single boaster dose every year for 3 years to get permanently protected for their progeny.

Clostridium perfringens oriented enterotoxemias (Indian Scenario)

Enterotoxemia caused by *Clostridium perfringens* type D in sheep and goats and their lambs and kids is prevailing in India since long time.

I.V.R.I. Mukteshwar/Izatnagar is producing an anaeculture bacterin using highly toxigenic Cl. welchii type D strain grown in anaerobic liquid medium containing P.B.S. (pH-8) for 24 hours at 37⁰C with subsequent addition of trypsin to ensure maximum toxin production. This converts prototoxin to active toxin. The culture is checked for purity and toxicity as tested in mice. Culture is then formalized (0.05% final concentration) and inactivated at 37⁰C till product is sterile and non-toxic. This product is used for prophylaxis of enterotoxemia in sheep and goats since early fifties of 20th century in India.

However, during early seventies presence of lamb dysentery in lambs and kids was diagnosed in the State of Jammu and Kashmir which was due to Enterotoxaemia caused by *Cl. welchii* type B and C (with l and b toxins). No vaccine was available for this disease upto early eighties. Similarly enterotoxamia of calves' dues of Cl. Welchii type C and D was also diagnosed in Maharashtra in seventies.

BAIF, Wagholi Scientists (including the author S.V. Pandit) developed Multi-component clostridial vaccine (s) including Cl. Welchii types B, C and D which was adjuvated with aluminium hydroxide gel for better immunization during early eighties this vaccine was found useful for sheep & goats in J&K states.

Suggested Reading

Finnie, J.W. Pathogenesis of brain damage produced in sheep by *Clostridium perfringens* type D epsilon toxin: A review. (2003). *Aust. Vet. J.*, 81: 219–221.

Rood, J.I. and Cole, S.T. (1991). Molecular genetics and pathogenesis of *Clostridium perfringens.* Microbiol. Rev. (55): 621-648.

Sakurai, J.; Nagahama, M.; Oda, M. (2004). *Clostridium perfringens* alpha-toxin: Characterization and mode of action *J. Biochem.* 136: 569–574.

Songer, J.G. (1996). Clostridial enteric disease of domestic animals. Clinical Microbiology Reviews, (9): 216–234.

Wierup, M. (1977). Equine intestinal clostridiosis. An acute disease in horses associated with high intestinal counts of Clostridium perfringens type A. Acta Vet Scand Suppl: 1–182.

□□□

Chapter 28

Colibacillosis of Newborn Calves, Piglets, Lambs, Kids and Foals

Colibacillosis is an infectious bacterial disease of newborn young ones of domesticated farm animals, including calves, piglets, lambs, kids and foals characterized by either enteric disease or septicaemia caused by enteropathogenic or invasive serotypes of *Escherichia Coli* (*E. coli*) organisms respectively.

The disease occurs all over the globe and produce huge economic losses in animal industry, including dairy, meat, wool, piggery and horse farming industries due to the high mortality in newborns. Practice of non-feeding of colostrums to newborn male calves of cows and buffaloes is responsible for very high calf mortality in India due to subsequent colibacillosis in them.

About the causative organism

Pathogenic sero-types of *E. coli* causing coli bacillosis are gram negative small or slender rod shaped non-spore forming vegetative motile organisms with flagella with capsular presence significantly or insignificantly.

E. coli serotypes in domestic animals possess somatic "O" antigens Varing from O_1.... O_3, O_9... O_{20}....O_{45} ....O_{101} ....O_{138} ....O_{145} ,O_{147} ....O_{149} ....O_{157} in pig lets O_{111} ....O_{103} ...O_5 ....O_{26} in calves and O_{101} in foals and flagellar antigens H-1 to H-7 as well as capsular antigens K-1 to K7 as well as capsular antigens K-1 to K-81 .... K-85 .... K-89 ....K91 and K-99, etc. Enteropathogenic *E. Coli* serotypes also possess processes known as pili or fimbriae containing adhesive factors known as Adhesins designated as K^{99+} or K^{88+} or 987 P, which are also known as F-4, F-5 and F-6 respectively (F stands for Fimbriae). Some other surface adhesive antigens are F-41, F-17 and 25 present on some enterotoxogenic strains of E.Coli. Some enteropathogenic *E. coli* posses enterotoxins in their body which are endotoxins and are designated as either heat stable enterotoxins (ST) or heat labile endotoxins (LT). The most common enteropathogens which cause diarrhoea in newborn farm animals are enterotoxigenic *E. coli* (ETEC) which are not invasive and cause diarrhoea by adhering to the wall of small intestine, colonize and produce enterotoxins in small intestine.

Less common cause of the disease of newborn farm animals are Enterohaemorrhagic *E. coli* (EHEC) which are attaching and effacing *E. coli* also known as (AAEC) which produces haemorrhagic colitis. They are also known as verocytotoxic *E. coli* (VTEC) because they produce verocytotoxins. Necrotoxogenic *E. coli* (NTEC) produce cytotoxic Necrotising factor-1 (CNF-1) or factor-2 (CNF-2). NTEC-2 isolates are restricted to calves and lambs with diarrhoea and septicaemia. (Mainil, *et al.*, 1997). Some "EHEC" found in cattle are of Zoonotic importance, such as *E. coli* serotype 0157H:7 of cattle causes haemorrhagic colitis and haemolytic uremic syndrome in humans (Dorn, 1993).

Epidemiology and disease transmission

The primary source of infection is the faeces of infected calves shedding huge load of enterotoxigenic *E. coli* in diarrhoeic faeces. The mother cows of the infected calves also act as the reservoirs, shedding the enterotoxigenic *E. coli* in their normal faeces. In case of colibacillosis of newborn piglets, lambs and kids also source of infection is the infected newborns as well as their mothers shedding the infected organisms.

The unhygienic management of the calving sheds, piglet barns, lambing/kidding pens increase the concentration of the *E. coli* enterotoxigenic serotype organism population especially during winter or rainy season. Newborn calves/piglets/lambs/kids acquire the infection from contaminated bedding, calf pails, dirty calf pens, nearby diarrhoeic calves/piglets/lambs/kids, overcrowded calving/furrowing/lambing/kidding grounds and from the skin of the perineum and udder of the parturient dam/cow/eve, within few minutes after the birth.

Habbit of licking of newborns after giving birth by the mother animals helps in transmission of the pathogenic *E. coli* from the flooring or from the soiled feeders, waterers and other formites in the parturition sheds. This is how the newborns get the dose of infection of enterotoxigenic *E. coli* including those with K99+ piti, K 88+ pili or

987 P adhesions in case of piglets and with K99+ ETEC or with Art 25 and F-17 in case of calves producing enteritis and with K88+ fimbriad adhesion in case of calves with enteritis and septicaemia (Lintermans, *et al.*, 1988). The newborn young ones get infection through ingestion orally and in the absence of feeding of colostrums or inadequate quantity of feeding of colostrums or in the absence of antibody in the colostrums against a specific enterotoxigenic *E. coli* infection the pathogenic organisms react the site of predilection for the specific pathogen in the intestine namely illium without resistance where they can act to produce pathogenic effect.

Pathogenesis Enterotoxigenic Colibacillosis

Adhesions in the pili or fimbriae of enterotoxigenic *E. coli* allow them to adhere to the intestinal villous epithelied cells and prevent peristaltic elimination by the gut and the production of heat labile (LT) and heat stable (ST) enterotoxins. In case of calves K -99+ ahnesin and heat stable (ST-1) are the major virulence attributes of enterotoxigenic strains of E. Coli K-99+ adhesion has an ileum of calf as the site of predilection. While in case of piglets classical *E. coli* serogroups 08:K87, 045, 0138:K81, 0141:K85, 0147:K89, 0149:K91 and 0157:KV17 strains usually express and produce K88+, 987P+ and K99+ pilus antigens which adhere to ileal villi, colonise intensively and cause profuse diarrhoea (Casey *et al.*,1992). Some other strain of *E. coli* produces heat stable enterotoxin (ST). Some serotypes of *E.Coli* of calves' also elaborate F-41 adhesin to K99 and other surface adhesions, such as Att 25 and F-17, these *E. coli* produce enteropathogenic as well as septicaemic effect (Lintermans *et al.*, 1988).

The heat stable enterotoxin (ST) which is common to bovine, porcine and human strains of enterotoxigenic *E. coli* is an endotoxic product from *E. coli*. Enterotoxins are secreted in the upper small intestine ilium after the colonization of the *E. coli* organisms due to adhesions of the same with the help of adhesion factors of pili. These powerful endotoxins allow the net secretion of fluid and electrolytes from the systemic circulation into the human of the gut resulting in varing degree of diarrhoea, dehydration and electrolytic imbalances, acidosis and hyper kalemia. When the acidosis is severe, circulatory failure, shock and death takes place. This hyperkalemia in newborns with neonatal diarrhoea and acidosis also results into cardiac rate and rhythum abnormalities like bradicardia and atrial stand still. The response to enterotoxin in calves and piglets is similar to cholera enterotoxin in man (Wilson *et al.*, 1992).

Septicaemic Colibacillosis (Pathogenesis)

This occurs in all the species of domestic young ones due to invasive *E. coli* serotypes by invading the circulatory system (followed by invasion of the tissues) via intestinal mucosa tonsillar crypts, nasopharyngeal mucosa or via umbilical cords vessels. The invasive strains of *E. coli* are able to invade extra intestinal tissues to resist the bactericidal effects of complement to survive and multiply in the body tissues and fluids to escape phagocytosis and intracellular killing by the phagocytes and to induce tissue damage by release of cytotoxins. Thus, calves and piglets deficient in colostral immune globulins are highly susceptible to septicaemia. In animals, which do not die after septicaemia, localization of bacteria takes place in joints and other organs and tissues. *E. coli* serotype 0115: K"V" 165 can cause either diarrhoea or septicaemia in piglets and calves.

The clinical lesions in septicaemia are attributable to the effects of endotoxin which causes shock. The general effects of such endotoxin are hypothermia, low decreased blood pressure, low heart beats and decreased cardiac output, hyperglycemia followed by hypoglycemia and depletion of liver, glycogen and arthritis is a common sequel of the septicaemia in calves, foals and lambs, meningitis is common in calves. *E. coli* strains of serotype 0-78 are invasive and cause septicaemia in calves, piglets and lambs. Their powerful endotoxins cause endotoxic shock with high mortality rate (Gyles, 1992).

Zoonotic Implications of *E. coli*

Cattle have been incriminated as a source of *E. coli* which produces food born disease in humans (Whipp *et al.*, 1994).

E. coli associated with enteric disease in humans produce "Verotoxin" also known as a "Shiga like toxin" (Blanco, *et al.*, 1993). Most prevalent serotype in North America, Europe and U.K. is E. coli, serotype 0157 H: 7 which is verotoxigenic *E. coli* (VTEC), causes haemorrhagic colitis and haemolytic uremia syndrome in human being. This is attributed to the consumption of uncooked ground beef and raw milk. Cattle in Spain are reported to have infection of verotoxigenic *E. coli* of serotype 0157 H: 7 and were isolated from beef calves 8 weeks of age.

Symptoms and postmortem findings

Calves show 2 different menifestations of coli bacillosis, namely, coliform septicaemia and Enterotoxigenic colibacillosis.

Coliform septicaemia

This is most common in first 4 days of neonatal life of calves which have low levels of serum colostral immunoglobulins because of inadequate passive transfer of colostred immunoglobulin (Aldridge, *et al.*, 1993). These calves show a course of disease 24 to 96 hours with high mortality upto 88%. The common symptoms include initial high temperature followed by subnormal temperature, recombancy, dehydration, tachycardia, weakness and calf becomes moribund before death. The few surviving calves may develop localization of *E. coli* after speticaemia in joints to produce weak authritic calves. This may also develop meningitis with opithotonus, convulsions and tremors. Few calves may also develop diarrhoea with dysentery.

Enterotoxigenic Colibacillosis

In this form of the disease, few calves 3 to 5 days of age may develop per acute enteric toxemia with severe weakness, subnormal temperature, cold elamony skin, pale mucosal collapse of superficial veins and death within 2 to 6 hours after showing convulsions. But majority of calves develop diarrhoea with profuse watery faeces to pasty pale yellow to white faeces with blood flakes and extremely foul smell. Calves under 8 days of age may stop sucking milk and drinking, become severely dehydrated with extremely distended abdominal to fluid filed intestines. The recession of eyeball is the reliable indication of the degree of dehydration. Death usually occurs in 3-5 days. The hyperkalemia in calves due to dehydration with neonatal diarrhoea and acidosis is associated with bradicardia (increased heart beats) and atrial stand still. Some verocytotoxigenic *E. coli* (VETEC) strains produce disease in Veal calves with haemorrhagic enteritis with anorexia, fever diarrhoea with blood and mucous in faeces, haemorrhagic diasthesis on conjunctivae and mucous membranes of the mouth and nose.

Colibacillosis in Porcines

Coliform septicaemia occurs in Piglets within 24 to 48 hours of age. Piglets become weak, almost comatose with subnormal temperature.

Enterotoxigenic colibacillosis in newborn piglet's upto 3 days of age

The faeces vary from pasty to watery consistency diarrhoea is profuse, staining tails which become straight and wet. Temperature is normal to subnormal. They become recombant and show paddling movements. The dehydration leads to death in 24 hours.

Colibacillosis of lambs and goat kids

It is generally of septicaemic type showing symptoms similar to the calves lambs and kids aged 1-2 days or 3-8 weeks of age are affected. Acute meningitis with stiff gait followed by recombancy and convulsions are observed. Chronic cases become arthritic.

Postmortem lesions of colibacillosis in calves, lambs, kids and piglets are characterized by absence of lesions in peracute septicaemia while in acute cases, subserosal and submucosal haemorrhages are common. Sometimes, a degree of enteritis and gastritis is observed in septicaemic form but commonly this may be absent. Fibrinous exudates may be present in joints with artiritis. Omphaloflabitis, pneumonia and meningitis may also be evident.

In enterotoxigenic colibacillosis, intestines may be filled fully with fluid and abdomen distended with fluid and milk clot. Abomasal mucosa may have haemorrhagic spots, intestinal mucosa may be hyperemic or normal and mescentric lymph-nodes may be oedematus jejuna and ilial villi may be atrophied or fused. In histopathological sections of enteric lesions containing areas of intestines, the presence of large number of bacilli adherent to the brush borders of enterocytes is quite predominant.

Diagnosis

Blood culture from suspected septicaemic form of colibacillosis affected animals (Young ones) is carried out using blood collected from Jugular Vein of suspected animal by direct inoculation of brain heart infusion medium and further isolation on mackonkey agar plates for isolation of "invasive serotype" *E. coli* and their identification require serotyping of "O" (somatic) antigen e.g. 0:78 serotype is invasive produces septicaemia in calves, piglets and lambs. Similarly serotype 0157H: 7 causes both enteritis as well as septicaemia in cattle and in human cases. Somatic "O" antigens can be detected by plate agglutination test after "heat treatment" of *E. coli* blood isolate as heat treatment destroys "H" flaggelar and "K" antigens (Capsular antigens). The definitive etiological diagnosis of enteric colitacillosis requires isolation of *E. coli* from intestinal wall using enrichment broth media followed by final isolation on solid mackonkey agar plates. But simple isolation of *E. coli* from faeces is not confirmative, as normal animals can also carry *E. coli* in their intestinal contents. Demonstration of specific "enterotoxigenic" nature of the faecal isolate is needed for final etiological diagnosis along with demonstration of specific adhesions from their pili/fimbriae to show their ability of colonization and adhesion to intestinal wall.

The laboratory tests to identify enterotoxigenic K99$^+$ *E. coli* include all direct fluoroscent antibody technique (FAT) using fluoroscent dye tagged monoclonal or polyclonal antibody against K99$^+$ antigen. ELISA test kit is also available with monoclonal/polyclonal antiserum for detection of enterotoxin or the organism in the faeces. Similar diagnostic kit using Latex Agglutination test technique for detection of enterotoxin/organism is also available.Several ELISA tests are available with monoclonal antibodies against VT-1 and VT-2 "Verocytotoxins" for examination of diarrhoeic faeces containing the "VETEC" organisms.Property of specific *E. coli* isolates of fermentation of sorbital for identification of 0157H7 zoonotic *E. coli* is used for diagnostic purposes. Determination of "drug sensitivity" of enterotoxigenic faecal isolate of *E.coli* from the faeces of animals affected with colibacillosis after specific identification as the "etiological agent" responsible for the outbreak, is useful for undertaking specific antibiotic treatment of colibacillosis outbreak cases.

Treatments

Intravenous broad spectrum antibiotic treatment (Terramycin or tetracyclins) and intravenous fluid and electrolyte treatment for few days is required for treatment of septicaemic colibacillosis. For enteric coli bacillosis, fluid and electrolyte replacement (oral therapy), Antimicrobial and immune globulin therapy, Antimortility drugs including kadin and pectin, Clinical management of outbreak, etc. are useful points for controlling the therapeutic aspect of the outbreak.

Protective measures

Feeding of adequate quantum of colostrums is the most important point in saving the newborns from falling prey to colibacillosis just after the birth. Sucking of colostrums from mother within one hour after birth is more effective than feeding the colostrums or milk replacers artificially.

Increasing specific Resistance of the newborns by vaccinating the pregnant dam or newborn

This type of immunization of dams by vaccination with vaccines containing enterotoxigenic strain of *E. coli* (ETEC) is a new concept which has received considerable research attention in recent years and the results are quite promising. (Moon and Bunn, 1993). Such vaccines are practical and effective because 1) ETEC infections occur in early neonatal life (24 hrs to 3-4 days), when antibody titres in colostrums and milk are highest, 2) Most of ETEC infections in farm newborns belong to a small family of "Pili" antigens, 3) Pili consist of good protein antigens on bacterial surface where they are readily accessible to antibody, 4) Pili are required for adhesion colonization which is a critical step in early pathogenesis of colibacillosis.

The pregnant dam is vaccinated 2 to 4 weeks prior to parturition with vaccine containing inactivated *E. coli* organisms containing specific pilus antigen. The colostrums of such dam contain high titre of antibodies against the specific pilus antigen. This colostrum is fed to the newborns, thus passively transfer of antibodies against specific ETEC pili takes place from the dam to its newborns. This antibody specifically inhibits the adhesion of ETEC to the intestinal wall of the newborn (colonization of ETEC) so that early pathogenesis of the ETEC in development of Enteropathogenic effect is halted and thus, the newborn is prevented from development of colibacillosis. Such vaccines containing *E. coli* with F-1, F-4, F-6 and F-41 adhesins or purified *E. coli* with K-99^{+} pili are used commercially for prevention of colibacillosis in calves and piglets. These vaccines are used in pregnant cows/sows, 2-4 weeks prior to parturition and colostrums of these dams is fed regularly after parturition for 4-5 days to their calves/ piglets for protection against colibacillosis.

Vaccine containing *E. coli* 0111: B4 (J-5) either modified live strain or inactivated strain is used to immunize calves at 1 to 3 days of age and booster vaccination of these calves 2 weeks later is used to immunize calves by active antibody production in them for controlling calf mortality/morbidity upto 60 days.

Passive immunotherapy of calves under 2 days of age with J 5 *E. coli* hyperimmune plasma given subcutaneously at a dose of 5 ml/kg body wt. has been found useful for treatment of calf morbidity and mortality. The protective effect of egg yolk powder prepared from eggs of hens vaccinated with heat extracted antigens from K-99+ piliated ETEC strain 431 have been evaluated in calves which were feed with milk replacer containing such hyperimmune egg yolk powder which protected them against ETEC induced diarrhoea.

Colibacillosis of "Newborn" animals (Indian scenario)

Authors have observed calf mortality of newborn buffalo calves in Bombay suburban district including at Arey Milk Colony since the time of early sixties of 20th century due to enteritis and septicaemia due to *E. coli* and salmonellosis infections especially in male calves which were deprived of colostrums feeding. Similar mortalities are reported in village cattle and buffalo calves since ancient times. But such mortalities are neglected due to commercial reasons. There was a research scheme sponsored by ICAR on the same subject in early sixties but only survellance work was undertaken under this scheme but the basic research on serotying of ETEC and subsequent development of protective vaccine development is lacking in India.

The author (Pandit, S.V.) while working for short duration at Agriculture University, Kolhapur tried to use random Adult Buffalo serum for subcutaneous inoculation in buffalo calves which were suffering from neonatal calf diarrhoea simulating enterotoxigenic colibacillosis (However, isolation of *E. coli* was lacking in those cases) and could successfully save them from death (There was a history of calves continuously suffering from diarrhoea with significant calf mortality prior to our experimentation). Idea of using adult buffalo serum was based on the assumption that adult buffalo on this farm might have exposure to Enteropathogenic *E. coli* which must have immunized them against the etiological agent on the farm responsible for calf diarrhoea.

The author (S.V. Pandit) while working at BAIF, Wagholi (FMD vaccine project) was producing non-specific immunoglobln free serum from blood received from Deonar slaugher house, Bombay for use in fermentor cell culture of BHK-21 cells for FMD vaccine production on large scale. Huge quantities of non-specific immunoglobulin were being produced every week as a "Waste" by-product in this process. The author was interested in production of purified gamaglobulin from this waste product which he presumed to contain large quantum of specific gamaglobulins against number field infections including *E. coli,* rotavirus and coronavirus infections responsible for calf diarrhoea and calf mortality. The author thinks that such gammgobulin fraction will be useful for treatment of calf mortality including coli bacillosis and rota/caronavirus infection. However, he had to shelve out this idea as he left BAIF due to some reason subsequently. Scientists at Poultry Diagnostic and Research Centre of Venkateshwara Hatchey Group, Pune were working on a project on development of egg yolk powder from immunized hens for feeding in calves for treatment of calf mortality/colibacillosis.

Suggested Reading

Aldridge, B.M., Garry, F.B., & Adams, R. (1993). Neonatal septicaemia in calves: 25 cases (1985-1990). Journal of the American Veterinary Medical Association, 203(9): 1324–1329.

Blanco, M., Blanco, J., Blanco, J.E. and Ramos, J. (1993). Enterotoxigenic, verotoxigenic and necrotoxigenic Escherichia coli isolated from cattle in Spain. American Journal of Veterinary Research 54: 1446–1451.

Casey, T.A., Nagy B., Moon H.W. (1992). Pathogenicity of porcine enterotoxigenic Escherichia coli that do not express K88, K99, F41 or 987P adhesins. Am J Vet Res 53: 1488–1492.

Dorn, C.R. (1993). Review of foodborne outbreak of Escherichia coli O157:H7 infection in the western United States. J. Am. Vet. Med. Assoc. 203: 1583–158.

Gyles, C.L. (1992). Escherichia coli cytotoxins and enterotoxins. Can.J. Microbiol. 38: 734-746.

Mainil, J.G., Jacquemin, E., He´rault, F., Oswald, E., (1997). Presence of pap-, sfa-, and afa-related sequences in necrotoxigenic Escherichia coli isolates from cattle: evidence for new variants of the AFA family. Can. J Vet. Res. 61: 193–199.

Lintermans, P., Pohl, P., Deboeck, F., Bertels, A., Charlier, G., Vandekerckove, J., Van Damme, J., Schoup, J.,Schlicker, C., Korhonen, T., De Greve, H., Van Montagu, M., (1988). Characterization and purification of the F17 adhesin on the surface of bovine enteropathogenic and septicaemic Escherichia coli. Am. J. Vet. Res. 49: 94–1799.

Moon, H.W., Bunn, T.O. (1993). Vaccines for preventing enterotoxigenic Escherichia coli infections in farm animals. Vaccine 11: 213–200.

Whipp, S.C., Rasmussen, M.A. and Cray, W.C. (1994). Animals as a source of Escherichia coli pathogenic for human beings. Journal of the American Veterinary Medical Association, 204: 1168–1175.

Wilson, J.B., S.A. McEwen, R.C. Clarke, K.E. Leslie, R.A. Wilson, D. Waltner-Toews, and C.L. Gyles. (1992). Distribution and characteristics of verocytotoxigenic Escherichia coli isolated from Ontario dairy cattle. Epidemiol. Infect. 108: 423-439.

□□□

Chapter 29

Salmonellosis in Cattle, Sheep, Goats, Pigs and Horses

Salmonellosis or paratyphoid is a baceterial disease of domesticated animals caused by *Salmonella* species other than *S. typhosa* and is characterized by transient septicaemia and enteritis in general and abortions occasionally. However. abortion is a predominant symptom caused by some host adapted salmonellae especially in equines and ovines. This animal infection has zoonotic importance, as it causes a food poisoning through contaminated meat and milk products of animal origin.

About the Causative Organisms

The disease is caused by the genus *Salmonella* belonging to the family *Enterobacteriacae*. They are gram negative short and slender rod shaped non-spore bearing organisms found in single, pairs or short chains in cultures. They produce rounded smooth colonies without haemolysis on blood agar and colourless colonies on Mackonkey agar and do not ferment glucose lactose, trehalose, manitol and other sugars. They produce pink red colonies on brilliant green methyl red agar medium and purple colonies with metallic shine on crystal violet agar. At least 2200 serotypes exist based on 670 antigen groups and numerous H-antigens recognized.

Salmonellae are classified into 3 major groups depending on their animal and human hosts as follows:

The first group includes salmonella species which are exclusively adopted to human, including *S. typhi* and *S. paratyphi* A and C organisms. The second group consists of salmonella organisms specifically adapted to animals of particular species exemplified by *S.abortus equi* which specifically produces abortions in equines (Horse and Donkeys) only and *S. abortus ovis* which produces abortions in sheep only. The third group salmonella organisms are not adapted to any specific animal species but produce infections/disease in any species of animals as well as human being, such as *S. typhimurium* produces infections in cattle, sheep, goats, pigs, horses, rats and human. This organism produces cross infections from one species of animal to another and also from animal to man or vice-versa.

Incidence

The disease is widespread in the world. Infection rate in New Zealand is 13 to 15% in dairy cows and calves and 4% in beef cattle. *S.dublin* and *S.typhimurium* account of nearly 90% of bovine salmonellosis in U.K.In USA, 16 to 22% calves shed organisms with *S. dublin, S.typhimurium* and *S. enteritidis* being predominant species involved. Australia had *S. dublin* incidence before 1983, but outbreaks of abortions, gastroenteritis and calf deaths due to *S.dublin* increased in Queensland after 1983. Great Britain, South America and South Africa had *S. dublin* as predominant salmonella incidence in addition to abortions due to *S. abortus ovis* in sheep. In Denmark, pigs have incidence of 22% salmonella subclinical infection with *S. typhimurium, S. infeutis* and *S. panama* as predominant species involved. This has made a major source of human infection in Denmark. A high frequency of antibiotic resistant phage type of *S.typhimurium* has been reported from Australia in cattle. In mid-Western U.S.A. salmonellosis caused by *S. Cholere suis* i.e. mainly swine host adapted infection with 95% incidence in pigs was recorded in outbreaks, in Iowa. Sheep assembling at high stocking rates increases the incidence of salmonella infection in Middle East during importation of sheep from Australia.

Epidemiology and Disease Transmission

Infected animals are the source of organisms for spread of salmonellosis by direct or indirect means. Organisms excreted by infected animals contaminate the environment, primarily feed and water supplies. The farm animals get infected in different ways by animal to animal transmission especially in case of host adapted serovars by contaminated animal feeds and by contaminated soil, birds, rodents, insects, water supplies. Liquid wastes from infected animals may contaminate streams, rivers and pastures directly. Bacteria may be disseminated during the transport of infected animals or during holding of animals in large numbers prior to slaughter and excretion of organisms is increased due to stress factor during both of these situations. The organisms survive for about 14 months in stables where calves are reared and survive for upto 6 years in dried faeces of bovine as compared to wet urine mixed faeces, where they survive only for 5 days. (McLaren and Wrey, 1991; Plym Forshell and Ekesbo, 1996). Piggery waste water and its re-circulation is a major source of continued cycling of salmonella infection (Henry *et al.*, 1995).

S. dublin is excreted in milk and is a source of infection to other animals in the herd and to the milkmen (Wood *et al.*, 1991). In case of *S.abortus equi* natural infection may be due to the ingestion of food-stuffs contaminated by uterine discharge from carrier or recently aborted mares. Transmission from the stallion at the time of service is also thought to occur. Infection persists in uterus and causes repeated abortions. In case of Sal. abortus ovis also venereal infection is presumed but doubtful.

Salmonellae are facultative intracellular organisms that survive in phagolysosome of macrophages and can evade the bactericidal effects of antibody and complement which makes then to persist is infected animals and in the environment. This is an important epidemiological feature of salmonellosis.

Infection of *S.dublin* in cattle becomes either a "clinical case" or becomes "Active carrier" and sheds the organisms constantly or intermittently. It can also become "latent carrier" when infection persists in lymph-nodes and tonsils but shedding in faeces is absent. It even become "Passive carrier, if animal constantly acquires infection from pasture or floor of calf pen but tissue invasion may not occur and after removal of this animal from infected environment, infection disappear suddenly."Latent carrier" can become "Active carrier" under conditions of stress, permanently. *S. dublin* causes a persistant infection in herds while *S.typhimurium* causes "sporadic" cases in cattle due to occasional exposures of animals to rodents faecal contaminated pastures/feedstuffs.

Pathogenesis

After ingestion of *S. dublin*, invasion of the organisms occur through the intestinal wall in the terminal lieum and caecum and progress as far as mescentric lymph-nodes. Beyond this point spread of infection in the animal depends on immunological status and age of the animal and the virulence of the organisms as well as the exposure of the animal to stress factors. Virulence of the organisms depends on presence of adhesion pili and flagellae, cytotoxin, enterotoxin, lipo polysaccharide and the inflammatory response they initiate in the intestinal wall. The influence of some of these factors not only contributes to the intestinal invasion but also to the systemic invasion of salmonellosis. Sal.dublin virulence plasmid mediates systemic infection in mice and cattle by causing macrophage dysfunction (Guilloteau *et al.*, 1996).

If the resistance of the animals is lowered and/or virulence of the organisms is higher due to above mentioned factors from the organisms bacteremia/septicaemia occurs and this leads to either clinical disease including enteritis, pneumonia or abortion and fever. If the animal's resistance is higher and/or the virulence of the salmonella organism is lower, the disease takes chronic course or even the animal becomes the "carrier" of the disease organisms and only "Shedding of the organisms" can occur either animal becomes "active" or "latent" shedder of organisms.

Disease symptoms

In acute salmonellosis, the disease is characterized by Septicaemia, acute enteritis and Chronic disease. Septicaemia is the characteristic form of the disease in newborn foals, calves and young pigs upto 4 months of age with profound depression, dullness, prostration high fever (105-107^{0}F) and death within 24-48 hours. Acute enteritis is a common form in adult animals of all species. It starts with high fever upto 105-107^{0}F for 24 to 48 hours followed by diarrhoea with blood and mucous, and intestinal mucosal casts in faeces which have putrid smell. Pregnant animals may abort and case fatality rate may reach 75%. This form can also occur in calves, foals and piglets, if they survive the septicaemic disease.

Chronic enteritis is a common form of the disease in pigs following severe outbreak. It also occasionally occurs in cattle and adult horses. There is persistent diarrhoea with blood and mucous for long periods leading to emaciation. Calves may show terminal dry gangrene of the extremities, swelling of hind limbs below fetlock joints and separation of skin above fetlock. Ovine and caprine salmonellosis is characterized by Acute enteritis as well as Septicaemia. Abortion is also common which is caused by salmonellae other than sal.abortus ovis in U.K. some cows die after abortion and many of the lambs born above die subsequently. In pigs, septicaemic form occurs, when affected by *S. Cholerae suis*, with a dark red to purplish discolouration of the skin is evident. Nervous signs including tremors, weakness, paralysis and convulsions may be prominent. Case fatality can be upto 100% Bronchopneumonia and pleural pneumonia can occur in pigs with *S. cholera suis* infection.

Postmortem findings

Peracute death due to salmonella infection may not show any evidence of lesion during postmortem. Animals died of septicaemic form will show extensive submucosal and subserosal haemorrhages.

Pigs with *S.cholerae suis* infection produce septicaemic lesions and the characteristic lesions is "turkey egg" appearance of kidney usually associated with hog cholera. A rhomboidal area of infarction is also present in swine. Moreover, "hepatization" and congestion of lung is quite common due to pneumonia in pigs and typical purple discolouration of skin with extreme erythema with haemorrhages to the plaques and circumscribed scabby lesions similar to swine pox are detected on white skin.

Zoonotic Implications

Salmonellosis is a common human intestinal disorder primarily caused by salmonella contaminated meats and poultry. Transmission of Salmonellosis to human occurs via contaminated raw milk and meat, particularly sausages, eggs and poultry products. In Denmark, Pork is a major source of human Salmonellosis (Baggesen *et al.*, 1996). Total cost of Salmonellosis in man, in Canada goes upto U.S. Dollars 100 million and in USA, it is upto 1 billion U.S. dollars which is mostly due to meats and poultry (USA) and poultry (Canada) contaminated with salmonella serotypes as reported by Khakkria R. *et al.* (1991).

The increasingly common isolation of Sal.typhimurium (DT 104 phage type) is of major concern for the world health officials. This phage type was first reported in UK, in 1984 and emerged as an increasing cause of salmonella infections in human and animals in England, Wales, Scotland, Germany, France, Austria and Denmark by 1990's. It was the predominant salmonella isolated from 9 species of animal including poultry, cattle, sheep, pigs, pigeons, horses, cats, dogs and rabbits as well as from human in contact with them and their meat products. Important finding was that all these isolates were resistant to one and 98% isolates were resistant to multiple antibiotic including ciproflaxin which was more serious in zoonotic point of view, as these antibiotics are the last resort for current human treatment.

Shedding of salmonellae in cow's milk and consumption of such raw milk is also major source of human infection which can be reduced by pasteurisation / boiling of milk. Veterinarians handling salmonella abortion cases may get infection via cutaneous wound contamination or through contamination through faecal shedding by enteritis cases in animals due to salmonella infection. This needs proper handling of animals infected with salmonellosis by veterinarians (disinfection).

Spleenomegaly and necrotic white foci and liver (paratyphoid nodules) may be present in animals died of septicaemic form. The placentas of cows and eves aborting EUW to salmonella species may contain very large number of intravascular bacteria. Acute interitic form of salmon salmonellosis brings about intestinal lesions varying from mucoenteritis with submucosal petechae to diffuse haemorrhagic enteritis, similar lesions may also be seen on abomasums. Multiple mucosal erosions of abomasal wall may be present in case of *S. dublin* infection in calves. Severe necrolic enteritis in ileum and large intestine may also be present with watery intestinal constraints having putrid odour and with mucous and whole blood. Mescentric lymph-nodes are enlarged oedematous and haemorrhagic.

In chronic enteritis, discrete areas of necrosis of caecal and colon wall which is thickened and covered with diptheratic material overlying a red, granular mucosal surface. Button ulcers in caecum and around illio-caecal valve in pigs with *S. cholera suis* infection of chronic nature may be seen.

Diagnosis

For definitive diagnosis of salmonella infection in animals, isolation of organisms from heart, blood, liver, gall bladder, spleen and mescentric lymph-nodes or from bone marrow should be attempted. Typical non-lactose fermenting colourless colonies of Mackonkey Agar and their further serotyping as per Kofmans whites schema using H and O type sera is needed for confirmatory diagnosis of salmonellosis Faecal culture is not useful for diagnosis of clinical disease but it is used in studying of shedding patterns of carrier animals. Isolation of salmonella is done from uterine swabs and placenta for diagnosis of abortion due to salmonellosis. Use of liquid enrichment media like salenite broth/tetrathionate broth before final culturing on solid Brilliant green agar or Mackonkey Agar plates increases the chances of positive isolation of salmonella organisms (Duijkeren E. Van *et al.*, 1995). An antigen capture ELISA with enrichment culture for detection of salmonellae from faecal samples is more rapid compared to routine techniques. PCR is highly specific and sensitive for faecal sample examination and is genotype specific (Cohen *et al.*). Serological testing using ELISA test on serum/milk sample can be used for herd testing of sal. dublin carriers for culling of positive reactors. It is based on antibody to O antigen of lipopolysaccharide of organism.

Treatment

Sulphoxine trimethoprim given parentarlly as well as ampicillin and amoxicillin are useful antimicrobials for *Salmonella dublin* infection. Chloromysin and Nitrofurazones are now banned in Europe which were used extensively in past for salmonellosis treatment. Gentamycine at 3 mg/kg B.W. combined with ampicillin 20 mg/kg B.W. given at 8-12 hours interval is recommended for treatment of horses against salmonella infections. Chlortetracycline and Sulphamethazine were used for swine treatment. Supportive fluid eletralyte treatment is given for checking of diarrhoea and dehydration.

Control

1. Identification and culling "or" isolation and treatment or carrier animals.
2. Prophylactic use of antimicrobials
3. Restriction of the movement of the animals around the farms.
4. Providing water supply through troughs which are not at the reach of the faecal contamination.
5. Rigorous disinfection of building with phenolic disinfectants.
6. Suitable hygienic construction of stables/housing of animals.
7. Heat treatment of feed.Careful disposal of infective materials.
8. All persons working on infected premises should take care of their personal hygine suitably.

Above 8 points should be carefully followed for control of salmonellosis, though the eradication of salmonellosis is extremely difficult.

Immunization

Vaccines of different types are available commercially or even autogenous vaccines are used for prevention of clinical salmonellosis symptoms and deaths in domesticated animals. However, even though there is a reduction of shedding of organisms by the "affected animal or the carrier" animal in vaccinated herd, the total shedding of salmonellae from them is impossible. Hence, total dependence on vaccines for eradication of the disease is not practicable. Following information on vaccines is available from the literature.

Both live avirulent or attenuated vaccines are available as well as killed oil or aluminium hydroxide gel adjuvanted. Vaccines are commercially produced/experimentally produced as below:

1. Calves vaccinated at 1-3 weeks of age with a modified aromatic dependent sal. dublin bacterin produce detectable anti-polysaccharide immunoglobulins after immunization (Roden *et al.*).
2. Live oral vaccine against S. typhimurium and S. dublin is designed and showed to confer protection experimentally.
3. "Genetically altered S. dublin" vaccinated calves responded with increased Humoral mediated as well as cell mediated immunity as measured by ELISA and skin test respectively (Smith. *et al* 1993).
4. Genetically hybridized (derived) strain from S. dublin and S. typhimurium was being evaluated (Lindberg *et al.*, 1993).
5. Strain 51 "Rough variant of S. dublin was found to be safe and effective against both S. dublin and S. typhimurium in calves, in U.K.
6. Attenuated *S. dublin* (SL 1438) and *S. typhimurium* (SL 1479) given orally or by IM routine was found effective.
7. *S. Cholerae suis*, attenuated live vaccine is available for protection against abortions and protection of neonates in pigs (Kramer *et al.*, 1992).

However, number of salmonella surveillance reports is available with IVRI and Kasauli salmonella typing laboratories.

Sharma, V.K. and Patil, R.G. from Mathura Vet. College undertook surveillance programme by examination of survage samples and isolated number of salmonella species and their phages in 1962-63.

Review on recent advances in the diagnosis of salmonellae along with other members of Enterobacteriae is presented by Thapliyl at BM-4, pp.22 in report on IAVMIS XIV Annual Conference and National Symposium on "Recent advances in production and testing of Vet. Biological" at Pune, in Jan., 1994.

The author (S.V. Pandit) while working at Veterinary Disease Investigation Centre, M.S. Poona investigated sheep mortality in exotic farm at Thathawade, near Pune in 1964-65, with pneumonia and enteritis. He could isolate *S. typhimurium* along with pasturella multoceda from heart blood, bile duct and Mesenteric lymph-node and liver samples from this outbreak in sheep. This isolation of salmonella was confirmed by Salmonella reference laboratory at Kasauli, in U.P. The author (S.V. Pandit) also isolated *S. dublin* (as confirmed by Kasauli Lab) from Gir calf died of enteritis during calf mortality outbreak in 1965-66.

Suggested Reading

Baggesen, D.L., H.C. Wegener, F. Bager, H. Stege, and J. Christensen. (1996). Herd prevalence of Salmonella enterica infections in Danish slaughter pigs determined by microbiological testing. Prev. Vet. Med. 26: 201-213.

Cohen, N.D., Martin, L.J., Simpson, R.B. (1996). Comparison of polymerase chain reaction and microbiological culture for detection of salmonellae in equine faeces and environmental samples.Am J Vet Res. 57: 780–786.

E. van Duijkeren, C. Flemming, M. Sloet van Oldruitenborgh Oosterbaan, N.C. Kalsbeek & J.W.B van der Giessen (1995) Diagnosing salmonellosis in horses culturing of multiple versus single faecal samples, Veterinary Quarterly, 17(2): 63-66.

Guilloteau L.A., Wallis T.S., Gautier A.V., MacIntyre S., Platt D.J., Lax A.J. (1996). The Salmonella virulence plasmid enhances Salmonella-induced lysis of macrophages and influences inflammatory responses. Infect Immun. 64: 3385–3393.

Henry, D.P., Frost, A.J., O'Boyle, D. and Cameron, R.D. (1995) The isolation of salmonellas from piggery waste water after orthodox pondage treatment. Australian Veterinary Journal 72: 478–479.

Khakhria, R, Duck, D, Lior, H.(1991). Distribution of Salmonella enteritidis phage types in Canada. Epidemiol Infect. Feb; 106(1): 25–32.

Kramer, T.T., Roof M.B., Matheson, R.R. (1992). Safety and efficacy of an attenuated strain of Salmonella choleraesuis for vaccination of swine. Am J Vet Res. 53: 444–448.

Lindberg, A.A., Segall, T., Weintraub, A., and Stocker, B.A. (1993) Antibody response and protection against challenge in mice vaccinated intraperitoneally with a live aroA O4-O9 hybrid Salmonella dublin strain. Infect Immun 61: 1211-1221.

McLaren, I.M.and Wray, C. (1991). Epidemiology of Salmonella typhimurium infection in calves: persistence of salmonellae on calf units. Vet Rec. 129: 461-462.

Plym-Forshell L., Ekesbo I. (1996). Survival of Salmonellas in urine and dry faeces form cattle-an experimental study. Acta Vet Scand 37: 127–131.

Roden, L., Smith, B.P. Spier S.J., Dilling, G.W. (1992). Effects of calf age and salmonella bacterin type on ability to produce immunoglobulins directed against salmonella whole cells or lipopolysaccharide.Am J Vet Res; 53: 1895-1899.

Smith, B.P., Dilling, G.W., Roden, L.D. (1993). Vaccination of calves with orally administered aromatic-dependant Salmonella dublin. Am J Vet Res 54: 1249-1255.

Wood, J.D., G.A. Chalmers, R.A. Fenton, J. Pritchard, M. Schoonderwoerd, and W.L. Lichtenberger.(1991). Persistent shedding of Salmonella enteritidis from the udder of a cow. Canadian Veterinary Journal. 32: 738-741.

❑❑❑

Chapter 30

Leptospirosis in Cattle, Sheep, Goats, Pigs and Horses

Leptospirosis occurs in cattle, sheep goats, pigs, horses and rats and is caused by leptospira in terrogans species of bacteria with many distinct serovars, some of which are host adapted (maintenance host adapted) and some are non-host adapted (accidental host adapted). Infection of leptospirosis infections is having a worldwide distribution, mostly in warm and wet climate.

About the Causative Organisms

Leptospira organisms are spiral shaped organisms belonging to the class *Spirochaeta* which are motile which are fastredious in their growth requirements and hence, extremely difficult to isolate and maintain on artificial media. They can be demonstrated in septicaemic blood or urine. Samples by using dark field microscopy techniques. *Leptospira* organisms belong to the genus with single species *Leptospira Interogans* containing 212 serovars arranged into 23 serogroups.

Differentiation between serovars (serotypes) belonging to a particular serogroup is by cross agglutination tests Another system of Restriction Endonuclease Analysis (REA) is less time consuming which analyses DNA of Leptospira organism as a genotyping taxanomic tool (Woodword *et al.*, 1991).

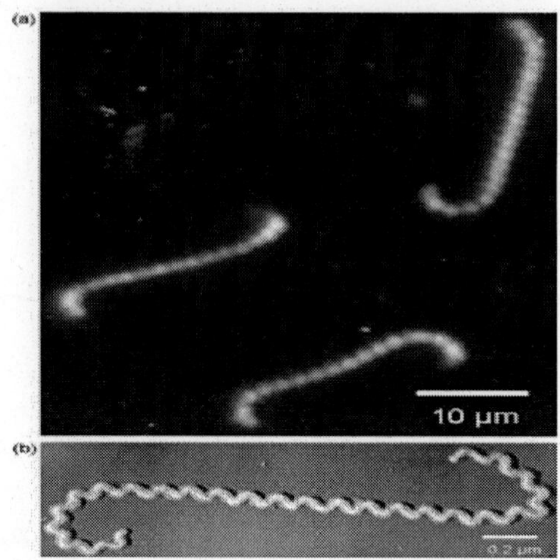

Fig. 1: (a) Dark filled microscopy (b) Electron micrography of Leptospira

Disease Leptospirosis is classified into 2 broad categories, namely host adapted and non-host adapted Leptospirosis. An animal infected with host adapted serovars of the organism is a "Maintenance" or "Reservoir" host while an animal infected with non-host adapted serovars of the organism is an "incidental" host. The following is the list of Leptospiral serovars and their respective "maintenance/ reservoir" hosts and "incidental" hosts.

Sr. No.	Name of organisms serovar	Maintenance / Reservoir	Incidental host
1.	*L.hardijo-bovis* (North America)	Cattle	Sheep, Man
2.	*L. hardjo-prejitno* (Europe)	Cattle	Sheep, Man
3.	*L. Bratislava*	Pig & Horse	Man
4.	*L. pomana*	Pig, Sknk, Racoon, Opossum	Sheep, cattle, man
5.	*L.Grippotyphosa*	Racoon, opossum squirrel	Sheep, cattle
6.	*L.ictero haemorrhagica*	Brown Rat	Cattle, pig, man

Leptospira pomona is the commonest infection in all farm animals, but its international distribution is unpredictable. It was not present in U.K. but recently only sporadic infection is recorded in U.K.

L. Canicola is recorded in cattle and pigs but only sero prevalence in horses without isolation of organisms is detected in horses. *L. icterohaemorrhagica* is isolated from cattle and pigs while its only seroprevalence is detected in horses.

L. grippotyphosa is isolated from cattle and goats, and seroprevailing in horses. *L. Sejrae, L. hebdomadis* and *L. australis* infections are detected in cattle. *L. Szwajizak* is predominant in Israel.

Epidemiology and Mode of Transmission

The source of leptospiral infection is mainly an infected animal which contaminates the pasture, drinking water and feed by infective urine, aborted factus and uterine discharges. Viable infected newborn neonate harbour the infection for several weeks after birth. Infected semen is a possible source of infection through natural or artificial insemination but is rare. No incidence of coital infection through boars is recorded while such venereal infection is possible in cattle. High intensity and long duration of leptospiral infection in pigs is responsible for their important role in epidemiology of leptospirosis.

All animals during their period of affection as well as for long duration of recovery period can shed laptospirae in urine and act as "Carriers" of infection. Pigs and rats are important carriers of *L. pomane* and *L. icteohaemorrhagiae* through urine to human infection via intact skin and cornea getting infected by splashing of urine (droplet infection).

Survival of leptospirae on wet ground especially during rainy season in ponds and ditches/trenches is very much favourable for spread of leptospiral infection from animal to animal of the same species as well as from one species to another as well as from animals to human beings. Leptospiral survive for 183 days in water saturated soil while they survive only for 30 minutes, when soil is air dried. They survive better on soil with pH between pH 6 and pH 8 but pH above and below this range is detrimental to this infection.

Pathogenesis

Leptispires invade the host across mucosal surfaces or softened skin by attaching to the constituents of the extracellular matrix through an active process involving surface proteins. After entering the skin they are found in liver and kidney via septicaemia. Leptospires release lymphokines, such as Tumour Necrotis Factor (TNF) from monocytes through the endotoxic activity of the leptospiral LOS may be an important virulence mechanism which impart damage to endothelial cells resulting into haemorrhages in liver and kidney tissues, septicaemia and endotoxemia, causing haemorrhages, hepatitis, nephritis, meningitis and icterus during acute disease and abortion, still birth and infertility in chronic disease.

Disease symptoms and lesions

The clinical findings in leptospirosis in all species of animals are similar with any species of Leptospira except in case of *L. ictero* haemorrhagica which causes septicaemia. The incubation period is 3-7 days in all animals. The disease caused by Leptospiros Pomona in cattle is described here as a representative example.

Acute and Subacute Leptospirosis

This form is most common in calves upto one month old. Septicaemia with high fever upto 105 to 107^{0}F, anorexia mucosal petechiation, depression and acute haemolytic anaemia with haemoglobinuria, Jaundice loud heart beatings, and dyspnea are the characteristics symptoms with high mortality. In adult, cattle abortion and drop in milk production is present. Necrotic dermatitis with severe lameness and mastitis are some other symptoms. In subacute form of the disease above symptoms in milder form are observed. Blood stained or yellowish orange milk is present. Not all symptoms are present in every affected animal.

Chronic Leptospirosis

The disease may be restricted to the "storm of abortions" in groups of cows at the same stage of pregnancy. Abortion occurs during last trimester of pregnancy.

Disease in pigs

Chronic form is the most common in pigs with abortion and still births while acute form is rare which shows septicaemic form with high mortality rate which is caused by *L. icterohaemorrhagiae*. Disease in sheep and goats manifests abortions during acute form of the disease and agalactia is quite common. Horses also exhibit abortions and still births as major symptom. Periodic opthalmia and uveitis in horses also known as "Moon blindness" is characteristic.

Diagnosis and serological tests

During the septicaemic stage of the disease, leptospirae are present in blood with laboratory evidence of haemolytic anaemia and often haemoglobinuria. However, only positive diagnostic measure at this stage is culturing of the blood. In case of abortion, the kidney, lung and pleural fluid of aborted foetus be examined for the presence of organisms.

The examination of urine samples for the Leptospiral organisms probably offers the best opportunity of confirmatory diagnosis, as shedding occurs in urine for about 26-32 weeks after infection. Dark field microscopy or fluoroscent antibody stained urine samples for FAT microscopy can be used (Smith *et al.*, 1994). ELISA test on cervico-vaginal mucous for antibody testing or use of DNA probes provide more accurate diagnostic procedure (Smith, *et al.*, 1994). Acute and convalescent sera taken 7 to 10 days apart from clinically affected animal or from those with a history of abortion along with 15-25% of apparently normal animals on the farm for serological diagnosis.

For determination of infection status about Leptospirosis, 10 sera from each group of yearlings, the first calf dams, second calf dams and mature age groups on the big size farm as well as tissues and blood from rodents around the farm are taken for seralogy and microscopy and culture respectively. Rising titres in sera collected as above (paired sera) and high titres in sera randomly collected as above using the Microscopic Agglutinationlysis Test (MAT) is useful in diagnosis of Leptospira infection. Even the declining titres are also indicative of past infection 1 to 4 weeks prior to abortion because active infection occurs 1-4 weeks prior to abortion and titres may declines at actual abortion time. MAT titre ^{3} 1:100 is a diagnostic titre which is present at active infection phase.

It is necessary to keep a battery of Leptospiral serotype serovar (group culture) in the culture seed bank at the Leptospira typing and serodiagnosis Laboratory (Reference Laboratory) for conducting Microscopic Agglutinationlysis Test (MAT) on each serum sample using numbr of serotype cultures as litre antigens as this test is serotype specific and anyone or more out of large numbr of serotypes may be present on every farm. The ELISA test is much more accurate than any other test used for leptospira diagnosis and has many advantages in practical point of view in the laboratory handling (Smith *et al.*, 1994). Reciprocal titre of 3000 is proposed as a diagnostic titre for *L. Pomona* but no such "threshold" for any other species available for other Leptospirae.

Treatment

Use of Dihydro streptomycine (12 mg/kg body wt. intra-muscularly twice daily for 3 days) is effective in treatment of systematic infection for halting clinical symptoms as well as for halting shedding of leptospires in urine which is most useful to stop the lateral spread of infection. Antibiotic treatment adjuncted with vaccination of rest of the herd is useful in preventing new cases of abortions and still births occurring in the herd.

Control

On individual farm, leptospirosis can be eradicated or controlled by vaccination and antimicrobial treatment as above. However, new cases of disease can occur due to introduction of new "Carrier" animal or even introduction of rodent" carrier on the farm. Hence, eradication may be difficult on the farm. Hence, it is more practicable to detect the fresh "Carrier" introduction and treat the same with antibiotic and follow annual vaccination programme regularly. Use of "Leptospira free" certified semen is also necessary to maintain the "Leptospira controlled" status on the farm. Bulls destined for artificial insemination centres must be free of antibody to *L. hardjo, L. grippotyphase, L. canicola, L. Pomona, L. sejroe and L. icterohaemorrhagiae* at a final serum dilution of 1:100 in the MAT. But MAT is not a sure shot test for detection of Leptospira infection and hence, more reliable PCR assay is used for detection of Leptospires in semen.

In most of the countries, where dairy industry is predominant, the polyvalent bacterin containing Leptospiral serovars prevailing in the country (even upto 5 or 6 serovars) is used to protect the animals. Vaccinations are carried out annually, including calves above 3 months of age. Similar vaccines are also used for pigs. Development of carrier animals after vaccination as such animals harbor organisms in kidneys and become "Renal carriers" by shedding of organisms in urine. But still the only way to reduce the leptospira infection is to carryout vaccination and treatment of vaccinated animals with Residual antibiotic therapy which supposed to reduce human infection chances.

Zoonotic Implications

Leptospirosis is an important zoonosis and is an occupational hazard to butchers, farmers and Veterinarians (Heath and Johnson, 1994). Incidence of positive agglutination tests in humans in contact with infected cattle is low surprisingly and clinical cases in humans acquiring the disease from animals is not common. Human infection is most likely occurring by contamination with urine or uterine discharges from animals especially veterinarians get such infection.

Cow's milk is not much involved in human infection due to pasteurization of milk and practice of boiling of milk but milkers handling infected cows become prone to infection. In one survey in New Zeland, 34% milkers were affected. Human Leptospira infections are attributed to *L. icterohaemorrhagiae* infection, causing case of Jaundice and Brown rat infection is a source of such human cases which occurs through contamination of urine from rats especially during rainy season, labour camps/shanties in urban and suburban areas in developing countries. (Remember outbreaks of Leptospiral Jaundice in Bombay suburban district and in Tamil Nadu during few years back (late nineties recently).

Leptospirosis – Indian Scenario

There were only sporadic reports of Leptospira infections in cattle, sheep, goats and pigs in past, in India. Leptospirosis in dogs is known since 1916 in India *L.icterohaemorrhagica* reported by Ayyar (1932).

The author (Pandit, S.V.) while working at Disease Investigation Section, M.S. Poona while investigating the incidences of abortion and still births at dairy herd of Mahatma Gandhi Ashram's Goshala with Gir cows and heifers at Urulikanchan, Distt. Pune during 1972-73 collected some random and paired sera samples from aborted cows and these sera were submitted, after to reference Leptospira diagnostic laboratory at Groningen Amsterdam in the Netherlands for serodiagnosis. They reported presence of significant titres against a battery of leptospira live antigens including L.Pomona, *L. hebdomadis, L. Canicola, L. Grippotyphosa L. Sejroe,* etc. Some of these titres were in increasing range indicating the presence of these infections which might have been responsible for abortions and still births in Gir cows in that herd as possibility of Brucella abortus infections and vibrios in those abortion cases was ruled out serologically and by cultural examinations for Brucella and vibrio infections.

Facilities for Leptospira typing using a battery of Leptospiral serovar cultures including *L. ponona, L. Canicola, L. hebdomadis, L. ictterohaemorrhagica,* etc. was developed by Prof. Khera *et al.* at I.V.R.I., Mukteshwar. They demonstrated Microscopic Agglutinationlysis Test during summer Institute in immunology held at IVRI, Mukteshwar during 1971 (May-July). Similar facilities were also developed at Animal Research Institute of Tamil Nadu Agriculture University at Madhavaram during late nineties (1998). They helped even during investigation of Human Leptospiral Jaundice outbreaks in Tamil Nadu during late nineties. There is a description on recent advanced techniques, such as PCR, ESLIA and DNA Hybridization methods (DNA Homology studies as mentioned by Srinivasa, S.K. 1974 of IVRI, Izatnagar in report on XIV Annual Conference and National symposium on "Recent Advances in Production and Testing of Vet. Biological" by IAVMA at Pune pp. 23 (BM-5) and also mentioned by Ramdas P. and P. Richard Maillasami of Madras Vet. College, 1992, in the report on DAE symposium on vaccine Prod. and Animal Cell Bio-technology held at Pune. But in both of these reports, there is no mention whether they had developed these techniques at the respective institutes and studies any outbreaks of Leptospirosis.

Suggested Reading

Heath, S.E. and Johnson, R. (1994) Leptospirosis. J. Am. Vet.Med. Assoc. 205: 1518-523.

Smith, C.R., Ketterer, P.J., McGowan, M.R., Coreny, B.G. (1994). A review of laboratory techniques and their use in the diagnosis of Leptospira interrogans serovar hardjo infection in cattle. Australian Veterinary Journal 71: 290–294.

Woodward, M.J., and G.J. Sullivan. (1991). Nucleotide sequence of a repetitive element isolated from Leptospira interrogans serovar hardjo type hardjobovis. J. Gen. Microbiol.137: 1101-1109.

□□□

Chapter 31

Listeriosis in Sheep, Goats and Other Ruminants

Listeriosis is bacterial infectious disease of sheep, goats and other ruminants caused by *Listeria monocytogenes*, generally after introduction of animals to spoiled silage and is characterized by septicaemia resulting into encephalitis, abortions, mastitis and occasionally enteritis.

About the causative organism

Listeria monocytogenes is a gram positive rod shaped organism which grows aerobically between 30 to 37^{0}C and even between -0.4^{0}C to 45^{0}C at pH 4.5 to 9.6 and is susceptible to common disinfectants and antibiotics like Penicillin and Chlortetracycline. The organism is eubiquitous and present in soil which contaminates the silage which has pH above 4.5, which is poorly fermented and in which pockets of aerobic deterioration are present (Ash contents of greater than 70 mg/kg dry matter indicates soil contamination of silage). Moist preserved feeds like brewers grains wet spoiled hay bales and silage made from commodity by-products like orange and artichoke wastes are liable for listerial over growths.

L. Monocytogenes have 16 serovars on the basis of somatic and flaggellar antigens. Serovars 4b, ½ a, ½ b, and 3 are of most common occurence from disease of animals (Farber and Peterkin, 1991).

Virulent strains of L. monocytogenous multiply in macrophages and monocytes and produce "Liseriolysin O" an haemolysin which is a major virulence factor (Low and Donachie, 1997).

Epidemiology and disease transmission

The disease occurence is most common in Northern and Southern latitudes especially in temperate climate and less common in tropical and subtropical climate. In northern latitudes, it occurs distinctly in season between December to May in concurrence with feeding of silage time but not so in Australia. Disease occurs in North America, Europe, U.K., New Zeland and Australia. The Listerial Encephalitis occurs in sheep older than 6 weeks upto 12 weeks and ewes over 2 years of age while abortion occur sporadically in cattle but outbreaks of abortion occur in sheep and goats. Spinal myelitis occurs in sheep of all ages (Seaman *et al.*, 1990). While, septicaemic disease with high mortality occurs in lambs and kids, and periparturient ewes. The catarrhal conjunctivitis in both sheep and cattle occurs in outbreak form.

With septicaemic disease and abortion, the organism is transmitted by ingestion of contaminated gains or silage. Lambs may get infected with suckling of ewes with listerial mastitic teats or contaminated navel of does. The encephalitic form of the disease results from infection of the terminals of the trigeminal nerve consequent to abrasions of the buccal mucosa from feed or browse or from infection of tooth cavities.

Poor nutritional status, sudden weather change (cold or wet) stress of late pregnancy, transport, long flooding resulting into poor access to pasture are some stress factors which are responsible for increasing susceptibility of animals for precipitation of already infected status of animals. Carrier animals faeces contaminate the pastures which may alone act as risk factor. Several studies have shown that oral, conjunctival and parenteral challenge of pregnant animals results in more severe signs of septicaemia, followed by abortions.

Pathogenesis

The organisms penetrate the mucosa of intestine lead to sub-clinical infection with prolonged faecal excretion of the organism/ excretion of organisms in milk. If animals are pregnant, the stress converts subclinical disease into clinical disease and septicaemia occurs, resulting into abortion or encephalitis.

The organisms are facultative intracellular pathogens that can infect cells including intestinal cells by directed endocytosis. They can survive and grow in macrophages and monocytes (Low and Donachie, 1997) cell mediated immunity as well as humoral immunity is responsible for clearance of bacteremic infection (Miettinen *et al.*, 1990). In pregnant animals, invasion of placenta and foetus occurs within 24 hours of bactermia and oedema and necrosis of placenta leads to abortion/still births, metritis of the ewe also occurs.

Clinical symptoms and postmortem lesions

Fever (104^0 to 107^{0}F) followed by inco-ordination, head deviation, tilting of head, facial paralysis, dropping of ear, lip paralysis, keratitis, corneal ulceration, pan opthalmitis of both or one eye, paralysis of jaw muscles are the main symptoms. This is followed by ataxia, falling on one side and final recombancy may occur. Death due to respiratory failure occurs. Outbreaks of abortions occur in cattle but more frequently in sheep.

Infection of udder involves single quarter and poor responsive to treatment and becomes chronic. Histologically micro-abscesses in central nervous system can be shown (in brain stem and in cervical or lumber spinal cord). Multiple foci of necrosis in liver, spleen and myocardium are detected. Placentitis and endometritis are the lesions in cases of abortion.

Diagnosis

Half of mid-sagittaly sectioned brain, including brain stem, chilled or frozen for culturing or FAT is useful for diagnosis by bacteriological examination and rest of the half counter part for histopath examination by LM and IHC (Immuno Histo Chemistry) in case of encephalitic form of the disease. In case of septicaemic and abortion form, liver, spleen, lung, placenta, foetal stomach content by cultural and FAT exam is useful for diagnosis and similar portion of tissues fixed in 10% formation for histopathological exam (using LM and IMC techniques) are used for diagnosis.

Treatment

Chlorotetracycline (10 mg/kg body wt. per day for 5 days) is useful. Penicillin, (44000 IU/kg body wt. for 7 to 14 days) is used for therapeutic use.

Control

Eradication is not possible. Organisms are ubiquitous; control on silage is useful for avoiding infection through ingestion of contaminated feeding materials. Bactins and inactivated vaccines are commercially available in some countries.

Suggested Reading

Farber, J.M., and P.I. Peterkin. (1991). Listeria monocytogenes a foodborne pathogen. Microbiol. Rev. 55: 476–511.

Low, J.C., Donachie, W. (1997). A Review of *Listeria monocytogenes* and Listeriosis. Vet J. 153(1): 9–29.

Miettinen, A., Husu J., Tuomi, J. (1990). Serum antibody response to *Listeria monocytogenes*, listerial excretion, and clinical characteristics in experimentally infected goats. J. Clin. Microbiol. 28: 340–343.

Seaman, J.T., Carrigan, M.J., Cockram, F.A. and Carter, G.I. (1990) An outbreak of listerial myelitis in sheep. Australian Veterinary Journal 67: 142-143.

□□□

Chapter 32

Glanders and Farcy in Horses, Donkeys and Mules

Glanders is an infectious becterial disease of horses, donkeys and mules characterized by septicaemia with terminal nodular broncho-pneumonia in acute and chronic form of the disease in generalized form on nodular skin and nasal septal lesions with final ulcartion in localized form of the disease called as Farcy. The disease is caused by the organisms named *Peifferella mallei*. The disease has zoonotic importance due to its incidences in vets and studmen handling the affected horses. The disease is geographically restricted to Eastern Europe, Asia, Minor Asia and North Africa. The disease was wide-spread in later part of 19th century and even upto mid-20th century when horses and ponies were present in the cities and armies large concentrations.

After the extablishment of Indian Veterinary Research Institue at Mukteshwar, Kumaon, U.P. in 1898, within few years, diagnostic reagent "Mallein" was developed for detection of "Carrier" animals of glanders by intradermo-palpebral and subcutaneous allergic test. With extensive use of this test, the systematic eradication programme for glanders control was undertaken by army authorities and by civil veterinary departments in certain extent. The concentration of horses in cities was also reduced by early seventies of 20th century. Both testing programme and reduction in horse population in cities brought incidence of glanders in significant control but total eradication has not taken place as evident from reports of glanders in Satara district horses of studfarm in Poona and Satara district during 2006-2007. During this period, out of 402 horses involved in 2 outbreaks. 23 animals suffered, out of which 21 died.

About the causative organism

Pfeifferella mallei, the causative organism of glanders belongs to the family *Actinobacillacae*. Presently, the generic name is changed to *Pseudomonas,* thus it is renamed as "*Pseudomonas mallei*" (Radostits, 2000). *Pseudomonas mallei* is a gram negative slender rod shaped organism which is non-spore bearing, non-capsulate. It is an obligate parasite and is readily destroyed by light, heat and usual disinfectants. It can be cultured on Loffler's inspisated serum medium as well as on potato agar medium on which it produces mahogany brown coloured calonies which are mucoid in nature.

Epidemiology and Transmission

Apparently recovered animals from the disease are "Carriers" and they are the source of infection to the susceptible animals. Chronic nodular lesions of recovered carrier animals rupture into bronchi and infect upper airway passages and nasal/oral secretions which contaminate the feed or fodder in the stables of animals. The contaminated feed/fodder when ingested by animals in contact pass on infection to healthy stable-mets. Even communal watering troughs also spread the infection.

Cutaneous spread of the infection may be a source for skin infection through the abrasion of skin. During the actual outbreak, the spread of infective discharges from nasal septal ulcerative lesions or discharges from skin (farcy) nodular lesions easily make the "direct contact" as source of infection to the stable mets.

Pathogenesis

Invasion of the organisms through intestinal wall brings about septicaemia in acute cases and bactermia in chronic cases. Localisation occurs in lungs, skin and nasal mucosa or other viscera which becomes the typical site for "nodule" formation. Terminally broncho pneumonia develops which brings about death caused by anoxic anoxia.

Symptoms and postmortem findings

In acute disease, there is high fever, cough and nasal discharge, with rapidly spreading ulcers appearing on nasal septal mucosa as well as nodules on the skin of lower limbs or abdomen. Death due to septicaemia occurs in few days. In chronic forms of the disease, 3 types of manifestation can occur:

i) Pulmonary glanders in which chronic pneumonia with cough, frequent epistaxis and laboured respiration occurs.

ii) In nasal form of the disease, nodules of 1 cm size appear on turbinates and nasal septum which subsequently ulcerate. Serous exudates continuously run from ulcers, which becomes muco-purulent and blood stained as time goes on. Submaxillary lymph-nodes enlarge. Ulcers ultimately heal and stellate scars replace the ulcerations.

iii) Skin form of the disease known as "Farcy" is characterized by appearance of subcutaneous nodules on skin of medial aspect of the hock which ulcerate and show oozing of purulent discharge. The lymph-nodes of this area are swollen along with the connecting lymph vessels which are prominently apparent with fibrous consistency. Lymph-nodes may ulcerate and oozing pus.

The chronic form usually lasts for several months. Postmortem lesions of acute form of the disease are characterized by multiple petechial haemorrhages throughout the body. Severe catarrhal broncho pneumonia with "lead shot" like swollen lymph-nodes is characteristic of glanders. In chronic form, there are milliary nodules in lungs similar to tuberculosis milliary abscesses, scattered throughout the lung tissue. Ulcers are present on the mucosa of upper respiratory tract, especially on nasal mucosa. Few ulcerative lesions may be present on larynx, bronchi and trachea. Nodules and ulcers will be present on skin and subcuits of limbs. Lymph-nodes and lymphatic vessels draining the lower parts of the limb will be swollen and prominent.

Diagnosis

Demonstration of typical *Pseudomonas mallei* organisms in smears from oozing lymph-node ulcers is diagnostic. However, complement fixation test is confirmative for final diagnosis.

Treatment

Penicillin and streptomycin have no detectable effect on the progress of the disease. However, sodium sulpha diazine is useful which requires 20 days period for complete recovery upto 100%.Formalised preparation of Ps. mallei and sulphadiazine and sulphadiazine/sulphadiamidine are reported to be very effective in treating glanders cases.

Control

Even through treatment makes clinical recovery, the recovered animals are not solidly immune. Moreover, the recovered animals may remain as carriers. Hence, complete quarantine of affected premises, destruction of clinical cases and "mullein" testing of in contact animals at the interval of 3 weeks and removal/destruction of "positive" reactors is advocated as per "glanders and farcy act" which is in vogue since Britishers time (late 1890's time) in India.A vigorous disinfection programme for feed/water troughs, equipments and stable premises should be instituted to prevent spread while eradication is being carried out (Hickman J. 1970, Equine Vet J. 2.153).

Tests

For detection of the carrier animals, the CFT is the most accurate serological test as usual official test. Other tests available are an indirect haemagglutination test using "Mallein" as Antigen (Gangulee *et al.*, 1966,) and the conglutinins absorption test (Sen *et al.* 1968). A dot enzymelinked immunosorbant assay (ELISA) is suitable for use in all soliped species (Verma, *et al.*, 1990). Mallein intradermopalpebral test has largely displaced the ophthalmic and subcutaneous tests. 0.1 ml of mallein is injected intradermally into the skin of lower eyelid with tuberculin syringe and read at 48 hours. Positive reaction comprises of marked oedema of the eyelid with blepharospasm and severe purulent conjunctivitis (Hage back, 1993).

Mallein is produced at IVRI, Izatnagar by growing Pf. Mallei strain on synthetic medium for 15 days and steaming pure growth for 1 hour in a Koch's sterilizer. The filterate is evaporated in porcelain dish over steam to half of the original volume to which 5% phenol solution is added in proportion of 1 part phenol solution : 9 parts of conc. filtrate which is taken after Seitz filtration. The product is tested for starility and efficacy by actual testing.

Suggested Reading

Radostits, O.M., C.C. Gay, D.C. Blood, K.W. Hinchcliff (2000): Veterinary Medicine, 10th ed., W.B. Saunders Company, London.

❑❑❑

Chapter 33

Tuberculosis in Cattle, Pigs and Goats, Sheep and (rarely) in Horses and its Zoonotic Importance

Tuberculosis of cattle, pigs and goats, sheep and rarely in horses is chronic bacterial disease caused by *Mycobacterium tuberculosis* and is characterized by progressive wasting of the condition of the animal leading to death.

The disease is a global problem and even though it has come under virtual control in the developed countries for the number of years, the final eradication could not be achieved due to a number of problems like "No visible lesions" reactors, re-emergence of the disease in "accredited" herds because of energic carriers being left in those herds and presence of tuberculosis reactor animals in wildlife bovine species which is difficult to eliminate completely. While in developing countries, elimination of positive reactors by slaughter has religious limitations. Moreover, even though control programme of vaccination has shown good results in developed countries and treatment of animal and humans by use of antibiotics have shown good result. Re-emergence of tuberculosis has been observed due to newly evolved problems of immune-suppression occurring due to disease infections like HIV infections in man.

About the causative organism

Mycobacterium tuberculosis exists in 3 antigenic serovars, namely *Mycobacterium tuberculosis Var bovine* which is also named as *Mycobacterium bovis Mycobacterium tuberculosis var Avium* which is one of the group members of "Mycobacterium Avium - intracellular complex" which also include Mycobact intracellular and other well defined species like *M. Kansasii, M. fortuitum, M. flei* and other species and the most important serovar is *Mycobacterium tuberculosis var human* which is primarily a causative agent of human tuberculosis as well as tuberculosis of monkeys but also causes transient tuberculosis in bovines and pigs. Mycobacterium Avium – intracellular complex are ubiquitous opportunist organisms and in livestock have most importance in swine due to carcass condemnation. Tuberculosis produced by this complex group is not a major disease problem in animals but animals infected with these organisms react to the mammalian tuberlin test, creating difficulty in mycobacterium bovis tuberculosis eradication programme. *Mycobacterium avium* infected pigs also play a significant role in human zoonosis.

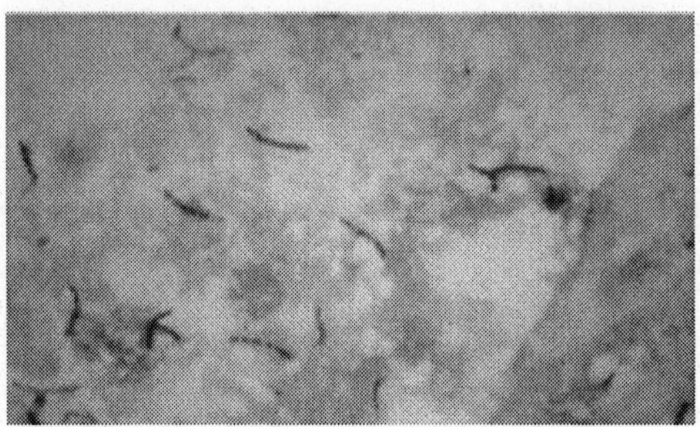

Fig. 1: M. tuberculosis (Z.N. stain)

Out of all the 3 serovars of the *Mycobacterium tuberculosis,* Mycobacterium bovis is the most significant organism which is responsible for the disease both in bovines as well as in humans and hence, we will discuss "tuberculosis" due to "bovis" infection in details in the chapter and refer to other species, whereever needed.

Epidemiology and disease transmission

Mycobacterium bovis causes disease in bovines, swines, caprines, ovines and equines. Organisms are excreted in sputum, faeces (from both from intestinal lesion as well as from swallowed sputum from pulmonary lesions) milk, urine, uterine and vaginal discharges. Animals with gross lesions that communicate with airways, skin or intestinal lumen are obvious spreaders of infection. Animals may even excrete bacteria before visible lesions appear as early as 90 days after infection (Mcilory *et al.,* 1986; Neill *et al.,* 1991).

Wildlife reservoirs including mule, deer, bisons, brush tail possum and badgers are incriminated as source of infection in cattle in North America, New Zealand and U.K. (Morris, *et al.,* 1994; Cheeseman, *et al.,* 1989; Whipple *et al.,* 1997).

The organisms excreted by the affected and carrier animals are transmitted to the susceptible cattle through injection via contaminated pasture or water though that contains contaminated water. However, this route of transmission is less frequent as the organisms contaminating pasture and water cannot survive longer due to their exposure to sun. However, major source of transmission is inhalation of contaminated air in confined animals in closed and crowded stables sheds, drinking of infected milk by calves and contaminated uterine discharges being leaked by neighbouring animals are some other sources of infection. Infection through intramammary route by using infected teacups of milking machine or by sitting of cows on contaminated bedding or flooring is also important source of tuberculosis of mammry glands. Feeding of offles from beaf of tuberculous cattle to pigs is important source of tuberculosis of pigs. Goats and sheep grazing with tuberculosis affected cattleherd on some pasture can contract tuberculosis. In horses, infection of tuberculosis is rare mainly due to their resistance (natural) to this infection.

In humans, zoonotic tuberculosis infection occurs through drinking of non-pasturised/raw milk without boiling from cows with tuberculosis of mammary lymph-nodes or with tubercular mastitis. This incidence is increased in developing countries recently due to increased incidence of HIV infection in human being which produces immune-suppression leading to increased susceptibility to tuberculosis in man inspite of BCG vaccination.

Pathogenesis

Tuberculosis spreads in the body of animal is by two ways. The "primary complex" consists of development of lesions at the portal of entry especially when infection enters the body via inhalation route. The first lesions develops at "caudal lobe of lung" and then in the regional pulmonary bronchial lymph-node. When infection occurs by ingestion, the primary lesions develops at tonsiliar site and at mesentric lymph-node tonsilar site and at mesenteric lymph-node but generally primary lesions may not be present in case of infection through intestinal mucosa.

The primary lesions in case of infection of calves through drinking of infected milk are pharyngeal lymph-nodes or mesenteric lymph-nodes.

The visible primary focus of infection develops within 8 days of infection, followed by "Calcification" of lesions occurring about 2 weeks later. The developing necrotic focus soon gets surrounded by "granulation" tissue, monocytes and plasma cells. Some of these cells fuse together to produce "Giant cells" with multiple nuclei. Soon the fibrous tissue is formed in the nodule which becomes tough due to fibrosis and infiltration and deposition of calcium salts make the nodule "Calcified". Before this to occur (calcification), the infection progress through the local lymphatics which produces similar foci of infection in regional lymph-nodes of the organs like lung, mesenteric lymph-nodes, liver, etc. which affect these organs with primary lesions.

This is followed by post primary dissemination of infection from "primary complex" to other organs to produce generalized "milliary" tuberculosis to produce multiple nodules in the body at various places or chronic organ tuberculosis caused by endogenous or exogenous re-infection of tissues rendered "allergic" to tuberculoprotein. In the later case, there may be no involvement of local lymph-node. As the disease is progressive, there is constant underlying toxemia which causes weakness, debility and eventual death of the animal. In pigs, localized non-progressive abscesses in neck's and head's regional lymph-nodes are most common. In cattle, peracute tuberculous pneumonia or chronic progressive generalized tuberculosis is noted.

Symptoms and postmortem lesions

Progressive emaciation and a capricious appetite and fluctuating temperature is commonly associated with disease but few animals may show no much symptoms inspite of generalized milliary type of lesions in the body. Animals are dosile, sluggish with rough or sleek hair coat but their eyes may be bright and alert.

The cattle may have subdued moist cough but it is easily stimulated by squeezing of pharynx or by exercising. Dyspnea with increased rate and depth of respiration is apparent in advanced stages. Tuberculous pleuracy without specific symptoms may be present.

Tuberculous ulcers in intestine may cause chronic diarrhoea. Enlargement of Retropharyngeal lymph-nodes may cause noisy breathing due to pharyngeal obstruction. In tuberculous metritis, infertility and recurrent abortions may occur. Tuberculous vaginitis may fail to conceive and may show chronic purulent discharge. In bulls, tuberculous orchitis may produce painless, testicles.

Tuberculous mastitis is of major concern due to danger of public health problems and spread of disease to calves. Enlargement of supra mammary lymph-nodes in palpable. Initially milk shows only few flakes which increase and finally the standing of milk may separate out amber coloured fluid with settled floccules at the bottom of milking vessel.

Generalized tuberculosis in pigs may be similar to cattle in symptoms. Broncho-pneumonia is common in sheep and goats and involvement of vertebrae is most common in horses. In cattle, sheep and goats, necropsy findings show identical lesions distributed in standard way.

Tubercular granulomas may be found in any of the lymph-nodes, particularly in bronchial, retropharyngeal, and mediastinal lymph-nodes (Conner *et al.*, 1994; Wipple *et al.*, 1996). In lungs, milliary abscesses may extend to cause of suppurative broncho-pneumonia with characteristics orange coloured thick to creamy plus. Tuberculous nodules may be present on pleurae and peritoneum. Localized tubercular nodules tend to stimulate development of enveloping fibrous capsule at various developing stages. Chronic tuberculous node will tend to show calcification at various stages. Generalized shot like milliary abscesses may be present, if generalized tuberculosis is present.

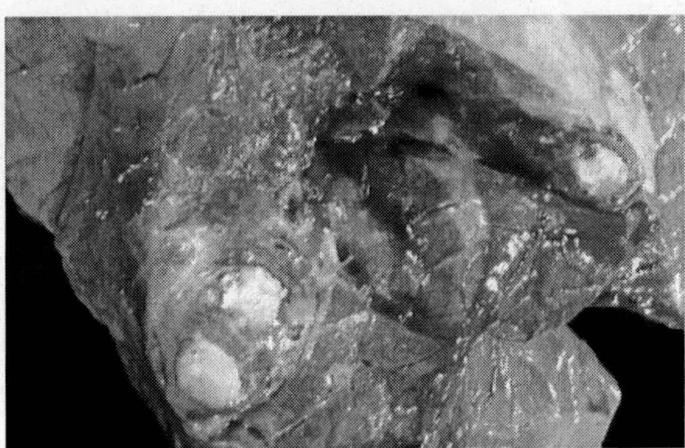

Fig. 2: Bovine tuberculosis

Histopathologically, presence of "Acid-fast" bacterial organisms showing pink colour, when stained with Zehil-neilsen staining procedure, are seen in the centre of tubercular nodule, surrounded by the necrosed tissue cells, with presence of multinuclear giant cells, mononuclear cells and fibroblast with various degrees of calcium salt deposits as per the age of the nodule is visible microscopically.

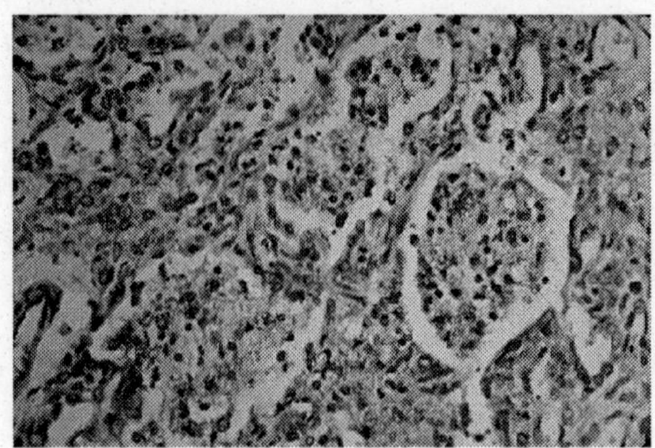

Fig. 3: Bovine tuberculosis (H.E. stain)

Diagnosis

Sputum or other discharges including uterine discharge, or milk sample, etc. are examined for presence of Acid fast slender rod shaped organisms in smears made from the same, using "Zieh Neelsen Staining" method followed by inoculation of these discharges into guinea pigs for confirmation of development of typical "Tubercular lesion" for diagnosis of "tuberculosis". This confirmation is carried out by histopathotogical examination of tubercular nodular lesion of guinea pig. Now improved cultural techniques and the use of nucleic acid probes are available for confirmatory diagnosis of tuberculosis in animals (Skuce, 2002). Detection of "Carrier of tuberculosis" by "Tuberculin Test" is the basis of all tuberculosis eradication programmes in the cattle and other animals. This is an "allergic reaction" to tubercular protein indicating prior sensitization of animal to the tubercular protein of mycobact tuberculosis infection prevalent in the animal body.

Production of Tuberculin Reagents for Tuberculin Tests

3 types of tuberculins are prepared as diagnostic reagents for tuberculin tests, namely 1) Tuberculin for subcutaneous test prepared from human strain bovine strain of mycobacterium tuberculosis, 2) Heat concentrated synthetic medium (H.C. S.M.) tuberculin and 3) Purified protein derivation (PPD) tuberculin. Both HCSM and PPD tuberculins can be prepared using either bovine or human strain of *M.tuberculosis.*

Tuberculin is prepared by growing desired strain(s) of *Mycobacterium tuberculosis* on Hanley and Dorset synthetic medium, after preparation of its seed on glycerol beef broth medium grown for

10 days and incubation of Hanley-Dorest medium at 37⁰C for 12 weeks. These flasks of production medium are steamed for 3 hours and contents filtered on fine meshed sieve and phenolised to final concentration of phenol to 0.5% and finally filtered through seitz filter. This is "Tuberculin" for sub cut test. The HCSM tuberculin is produced by addition of glycerol after heating the original tuberculin filterate mentioned above to evaporate the product to get 1/5th of original volume and they phenolise the same before seitz filtration. (Seetharaman, C. Sinha, K.C. Vet. Bio-Products and their uses ICAR, production, 1962). The PPD tuberculin is produced by extraction of the "protein" fraction of tuberculin using chemical method, leaving behind the residual ingredients of the growth medium which is responsible for "non-specific" allergic reaction which interfere with the specificity of tuberculin test.

Avian tuberculin is also used during tuberculin test for differentiation between "Mammalian tuberculosis and Avian tuberculosis" carrier animals. "Avian tuberculin" is produced on the same line as the production of Human/bovine tuberculins but using Avian strain of Mycobact tuberculosis instead of human/bovine strains during production.

Sub-cutaneous Tuberculin Test

This test is conducted by inoculation of tuberculin (Human/bovine) 1 ml quantity subcutaneously in the neck region of animal and observing the animal for rise of rectal temperature at 2, 4, 6 and 8 hours post inoculation. If temperature rises 2^{0} above normal 102^{0}F by 2 hours and > 104^{0}F upto 105-8^{0}F by 4 to 8th hours, the animal is regarded as positive reactor for tuberculosis.

Single Intradermal Test (SID)

This is regarded as more convenient test for diagnosis of "positive reactor" for tuberculosis 0.1 to 0.2 ml of tuberculin is injected by intradermal route in the cervical skin fold of neck which is measured for thickness prior to and after intradermal inoculation using vernier callipers. The reaction of rise in skin fold thickness is measured at 48 and 72 hours intervals again. If the "diffuse swelling" occurs at around the site of inoculation of tuberculin (doubling of the skin fold thickness), the test is read as positive. Bovine tuberculin is more potent and specific (Monagham *et al.*, 1994).

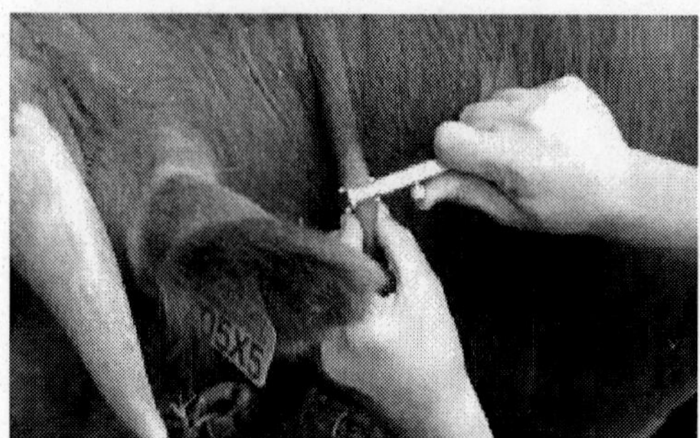

Fig. 4: Intradermal tuberculin test

In U.K. & Europe, SID is carried out in neck while in USA, Canada and Australia as well as in New Zealand, it is carried out on the skin fold (caudal fold) of tail. The test is regarded to be more "sensitive" on "cervical fold" as compared to the test on "caudal fold". It is more "specific" on "caudal fold" in comparison on "cervical fold".

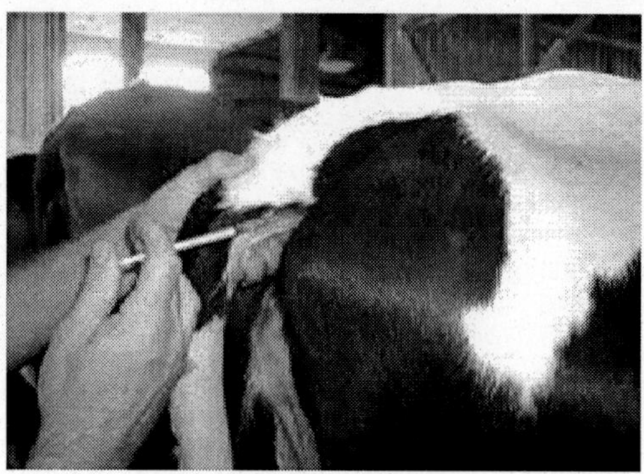

Fig. 5: Caudal fold test

Disadvantages of "SID test" are its lack of "specificity" as number of "No visible - lesion (NVL) reactor occur. Mammalian tuberculins are not sufficiently "specific" to differentiate between reactions due to infection with "mycobact bovis" and infection with "Mycobact avium" and mycobact paratuberculosis including vaccination with BCG and Nocardia farcinicus. Hence maximum permissible rate of NVL reactors due to tuberculin is 10%, beyond which if "NVL reactor" are recorded tests other than "SID" should be carried out. Even "Tuberculin test" is "less sensitive", when the tuberculosis infection has progressed upto "open thoracic/intestinal" case in the animal and the test in "negetive" in such cases. This needs more "clinical diagnostic" eye, when such cases occur to avoid failure of "tuberculosis eradication" programme.

In case of doubtful "SID" test results short thermal test using "subcutaneous test" with massive test dose of 4 ml and "Stormont" test using "second" intradermal dose at the same site of SID (Double Intradermal test) is carried out after 7 days of 1st test and 'reading" taken 24 hours after second injection. This needs 3 visits to the animals under test. For definite diagnosis and differentiation of tuberculosis from Johns disease (M. paratuberculosis) and Avian tuberculosis "Comparative test" is conducted on "Cervical site" at 3 different levels using all the 3 "Allergic test" antigens.

Phenomenon of desensitization occurs after "SID" test and animal is unable to react to SID carried out again for some time. It is, therefore necessary to wait upto 60 days at least for repeated test, if necessary in case of "doubtful" reaction recorded during the first SID test. Phenomenon of desensitition is also observed before parturition and after parturition in 30% cases upto 4-6 weeks.

In summary, false positive reactions occur in: 1) Animal sensitized to other mycobacterial allergens including those of avian or human tuberculosis or mycobact paratuberculosis (animals exposed to poultry differ or sheep/goat faeces in their feeds), 2) Animals sensitized to nocardia farcinicus (bovine farcy). 3) Animals sensitized to irritant injections for claiming for false compensation of rates during eradication programmes in developed countries.

False negative reactors occur when: 1) Cases of tuberculosis are in advanced stages, 2) Early cases until 6 weeks after infection, 3) Cows calved within the preceding 6 weeks, 4) Old cattle, 5) Low potency tuberculin or bacterially contaminated tuberculin is used, 6) Variable dose has been used in SID inoculation with multidose syringe and 7) Animals are desensitized by tuberculin administration during the preceding 8-60 days.

Other serological tests for diagnosis of tuberculosis

When more specific and sensitive test in required for diagnosis of positive reactor during eradication programme, serological tests other than SID or tuberculin subcut test are used in order to identify "energic" animals and cases sensitized by some other bacteria.

Complement fixation test (CFT), Fluoroscent Antibody Test (FAT), direct bacterial agglutination, precipitation and haemagglutination tests have been developed but have little potential value for routine diagnosis. ELISA which examines antibody to "defined antigen" of M. bovis before and after SID testing appears useful in detecting "non-specific" reactors (Lightbody *et al.*, 1998). However, SID read at 72 hours using injection in caudal fold with PPD (0.3 ml) dose is still the preferred method for all practical purposes in developed countries.

Control

Eradication of bovine tubercutosis has been virtually achieved in many countries by test and slaughter policy. Control on herd basis rests on removal of infected animals, prevention of spread of infection and avoidance of further new introduction of the disease.

For removal of infected animals, whole herd is tested by individual animals tested by "tuberculin test" using appropriate antigen and all positive reactors are slaughtered or removed from the herd. NVL reactors are tested by "comparative" test mentioned above to determine specificity of infection. Doubtful reactors are re-tested after 60 days of interval and confirmed for positive reactivity or "Anergy". Anergic animals are re-tested by appropriate serological tests mentioned above for confirmation.

Prevention of spread of infection should be instituted as soon as the first group reactor is removed. Feed troughs, waterers and shed as well as other equipments including milking instruments and utensils should be disinfected using hot 5% phenol or cresol disinfectants. Suspecious reactors are separated from main herd and re-tested and if negative, they may be mixed with main herd after proper interval of 60 days.

Calves reared on the farm should be fed tuberculosis free milk (Pasturised, if necessary). All other species of animals should be examined for tuberculosis by testing and removed from farm, if found positive. Human attendants should also be tested and only tuberculosis free attendants should be kept on the farm. Re-introduction of infection/infected animals should be avoided. It is necessary to educate the personals on hygiene and disease eradiation programme.

Vaccination

Bacillus of Calmetti and Guarin (BCG) vaccine contains naturally avirulent strain of mycolactrium which is a very "stable" strain and found to be safe while "vole acid - fast" vaccine is varing too much in virulence. Vaccine must be repeated annually after vaccination of calves as soon as possible after birth. However, vaccination makes the calves/animals "sensitive" to tuberculin test. It takes 6 weeks to produce immunity in animals/calves after vaccination and immunity is weak. Hence, the herd should be prevented from getting heavy exposure to tuberculosis after vaccination (Daborn and Grange, 1993).

Number of newer candidate vaccines including subunit vaccines and synthetic peptide vaccines, antigenically improved B.C.G. vaccine, attenuated mutants of mycobloto bovis, etc. have come but the results are yet waited for their conclusive file utility (Newell and Hewinson, 1995).

Problems of Tuberculosis Eradication

Even though test and slaughter policy is applied or vaccination is carried out in some countries, still complete eradication of tuberculosis has not been achieved even though virtual eradication has been achieved near completion. But during final stages of eradication, number of problems which have achieved great importance have arisen which are enlisted in the introductory paragraphs of this chapter in the beginning.

It is necessary to undertake intensive research work on the problem enlisted in order to achieve the final success in the eradication of this disease.

Tuberculosis Disease Scenario in India

Tuberculosis is most ancient disease of Bovines in India. Iyyar, 1940 detected tuberculosis in monkeys, Sengupta in 1974 and Verma, Bhardwaj, 1972 have similar observations in monkeys.

Rishender Verma (1999) detected 16% (163 Nos) monkeys, out of 1039 Nos tested at National Laboratory Animal Centre, Central Drug Research Institute, Lucknow, U.P. positive for tuberculosis after use of mammalian tuberculin for skin test.

Gajendra Singh worked on Bovine tuberculosis at IVRI, Mukteshwar during late nineteen fifties and early sixties. Marathe C.R. and S. Kumar at IVRI, Izatnagar worked on development of Purified Protein derivative (PPR) tuberculin for elimination of false positive reactors. Production of diagnostic agent for allergic test, namely tuberculin (Human and Avian strain) is one of the oldest product of

IVRI, Izatnagar at least since 1954. 3 types of tuberculins are produced including: a) Tuberculin subcutaneous; b) Heat concentrated synthetic medium tuberculin (HCSM), c) Avian tuberculin concentrated.

Tuberculin testing (Double intrdermal test) is carried out using HCSM tuberculin and Avian tuberculin on neck, one on each side respectively, on organized cattle and buffaloes as a routine exercise time to time to know the extent of positive reactors on the farms. Similarly tests are also undertaken on A.I. buffalo bulls as well as cow bulls for acceptance for use in A.I. work especially on Govt. and other valuable private/public sector farms.

It is the experience of the author (Pandit, S.V.) that positive tuberculin reactors many times turned out to be no visible lesion reactor (NVL reactor) on smear examination of slaughtered + reactor (superficial, inguinal and mammary lymph-node exam) carried out work during working at DIS, Pune from 1964 to 1974). As the treatment of tuberculosis using antibiotics/chemotherapeutic agents is costly, positive reactors are sold out for disposal by organized farms as slaughter of bovines is not preferred sentimentally in India. This keeps the focus of the infection continued at other place and purpose of testing is forfeited. Milk from positive reactor animals is dangerous for human use but fortunately such milk from stables around cities is used after pasteurization now-a-days.

Suggested Reading

Cheeseman, C.L., Wilesmith, J.W and Stuart, F.A (1989). Tuberculosis: The Disease and Its Epidemiology in the Badger, a Review. Epidemiology and Infection. 103(1): 113-125.

Daborn, C.J., Grange, J.M. (1993). HIV/AIDS and its implications for the control of animal tuberculosis. Br Vet J., 149: 405–417.

Lightbody, K.A.,. Skuce, R.A, Neil, S.D. l, and. Pollock, J.M. (1998). Mycobacterial antigen-specific antibody responses in bovine tuberculosis: an ELISA with potential to confirm disease status. Vet. Rec. 142: 295-300.

Mcilory, S.G., Neill, S.D., Mccracken, R.M. (1986). Pulmonary lesions and *Mycobacterium bovis*excretion from the respiratory tract of tuberculin reacting cattle. Vet. Rec. 118: 718–721.

Monaghan, M.L., Doherty, M.L., Collins, J.D., Kazda, J.F, Quinn, P.J. (1994). The tuberculin test. *Vet Microbiol* 40: 111-124.

Morris, R.S., Pfeiffer, D.U. and Jackson, R. (1994). The epidemiology of Mycobacterium bovis infections. Vet Microbiol 40: 153–177.

Neill, S.D., O'Brien, J.J. and Hanna, J. (1991). A mathematical model for Mycobacterium bovis excretion from tuberculous cattle. Vet Microbiol 28: 103–109.

Newell, D.G., Hewinson, R.G. (1995). Control of bovine tuberculosis by vaccination. Vet Rec. 136: 459–463.

Skuce, R.A., T.P. McCorry, J.F. McCarroll, S.M.M. Roring, A.N. Scott, D. Brittain, S.L. Hughes, R.G. Hewinson, and S.D. Neill. (2002). Discrimination of Mycobacterium tuberculosislosis complex bacteria using novel VNTR-PCR targets. Microbiology 148: 519-5.

Whipple, D.L., Clarke, P.R., Jarnagin, J.L., Payeur, J.B. (1997). Restriction fragment length polymorphism analysis of Mycobacterium bovis isolates from captive and free-ranging animals. J Vet Diagn Invest 9: 381–386.

□□□

Chapter 34

Johne's Disease (Paratuberculosis) of Cattle, Sheep and Goats

Johne's disease (Paratuberculosis) is a chronic bacterial disease of cattle, sheep and goats characterized by progressive emaciation of the affected animals, involving intestinal tract with chronic diarrhoeal disease and is caused by *Mycobacterium paratuberculosis*.

The disease is prevalent worldwide with widespread occurrence in Europe mainly in cattle and to a lesser extent in sheep and goats. It is common in sheep, in Iceland for long time and is recorded in sheep, in Australia. The disease in cattle is now being recognized with increased frequency in North America. It is prevailing in India since at least last decade of 19th century.

About the causative organisms

The causative organism *Mycobacterium paratuberculosis* is an acid fast slender rod shaped bacterium which is non-spore forming, facultatively intra cellular in character, when present in animal body. They can be stained by Ziahl-Neelsen acid fast staining. 3 distinct groups of strains of *M.paratuberculosis* have been identified. One wide-spread group caused disease in cattle and it can be easily cultured from infected faeces or tissues in 6-12 weeks incubation while second groups is found in sheep and goats which is difficult to culture from faeces inspite of presence of large number of organisms in faeces. Third group includes those identified from only sheep (not in goats) from Iceland, Canada and South Africa (Mc Nab *et al.*, 1991).

Epidemiology and transmission of the disease

The disease is transmitted by the ingestion of feed and water contaminated by the faeces of infected animals which are excreting the organisms. Because of the normally long incubation period of organisms, infected animals may excrete organisms in faeces for 15 to 18 months before clinical symptoms appear (Sweeney, 1996). The organisms are shed in semen of infected bulls (even survive antimicrobial treatment and freezing) and as a result intrauterine infection occurs commonly. The prevalence of foetal infection as high as 37% of cows with clinical disease and upto 8.6% of foetuses from injected cows without signs of the clinical disease was recorded (Sweeney, 1996). This occurs when infection of cows is in more advanced stages.

Calves could become infected by consuming colostrums and milk of infected cows soon after birth (Streter *et al.*, 1995). In calves reared on infected nurse cows, clinical disease occurs in 12-18 months of age (minimum incubation period). However, infection usually occurs in calves under 30 days of age and clinical disease is seen at as long period as 3-5 years of age, when the infection is already prevalent on the farm.

Size of infective dose, level of dilatory iron intake, age, stress and immune suppressive agents like Bovine Virus Diarrhoea (BVD) virus may affect the probability of development of clinical disease. Housed animals are subjected to a higher risk of infection because of heavy contamination by faeces and the long survival of the bacteria in protected sites. Increase in "cow-calf contact" is responsible for high incidence of the disease (Goodger *et al.*, 1996).

The organisms can persist in pasture for long periods without multiplication for upto 1 year. They survive better in "acid soils" as compared with "alkaline soil" (Johnson–Ifearulundu and Kaneene, 1997). Pasteurization of colostrums at 63^{0}C for 30 minutes is survived by the organisms. (Meylan *et al.*, 1996).

Pathogenesis

After oral ingestion, the organism localizes in the mucosa of the small intestine, its associated lymph-nodes and to lesser extent in the tonsil and supra pharyngeal lymph-nodes. The primary site of bacterial multiplication is terminal part of small intestine and the large intestine.

After primary multiplication in intestines, 3 possibilities can be shown by the infected animal, namely: 1) Animal can develop quick resistance and becomes "Infected Resistant" animal. 2) Some animals will partially control the infection and shed the infection intermittently

(Infected – Intermittant Shedders) or they become "Intermediate cases" incubating the disease for long periods and they will be "heavy shedders" of the organisms. 3) In some animals, the organisms persist in intestinal mucosa and from them clinical cases develop.

The organisms are phagocytosed by macrophages which is turn proliferate in large number of infiltrated intestinal submucosa, resulting into decreased abosorption, chronic diarrhoea and resulting maladsorption and leakage of proteins into hymen of the Jejunum. This brings about muscle wasting, hypoproteinemia and oedema. The blood derived macrophages are incapable of destroying the M. paratuberculosis organisms entrapped within them.

In case of "Infected Resistant" animals mentioned previously, the infection is controlled but the animals are unable to completely eliminate the organisms and hence, they do not "Shed" the organisms in faeces (faecal culturing cannot detected this group of animals) and the "Lymphocyte transformation test" response is absent in them, as their circulating lymphocytes are "sensitized". This "skin test" is also negative in this group.

In case of "Intermediate" cases mentioned previously, animals fail to control infection and antibodies appear in the circulation which are detectable by CFT or AGPT and the organisms are also shed in the faeces and are detected by microscopic examination of faeces or by cultural examination of faeces and "skin test" is positive and the circulating lymphocytes are sensitized.

In case of clinical disease, the organisms are detected by microscopy or by culture but the antibody responses and skin tests are viable. In sheep with Johne's disease, with or without clinical symptoms, a range of intestinal lesions are characteristic.

Two distinct histological types of granulmatous enteritis develop in sheep, such as: 1) "Tuberculoid" type with cell mediated immune response, consisting of "small granulomata" composed of epithetoid cells surrounded by many lymphocytes with "few" or "no" bacilli and number of glant cells and 2) Lepromatous type with a strong humoral response of lesions composed to accumulations of "macrophages" containing large number of mycobacteria (Clarke and Littke,1996). Most sheep with Johne's disease have multibacillary lesions (Lepromatous) with extensive diffuse microphage infiltration within the mucosa and submucosa.

In sheep, the local release of macrophages and other lymphocyte derived "cytokines" may exert an influence on the type of inflammatory and immune responses which develop during infection. The elevated production of cytokines along with a failure of clear heavy burden of bacteria may be one factor encouraging the chronic inflammatory lesion in paratuberculosis.

The paratuberculosis lesion is closely associated with organized lymphoid tissue of intestine which is abundunt in Payers patches especially in ileum of young animals and it explains why the adult animals lower susceptibility to Johne's disease, as they have reduced lymphoid tissue in their ileum (Juste *et al.*, 1994).

In young calves, organisms proliferate slowly in small intestinal site resulting into massive cellular infiltration of the intestinal sub-mucosa while in adult the bacteria are carried by macrophages to uterus, the faetus and mammary gland, testis and semen of bulls and small granulomata are produced in the lymph glands draining these areas. It is observed that the vaccination against Johne's disease cannot halt this process of progressive infiltration of mycobacteria upto uterus/mammary gland described above but it only stops the "cellular response" in these places which prevents the clinical disease.

Symptoms and post mortem lesions

Four stages of the disease occur progressively in cattle and sheep/ goats. During the initial phase of the silent carrier stage, the animals may not show any clinical sign but excrete the organisms in faeces, hence serological tests are negative but culture of the faeces in positive. This stage can last in calves' upto 2 years.

In second phase of the disease, carrier adults will not show clinical disease of the intestinal symptoms but may show "subclinical disease" with mastitis or infertility. However, faecal culture will be mostly negative but small percentage (15-25% of the infected animals) may become faecal culture positive but negative to serological tests.

Third stage is "Clinical Disease" which is seen in "Few animals" (Tip of the ice berg) only out of the total infected herd. This will occur 2 years after the initial infection in the herd of cattle. Gradual loss of body weight (inspite of abnormal appetite) and diarrhoea may develop while body temperature, heart rate and respiration is normal, fall in milk yield may occur and excessive thirst may be present. Diarrhoeic faeces may look like thick pea soup but without offensive odour. Fourth stage is the "advanced clinical phase" of the disease with extreme emaciation and intermandibular oedema fluid "water house" diarrhoea or pipe stream passage of faeces may be evident and "muscular wastage" of the body condition may necessitate "distraction" of the animal.

Even though infection rate may be as high as 100%, clinical disease may be evident in 5% of the herd in matured animals. In general incidence of disease was varying from 2.6 to 18% in some states while from 8 to 74% in other states in USA. Postmortem lesions in cattle are confined to the posterior region of the intestines, namely the terminal part of small intestine, the caecum and the 1st part of the colon. In advanced cases, even return and duodenum may also get affected. The ileo-caecal valve is always involved.

The lesion in the intestine of cattle consists of thickening of its walls 3 to 4 times with corrugation of its mucosa. The serosal lymphatics are also thickened. The ileocaecal valve is also thickened oedematous and initially reddened and gets corrugated later on the blood vessels of this region of viscera show atherosclerosis in advanced cases. The mesenteric lymph-nodes are oedematous along with those of iliocaecal region but there are no foci of necrosis and mineralization as in case of tuberculosis.

In cattle, the microscopic lesions of intestinal affected section consists of the infiltration of very large number of epithelioid macrophages and multinucleated giant cells within the lamina propria and submucosa and within the paracortical area of the draining lymph-nodes of the area with granulomatous lymphagitis. These lesions can be described as "Lepromatous type" The Ziehl-Neelsen staining of section of this area of intestine shows large number of mycobact paratuberculosis acid fast organisms in infiltrated macrophages and giant cells, under the microscope.

In case of sheep, the intestinal lesions can be of 2 types, namely: 1) Tuberculoid and/or 2) Lepromatous as detailed out under the section of pathogenesis in this chapter (see also: Pérez, *et al.*, 1996). The "lepromatous lesions" in cattle and sheep as detailed above described in old literature as "symplasma stage" (see old text book on Veterinary Bacteriology and Pathology by Gaiger and Devis chapter on Jones disease) which differs from "Tuberculoid" lesions, wherein distinct "Tubercles" i.e. typical cacaeated granuloma with minealisation occurs. The tubercles in tuberculosis disease is an "enclosed mass" of tissue reaction around focus of tubercular mycobacterial organisms which contains few epitheliod cells (macrophages), giants cells and fibroblasts while "Lapromatous lesion" is "non-enclosed" open "wide lesions" with thickened wall of affected intestine containing studed macrophages with mycobacteria and giant multinuclear cells infiltrated in submucosa and lamina propria.

Diagnosis

In "infected herd" with Johne's Disease, 4 types of animals may be observed, namely: 1) Animals with "Clinical" disease, shedding the organisms in their faeces, 2) Animals with subclinical infection (No visible symptoms) but shedding the organisms in faeces (Intermediate and incubating), 3) Animals infected but neither showing symptoms or shedding enough bacteria to be culturally detectable in faeces (Infected resistant), 4) un infected normal cattle.

For eradication of the disease, it is necessary to find out all "infected" animals and "normal" animals for their identification and elimination of the "infected" ones from the "normal" ones. This requires definite strategy for identification for each of the 4 types of animals mentioned above.

"Type-1" animals (clinical cases, shedding the organisms) can be easily identified by their typical symptoms and positive "acid-fast" staining of faecal sample smear examination (Zeihl-Neelsen staining) and the faecal culture of mycobacterium paratubercubses. "Type-2" animals (Intermediate and incubating) can be identified by positive "skin test" using "Johnin" and "Tuberculin" for comparison (Skin reaction to "Johnin" will be more pronounced than to "tuberculin") Type-2 animals will not have adequate humoral antibody response and hence, tests like CFT, serum ELISA are not so reliable in decting Type-2 animals but as Type-2 animals are shedders of organisms in the faces and hence, ZN staining/cultural/exam DOT ELISA for identification of organisms in faeces can be used for detection of Type 2 cases.

Type-3 animals (infected-resistant) which do not show symptoms and do not shed the organisms in faeces continuously (shed only occasionally, intermitantly) will be very difficult for detection, as they cannot be detected by ZN staining / cultural examination / DOT ELISA for identification of organisms in faeces all the time nor by CFT, serum ELISA as serum antibodies are not present to the reliable extent.

However, they can only be detected by "Skin test" using "Johnin" and "Tuberculin" for comparative allergic reaction. Type-4 animals (Normal) will be "negative" by all the test including serological tests like CFT, serum ELISA/AGID (in sheep) as well as faecal smcar exam/ cultural isolation from faeces/DOT-ELISA on faecal sample.

It can be noted from the above information that for purpose of detection of all type 1 to 4 categories of animals for elimination of "positive" infected Johne's diseased animals, no single test is reliable and hence, all above mentioned tests are required to be conducted, if eradication programme is to be undertaken. This sort of testing programme will require tremendous monetary expenditure for the Governments of states and the countries as well as huge manpower and management infrastructure and hence, the animal industry people from various developed and developing countries have not taken sufficient interest in eradication progrmmes for Johne's disease.

Production of "Johnin" reagent for skin test

Johnin is produced by growing selected strain of mycobact para-tuberculosis on synthetic medium after incubation at 37^{0}C for 10-12 weeks. The growth of culture is steamed for 3 hours and then the contents of culture flask are filtered through mesh sieve and concentrated over steam both to 1/10th of the original volume and stored for 14 days before Seitz filtration. After this, the product is distributed in ampules and sealed. The product is tested for sterility and potency in pre-infected cattle with Johne's Disease Sellharomanc and Sinha, K.C. (Vety Biological products ICAR, Publication, 1962).

Skin test of Johne's Disease

0.1 ml of Johnin reagent is inoculated by intradermal route in cattle/sheep/goat after shaving the skin of neck region as in case of tuberculin test and second dose of reagent (0.1 ml) is repeated at the same site by the same route. Thickness of skin is measured at inoculation site prior to 1st inoculation and after 48.72 hours of 2nd inoculation. Positive reactor will show at least 2 fold increase in the thickness of skin fold at inoculation site and diffuse oedematous swelling will be the indicator of specificity of reaction. The animal positive for tuberculosis will also show positive Johnin reaction. But the specificity of the test can be determined by comparative "Tuberculin" and "Johnin" testing simultaneously at respectable distance at the same time on neck of the test animal.

ELISA tests for Johne's Disease

Four different ELISA tests are developed for this disease. Serum ELISA test will be the 1st test to be used for detection of sero positive (cattle) animals above 2 years of age which are either clinically affected or some of the subclinically affected or some of the subclinically affected animals still incubating the disease (not yet shedding organisms) or some of the "Infected - Resistant" group of animals, though all animals in 2nd& 3rd category are not detected by this test. "Johne's" absorbed ELISA is the improved test (EIA) used for this purpose along with cultural exam of faeces which improves the positive detection of this 1st herd testing. Total test time is reduced to 2 hours by this test (Cox *et al.*, 1991). The"EIA" test is more sensitive than CFT as per Australian report (Ridge *et al.*, 1991). The DOT-ELISA is estimated to give sensitivity of 85% and specificity of 100% in clinical cases while sensitivity is 64% of specificity in sub-clinical cases. Milk ELISA is also used but the data on sensitivity/specificity is lacking. The sensitivities of the ELISA and AGID tests in sheep and goats is 62% and 78% respectively and hence, AGID is useful for flock - screening programme of sheep (Dubash *et al.*, 1996).

Treatment

Steptomycin (50 mg/kg b.wt) Isoniazid (20 mg/kg B.W.) and chofaziminae are the drugs which may give transient recovery from clinical disease but cannot cure the animal and its faecal sheding. Hence, treatment is not recommended.

Control

The control of Johne's Disease in cattle, sheep and goat herds/ flocks in which the clinical cases of the disease are present and sub-clinical infection is also present, is difficult to achieve because of the inaccuracy of the diagnostic tests available, as explained previously in this chapter. The next best option is the control of the disease at a very low level of prevalence. Only the farm specific recommendations for control are possible. This includes: 1) The identification and elimination of infected animals, using the tests and regiemes of the same described in this chapter. 2) The prevention of the new infections.

Overall hygienic measures including disinfection progrmmes, especially management of the faecal material and its disinfection is important. Rearing calves away from infected cows after removal of new born. Calves from their dams immediately after birth and feeding of Pasturised colosturm to them is useful. New replacement of animals should be undertaken only after through "testing" for absence of infection in them.

Vaccination

Vaccination provides a protection against "Clinical disease" only and not against shedding of organisms. Vallies vaccine contains paraffin oil-premic stone powder vehicle for live modified mycobact, paratuberculosis organisms or sigurds son vaccine containing killed virulent bacteria are the commercially available good vaccines. These vaccines are used in calves below one month of age only once without further repetition, as it is of no benefit to "infected" animal. The vaccinated animals develop "skin test" sensitivity for period upto 5 weeks post vaccination but it disappears, when calves are 18 months old. It is found 90% effective in avoiding clinical disease and continuous use may reduce the shedding of organisms though not completely (Gezon *et al.*, 1988).

Johne's Disease, Indian Scenario

This chronic malady is prevailing in India since long. There is mention about precipitation of acute form in goats probably due to the stress of faciolosis in liver on the experimental farm of IVRI Mukteshwar as long back as in early fifities (N.S. Datt mention in his articles in Pune symposium of IAVMI Jan, 1994). I.V.R.I. is producing "Johnin" an "allergic test" diagnostic agent since as long back as in 1954s. ADIO (CSG) - Dr. Shiraguppi came across incidence of Johne's disease in imported sheep and goats at sheep breeding farms in Maharashtra during late nineteen sixties and seventies. However, the statistical data is not available now.

Suggested Reading

Clarke, C. and Littke, D. (1996). The pathology of ovine paratuberculosis: gross and histological changes in the intestine and other tissues. J Comp Path 114: 419–437.

Cox, J.C., Drane, D.P., Jones, S.L. (1991). Development and evaluation of a rapid absorbed enzyme immunoassay test for the diagnosis of Johne's disease in cattle. *Aust Vet J.*; 68: 157–160.

Dubash, K., W.P. Shulaw, S. Bech-Nielsen, H.F. Stills, Jr., and R.D. Slemons. (1996). Evaluation of an agar gel immunodiffusion test kit for detection of antibodies to Mycobacterium paratuberculosis in sheep. J. Am. Vet. Med. Assoc. 208: 401–403.

Gezon, H.M., H.D. Bither, H.C. Gibbs, E.J. Acker, L.A. Hanson, J.K. Thompson, and R.D. Jorgenson. (1988). Identification and control of paratuberculosis in a large goat herd. Am. J. Vet. Res. 49: 1817–1823.

Goodger, W.J., Collins M.T., Nordlund K.V. (1996). Epidemiologic study of on-farm management practices associated with prevalence of Mycobacterium paratuberculosis infections in dairy cattle. J Am Vet Med Assoc. 208: 1877–1881.

Johnson-Ifearulundu, Y.J., and. Kaneene J.B. (1997). Relationship between soil type and Mycobacterium paratuberculosis. J. Am. Vet. Med. Assoc. 210: 1735–1740.

Juste, R.A., García Marín, J.F, Peris B., SáezdeOcáriz C., Badiola, J.J. (1994). Experimental infection of vaccinated and non-vaccinated lambs with *Mycobacterium paratuberculosis*. J Comp Pathol. 110: 185–194.

Meylan, M., Rings, D.M., Shulaw W.P., Kowalski J.J., BechNielsen, S., and Hoffsis, G.F. (1996). Survival of Mycobacterium paratuberculosis and preservation of immunoglobulin G in bovine colostrum under experimental conditions simulating pasteurization. Am. J. Vet. Res. 57: 1580–1585.

McNab, W.B., Meek, A.H., Duncan, J.R., Martin, S.W., van Dreumel, A.A. (1991). An epidemiological study of paratuberculosis in dairy cattle in Ontario: study design and prevalence estimates. Can J Vet Res. 55: 246–251.

Pérez, V., García-Marím J.F, Badiola, J.J. (1996). Description and classification 385 of different types of lesion associated with natural paratuberculosis infection in sheep. J Comp Pathol., 114: 107-122.

Ridge, S.E., Morgan, I.R., Sockett, D.C. (1991). Comparison of the Johne's absorbed EIA and the complement fixation test for the diagnosis of Johne's disease in cattle. *Aust Vet J*. 68: 253–257.

Streeter, R.N., Hoffsis, G.F., Bech-Nelsen, S., Shulaw W.P., Rings, D.M. (1995). Isolation of M.paratuberculosis from colostrum and milk of sub-clinically infected cows. Am. J.Vet. Res., 56.

Sweeney, R.W. (1996). Transmission of paratuberculosis. Vet. Clin.North Am. Food Animal Pract. 12: 305.

□□□

Chapter 35

Actinomycosis (Lumpy jaw) and Actinobacillosis (Wooden tongue) of Cattle

Actinomycosis and Actinobacillosis of cattle are infectious diseases of cattle caused by *Actinomyces bovis* and *Actinobacillus lignieressi* organisms respectively and are characterized by chronic granulomatous lesions developed in hard bony tissues and soft muscular tissues respectively.

About the causative organisms

Actinomyces bovis are filamentous organisms, stained readily with grams staining method and gram positive and have tendency for branching and produce "club" colonies (gramles) in the pus contained in "granulation tissue" lesions which are formed in bone tissue (hard tissues).

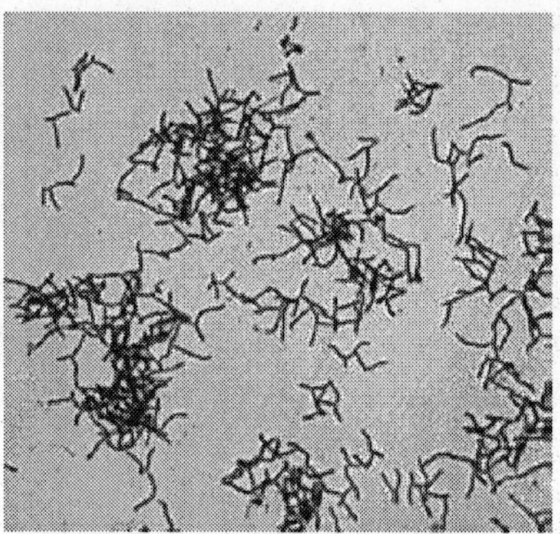

Fig. 1: *Actinomyces bovis*

Actinobacillus lignieressi are long bacillary organisms found in medium to long chains and are gram positive and produce "club colonies" similar to actimomyces bovis in the pus in granulation tissue lesions which (unlike actinomyces involving bony tissue) has tendancy to invade soft muscular tissue.

Epidemiology and Transmission

Both *Actinomyces bovis* and *Actinobacillus lignieressi* are the members of normal flora of mouths of cattle, the former is also found in oral flora of pigs while the later is found in oral flora of sheep. In case of *Actinomyces bovis* infection, infection is presumed to occur through injury to buccal mucosa caused by sharp objects (pieces of feed or foreign material). It can also occur through dental alveoli especially in young cattle, when teeth are erupted. Infection of alimentary tract is related to laceration by sharp foreign bodies.

In case of *Actinobacillus lignieressii*, the organism, living as commensal in oral cavity and rumen of ruminants (cattle and sheep), infection occurs through ulcerating or penetrating lesions to the sulcus of the tongue (This lesions occurs while cattle grazing "abrasive" pasture or pastures with spiny awns) and transmission may be enhanced by infected discharge contaminating these pastures or feeds. Similar high incidence is observed in sheep fed "Brickly" pear grass. Cattle feeding on pastures with copper deficiency has higher incidence of the disease.

Pathogenesis

In case of *Actinomyces bovis* rarefying osteomyelites is produced in jaw bone. The lesion is characteristically granulomatous both at primary Jaw bone site and where visceral involvement occurs. The lesion causes physical interference with prehension and mastication. Similarly physical interference of ruminal movement and digestion occurs, both resulting in starvation. Haematogenous spread occurs occasionally and localization of lesions also occurs in other organs.

In case of *Actinobacilbus lignieressii*, local infection of soft tissue of tongue or other muscular site, causes an acute inflammatory reaction and subsequent development of granulomatous lesions in which necrosis and suppuration occurs, often with discharge of pus to the exterior. Lingual lesion causes interference with prehension and mastication due to acute inflammation in early stage and due to distortion of tongue later on.

Symptoms and Postmortem Lesions

In case of *Actinomyces bovis* (Lumphy Jaw disease) both mandible and maxilla of jaw show bony swelling at the level of central molar teeth, which may be diffuse or discrete. These may increase slowly or faster within few weeks to months. Swellings are hard, immovable and painless in the beginning but painful in later stages. They usually break through skin and discharge pus through one or more openings. The pus may be sticky, honey like, containing yellowish white granules. Teeth embedded in affected bone may become malignated and painful, mastication becoming difficult. No involvement of local lymph-node occurs. Animal becomes emaciated and die eventually.

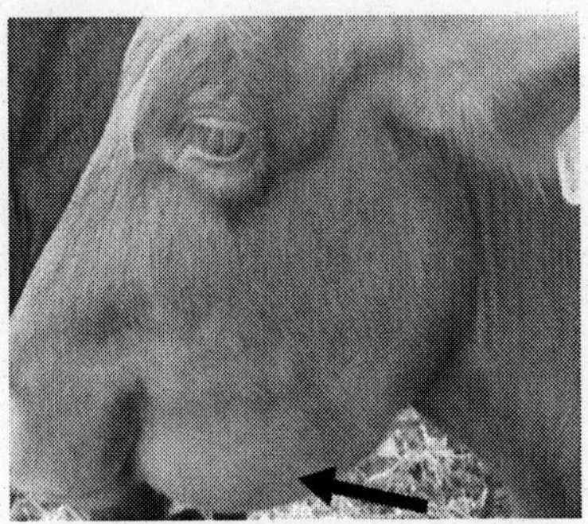

Fig. 2: Calf showing Lumpy jaw

Most commonly involvement of oesophagial groove region (soft tissue) occurs producing spread to lower oesophagus and reticulum which impairs digestion and cause diarrhoea. Sometimes orchitis and trachea may also be involved.

Postmortem lesions reveal rarefaction of bone and presence of loculi and sinuses containing thin, whey like pus with small gritty granules. Extensive fibrosis around the lesion occurs. The presence of "club" colonies containing typical thread like bacteria is characteristic of the disease, which can be observed by crushing of granules between slides and examining under microscope.

In case of Actinobacillosis, when tongue is involved, the disease is acute and animal is unable to eat for 48 hours. There is excessive salivation and animal chews the tongue gently as if chewing foreign body. Tongue is swollen, hard at base (tip normal). It is painful on palpation, nodules and ulcers present on sides of tongue. Later on tongue becomes fibrous, shrunken and immobile, with affected prehension. Lymphedenitis is common (as opposed to no involvement of lymph-nodes in Actinomycosis). They become swollen, especially submaxillary and parotid lymph-nodes are visible, often get ruptured with oozing pus (which is non-odourous). Retropharyngeal nodes are swollen and cause interference in swallowing and produce loud snoring respiration, Granulomas on external nares and skin and eyelids bleed easily. The granulomas show club like rosettes similar to actinomyces bovis granulomas, containing mass of bacteria.

Treatment

In both actinomycosis as well as actinobacillosis, oral or intravenous dosing of iodides is useful. Potassium iodide 6-10 g/day for 7-10 days given orally or sodium iodide 1 gm/12 kg body wt. given intravenously as a 10% solution, only once is enough for curing soft tissue lesions. Two more oral courses/intravenous single injection two more times is needed to cure bony lesions sulphonamides have better curative effect (Anderson *et al.*, 1990). Streptomycin (5 g/day for 3 days) along with iodide treatment is also better (Peel, *et al.*, 1991).

Actinobacillosis / Actinomycosis Indian Scenario

No much information about the extent of incidence of these infections in India is available. Actinobacillosis in Bullocks buffaloes and cows is described by Manjrekar (1938). Cutaneous actinobacillosis in balls is recorded by Parihar, *et al.* (1977).

However, the Author (S.V. Pandit) while working under Rinderpest eradication scheme in Dhulia district of Maharashtra came across very significant incidences of both of these diseases, predominantly actinomycosis in that area in indigenous cattle. Involvement of maxillary and mandibular regions showing extensive granulomatous lesions with oozing pus from those bone sinuses and containing typical gritty granules were observed in large numbers of village cattle used for bullock carts. Use of iodides (mostly oral and in few cases by intravenous route) showed variable results of recovery rate, probably due to insufficient repetition of doses.

Suggested Reading

Anderson, K.L., Fairley, R.A., Duncan, D. (1990). Suspected actinobacillosis manifested by facial enlargement in a heifer. Journal of American Veterinary Medical Association 197: 1359-1360.

Peel, M.M., Hornidge, K.A., Luppino, M., Stacpoole, A.M., Weaver, R.E. (1991). Actinobacillus spp. And related bacteria in infected wounds of human bitten by horses and sheep. Journal of Clinical Microbiology 29: 2535-2538.

□□□

Chapter 36

Bovine Mastitis of Infectious Origin

Bovine Infectious Mastitis is the inflammatory disease of the parenchyma of the mammary gland of cows, caused by infectious agents and is characterized by a range of physical and chemical changes in the milk and the pathological changes in the glandular tissue.

The most important changes in milk include discolouration, the presence of clots and large numbers of leukocytes while the pathological changes in glandular tissue include swelling, heat, pain and in duration in the gland in clinical cases while sub clinical cases can be identified only by above mentioned changes in the milk in addition to presence and rise of bovine serum albumin, sodium chloride contents of milk.

About the infectious agents causing mastitis

Bovine mastitis is caused by many different infectious agents, commonly divided into: 1) Those causing contagious mastitis (contagious pathogens) which include coagulase positive *Staphylococcus aureus, Streptococcus aglalatctiae, Corynae bacterium bovis* and *Mycoplasma bovis*. 2) Environmental pathogen which include *Streptococcus uberis* and *Streptococcus dysgalactiae* which are most prevalent while less prevalent are *Strept. bovis* (now equines) and environmental coli form (gram negative *E.Coli, Klebsiella* and *Citrobacter* species, *Enterobactor* species and *Pseudomonas* species). 3) Minor pathogens which include coagulase negative *Staph.albus, Staph citrus* and *Staph epidermidis,* etc. which are commonly present on skin and teats and 4) uncommon pathogens including *Actinomyces pyogenes, Nocardia* species *Mycobacterium bovis, Pasturella* species, anaerobic bacteria, fungi and yeasts.

Usually, the source of contagious pathogens is the infected glands of other cows in the herd and method to eliminate infected cows involve antimicrobial therapy and culling of chronically infected cows. The conscientious mastitis control programme can eradicate *Streptococcus agalactiae* from dairy herds easily while it is much more difficult to deal with a herd with high prevalence of staph. It is difficult to control *Mycoplasma bovis* mastitis, as this organism does not respond to antibiotic therapy.

Environmental pathogens involve 2 groups, namely coliforms and streptococci (coagulase negative), the main source of which is the environment of cow, including bedding, contaminated hard flooring of stable, milking of wet udders and test preparation and housing system. It is found that contagious pathogens like *strepto agalactiae, Staph aureus* are on reducing side progressively now-a-days due to antibiotic treatment but environmental pathogens are on increase, such as coliforms and streptococci, as they are aportunistic organisms and when defence system of cows is compromised due to milking machine stresses, they get upper hand.

Minor pathogens and uncommon pathogens are involved more in sub clinical mastitis. Fungal infections and Leptospira organisms are more of systemic infections or more generalized infection in cows and mastitis is only a part of their manifestation.

Epidemiology and Transmission

Surveys in dairy herds indicate that the prevalence of infection of mastitis pathogens is about 50% of cows and a quarter infection rates of about 25% in general. The prevalence of infection with *Staph aureus* in cow's ranges between 7 to 40% and in some herds is even higher. The *Streptococcus agalactiae* infection of cows (Mastitis) ranges from 1 to 8% of cows with relative incidence of str. agalactiae other streptococci and staph.aureus of 1:1:2 is a common finding. *Staph aureus* may still assume some importance as a cause of subclinical mastitis but its prevalence has been reduced by modern mastitis control programme leading to a higher proportion of culture negative mastitis quarters and perhaps consequent, increase in infections by *E. coli, Pseudomonas* and *klebsiella* species (Fox and Gay, 1993).

From 171 randomly selected herds, average annual incidence rate of clinical mastitis was 12.7 quarter cases per 100 cows per year. The most frequent isolates from clinical cases were *E. coli* (16%), *Staph aureus* (14%), *Strep. uberis* (11%), and *Strep. dysgalactiae* (8%) (Miltenburg *et al.*, 1996).

Infection of each mammary gland occurs via teat canal, the infection originating from either an infected udder or the environment in dairy cattle. The infection originating from infected udders is transmitted to the teat skin of other cows by milking machine liners, milker's hands, wash clothes and any other material that can act as an inert carrier.

Most new infections occur during the early part of the dry period and in the 1st two months of lactation, especially with environmental pathogens. The overall prevalence of infection of coagulase positive Staphylococcal infection in primiparous cows at parturition was 8.1%. *Primiparus* cows with these infections may represent significant reservoirs of infection to uninfected animals in the herd.

Corynaebact bovis grow best in milk secreted in the middle of lactation, whereas dry period secretion inhibits growth (Oliver and Juneja, 1990). Cows with a history of mastitis in preceding lactation may be almost twice as susceptible to clinical mastitis in current lactation as those without mastitis in preceding lactation. The high milk yielder cows are more susceptible for mastitis (Grohn *et al.*, 1995).

Factors, such as climate, housing system, type of bedding and rainfall influence the degree of exposure of teat tips to mastitis pathogens. Environmental pathogens multiple in bedding materials and have more chance to infect teat tips. The hygiene and negligence in bedding maintenance increase the chances of environmental pathogen causing mastitis. Efficiency of milking personal, milking machines, high milking speed and hygiene in milking parlour influence the incidence of mastitis (Bartlet *et al.*, 1992).

The ability of the pathogens to colonize the teat duct then to adhere to mammary epithelium influence the pathogenicity of the mastitis casusing pathogenic bacteria E. Coli isolates causing mastitis produce lipopolisaccharide endotoxins which are responsible for pathogenicity of mastitis. Staph aureus isolates produce many potential virulence factors including coagulase enterotoxinl, b toxins haemolysins, hyaluronidase and leukocidins which are responsible for characteristics inflammatory reactions of staph mastitis.

Pathogenesis

Infection of mammary gland always occurs via the teat canal and development of mastitis takes place through 3 stages, namely: invasion, infection and finally inflammation.

During invasion, pathogen moves from exterior of teat to the milk cistern via. milk in teat canal. During infection, pathogens multiply rapidly and invade the mammary tissue. Multiplication of certain organisms results in release of endotoxin as in coliform mastitis which causes profound systemic effects with minimal inflammatory effect.

Infection is followed by inflammation, when clinical mastitis occurs with variable clinical/subclinical abnormalities in udder and systemic effects (mild to severe). Swelling, hotness of udder and sometimes gangrene of udder tissue as well as abscess formation and atrophy of glandular tissue during chronic stages of mastitis are some of the final sequale of the whole process.

The most significant subclinical abnormality of the milk is the increase in the somatic cell count (SCC), which is the most important measurement of the milk quality and udder health. The total SCC when udder is in normal health, is $< 10^5$/ml of milk which can increase to more than 10^6/ml of milk in case of beginning of the mastitis. The bacteria release metabolic by-products like enterotoxin and cell wall components which induce chemotatctic influence to moblise leukocytes from blood circulation during mastitis, thus increasing the SSC in milk which is able to reduce bacteria which are inflammatory stimulasts, when they are reduced, the SCC naturally is reduced in the milk.

Neutrophils constitute 90% of mammary leukocytes and they phagocytose and kill bacteria during inflammatory reaction in the mammary tissue.

Symptoms and lesions of mastitis

Different pathogens can cause chronic, subclinical, subacute and peracute forms of mastitis. However, it is difficult to predict the involvement of specific pathogen as the causative agent of mastitis according to the symptoms/lesions they produce. It is, therefore, not possible to draw the line of treatment as per the causative agent, until the isolation of specific organism responsible for mastitis is completed and its antibiotic sensitivity is assessed.

The clinical findings in mastitis include: 1) abnormalities of secretion (milk), 2) abnormalities of the size, consistency and temperature of mammary glands and frequently a systemic reaction. The clinical forms of mastitis are usually classified as per severity and duration of mastitis.

Peracute inflammation is accompanied by swelling, heat and pain of the quarter, with severe systemic reaction. Acute inflammation is severe but without systemic involvement. Subacute inflammation is mild with persistant milk abnormality. Subclinical inflammation is manifested by high somatic cell count (SCC) without visible milk abnormality of udder. Duration of clinical and subclinical mastitis is short term (as in coliform mastitis) while duration of clinical mastitis is recurrent (as in *Staph aureus* and *strepto dysgalactiae*). Duration of clinical or subclinical mastitis is persistent (as in case of *Strepto agalactiae*).

The clinical abnormalities of milk during mastitis can be detected by observation of "milk strip" from each quarter of cow taken on the "Strip cup" with shiny black plate permitting the detection of discolouration of milk and milk clots, flakes and pus. If the wateryness of milk persists for more than 10 "streams" of milk from way quarter of udder, it is taken as significant "mastitis" quarter. This is accompanied usually by clot, flakes. The flakes at the end of milking may be indicative of mammary tuberculosis.

The physical abnormalities of the udder can be felt by palpation of udder, each pair of hind and fore quarters need to be palpated. Detection of fibrosis, oedematous inflammatory swelling and atrophy of mammary tissue can be detected in mastitis udder. The udder tissue may produce in duration and finally making the affected quarters blind or may produce sloughing of the affected parts occasionally. In last stages gangrenous feeling with cracking sound may be felt in case of staphylococcus or clostridial infection. The systemic reactions/ responses will include fever, tachycardia and ruminal stasis. Anorexia and recombany may or may not be present. This is usually associated with *E. coli, Klebsiella* and less frequently in case of staph aureus or strepto sp. Infection.

Diagnosis

Diagnosis of Mastitis is carried out at: 1) individual cow level or 2) at herd level.

Detection of mastitis at individual cow level

Culture and anti-microbiol sensitivity of milk sample can be done. ELISA may be used to detect antigens against *Staph.aureus, E. coli, Strepto dysgalactiae* and *Strepto agalactiae,* if cultural isolation in cases of clinical mastitis fail inspite of positive SCC (counts higher than 75,00,000 cells/ml of milk sample). Mastitis could be detected in such samples upto 50% level. Indirect tests for detection of subclinical mastitis include: 1) Somatic cell count (SCC), using "Automated Electronic counters" or using California Mastitis Test (CMT). Other indirect tests which measure antibody and "Increases in electrical conductivity of milk samples" can also be used for diagnosis of mastitis. CMT and other indirect tests are cheaper and quicker than "SCC" and equally accurate but require special collection of milk.

"CMT" reagent contains a "detergent" and "pH indicator". The detergent reacts with the somatic cells present in milk sample from "mastitis" positive quarters of udder and produces the varing quantity of gel which gets "stained" according to the pH of the milk sample. The gel produced is graded as Nil +, ++, +++ reactions and thus, milk samples are graded as negative/positive for mastitis from each quarter of udder of individual cow.

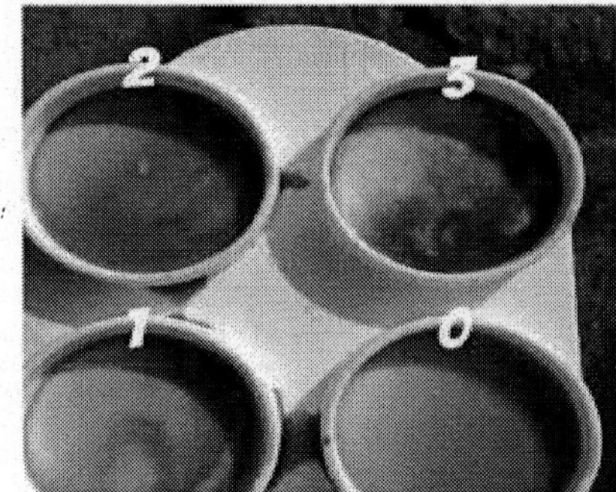

Fig. 1: California mastitis test with scores

There is a close relationship between "CMT reactions" and SCC as follows:

Test result	Reaction observed	Equivalent SCC
Negative (-)	No gel formation	0 to 200000 cell/ml
Trace (±)	Sligh "slime" when CMT paddle is rocked from side to side	1,50,000 to 5,00,000 cell/ml
1 (+)	Distinct "slime" immediately after mixing of solutions which disappear after some time. No doming up of peripheral "saline mass" (convening) by swirling of paddle	400000 to 5000000 Cell/ml
2 (++)	Distinct "slime" formation immediately after mixing of solutions fluid forms a peripheral mass when paddle is swirled exposing the bottom of cup of paddle	800000 to 5000000 Cells / ml
3 (+++)	Distinct "Slime formation" immediately after mixing of solutions which may dissipate by tinac. Surface of solution becomes convex or "domed up" by swirling of paddle	>5000000 cells/ml

Note: pH is usually highly alkaline but is acidic in some cases of mastitis

While considering cell counts/CMT results for diagnosis of mastitis, it should be noted that cell counts in first few days of lactation are exceptionally high which should not be mistaken for mastitis. Naturally CMT will also be positive during that period. Other reliable indirect test to know accurate estimate of cell counts is an ELISA of "Direct capture" type which measures elevated polymorphonuclear granulocyte antigen. This test provides accurate estimate of granulocytes as low as 1,00,000 cells/ml. An ELISA of myeloperxidase is almost as good as the capture ELISA, using monoclonal antibodies against neutrophil antigen. (Cooray, 1994).

Presence of sodium and chloride is increased in milk in mastitis problem which increases the "online" conductivity of milk during machine milking. A probe fitted in the milking cup of each quarter can measure and record these changes in conductivity during milking and detects the mastitis status of each quarter. (Milner *et al.*, 1996).

Detection of mastitis problem at herd level

The present day emphasis in mastitis control is to maintain a particular programme of hygiene and to monitor it by periodic examination of udder health by evaluation of milk at herd level. This is done by examination of "composite herd milk samples" (i.e. Bulk Tank Milk samples) which are already collected for butter fat testing at Milk collection centres using electronic cell counters. Dairy Herd Improvement Association (DHIA) in USA has adopted a SCC (Somatic Cell Count) scoring system with 10 catagories from 0 to 9, known as "Linear score" which is as follows:

Example: SCC = 200 (200,000 cells/ml)

1. Divide the SCC by 100 $\left(\frac{200}{100}=2\right)$
2. Determine the natural log (in) in 2 = 0,693147
3. Divide this value by 0.693147 0.693147 / 0.693147 = 1
4. Add "3" to the result 1+3 = 4 linear score

Thus, SCC = 200 (2, 00,000 cells/ml) is Equivalent with linear score 4

From this we can understand that linear score values are equivalent to SCC as follows:

Linear score	Somatic cell count
0.	12.5 midpoint (12500 cells/ml)
1.	25 (25,000 cells/ml)
2.	50 (50,000 cells/ml)
3.	100 (100,000 cells/ml)
4.	200 (200000 cells/ml)
5.	400 (400000 cells/ml)
6.	800 (800000 cells/ml)
7.	1600 (1600,000 cells/ml)
8.	3200 (3200,000 cells/ml)
9.	6400 (6400 000 cells/ml)

The counts are most useful in creating awareness in the mind of the farmer of the existence of a mastitis problem. It is not possible to determine the number of cows in a herd affected with mastitis by Bulk tank milk "Somatic Cell Count" (SCC) number but it is possible to know percentage of "quarters" of mammary glands of cows affected in a herd by knowing "SCC" number which is given below in tabular farm:

Bulk milk somatic cell count (cells/ml)	Per cent infected quarters in herd	Per cent production loss
2,00,000 cells / ml	6	0
5,00,000 cells / ml	16	6
10,00,000 cells / ml	32	18
15,00,000 cells / ml	64	29
20,00,000 cells / ml	80	Not calculated
30,00,000 cells / ml	96	Not calculated

The records of composite herd milk (Bulk tank milk) Somatic Cell Counts (SCC) can be used for planned hygienic (Sanitation) programme for control of mastitis problem in each herd.

Treatment of mastitis

However, it is time consuming to specific antibiotic therapy after conducting antibiotic sensitivity test on the mastitis causing bacterial isolate obtained by culturing the milk samples from affected quarter(s) of the cow is the most logical approach for treatment of clinical mastitis in individual cow. However, this process is time consuming but it has an advantage that use of "low spectrum" antibiotic can be made for treatment which avoids development of resistance in causative organism against broad spectrum antibiotic which may not be needed when short spectrum antibiotic would have been actually effective. Now-a-days, continuous use of penicillin and blactum antibiotic has resulted in development of resistance against the same in mastitis causing bacteria including staphaureus isolates for which cloxacillin may be effective or use of new generation antibiotics like cephalosporin may be required to be done. Most of the coliforms may require use of gentamycin or new generation ciprofloxacin use of intramarry infusions (commercial tubes) as local treatment of individual quarter through leat canal injection is useful in clinical acute/subacute form of mastitis. Tetracyclins/Terramycin, etc. have now-a-days reduced efficacy due to development of resistance by causative organisms because of continuous use. Use of oxytoxin by parenteral injection for flushing of udder by complete striping of milk before intramammary antibiotic treatment of individual quarter is effective in reaching of antibiotic to the interior of affected tissue of affected gland for efficient therapeutic effect of antibiotic.

Use of cobalt chloride along with antibiotic during intramammary treatment helps in penetration of antibiotic deeply. Similarly, addition of anti-inflammatory non-steroidal drugs, such as "ibuprofen" or "Phenyl butazone" with intramammary antibiotic preparations is also helpful in combating mastitis by reducing the cellular migration of granulocytes to the site of mastitis inflammation.

Dry cow therapy

This is one of the best methods to get rid of most of the mastitis problems from the affected cows because the treatment of antibiotic is more effective, when milk production is at halt during dry period rather than carrying out the same during lactation. Moreover, the problem of withdrawal of milk of antibiotic treated cow from the supply for human consumption because of fear of antibiotic sensitivity to human consumer is not there during "dry period" of such cows.

It is necessary to treat the cow immediately after drying, with very high dose of "antibiotic" by intramammary infusion containing "slow release" vehicle. This slow release of antibiotic removes the residual mastitis causing infectious agent effectively and it also "prevents" the "re-infection" of the mammary gland through teat canal. Use of antibiotics like cloxacilin (nafeillin) and cephalosporin in high dose (with slow release base) during dry therapy effectively act against b-lactum producing streptoylococcus aureus strepto agalactine, streptodysgalactiae and corynae bacterium pyogenes and have 80% curative effect on streptococcal infections and 60% effect on staph infections.

Use of adjuvants for non-specific immunity against mastitis

Cytokines are immunity stimulants which when combined with dry period antibiotic therapies have improved recovery chances of mastitis. Combination of commercial "Cephapirin" with recombinant interleukin-2 has improved the chances of recovery from mastitis by 20-30% as compared to cephapirin alone (Daley *et al.*, 1992).

Vaccines against mastitis

Not much progress in development of vaccines against mastitis has been achieved due to multiplicity of causative micro-organisms. However, vaccine against *E. coli,* namely R. mutane *E. coli* strain 0111: B4 (J5) was found to be useful in prevention of clinical mastitis produced by *E. coli* or many other gram negative mastitis producing organisms but it cannot stop sub clinical infections. This vaccine is commercially available in U.S. More than 50% of large herds and more than 20% of general size dairy herds are vaccinated by this vaccine in U.S.A. (Morin *et al.*, 1998).

Indian scenario

Even though, mastitis in cows and buffaloes was existing in India since ancient time no systematic records of its existence are available, as indigenous cows are poor milk yielders and dairy was not an organized business prior to independence. However, Govt. of India undertook crossbreeding programme and Dairy development programme during 1st and 2nd five year plan period and buffalo breeding was also undertaken at Arey Milk Colony was also undertaken at Arey Milk Colony systematically. Bombay Veterinary College developed its bacteriological laboratory facilities during early sixties. During this period, Disease Investigation Section M.S. Poona undertook Diagnostic centre for mastitis and some bacteriological investigation of mastitis was taken up under this scheme during mid-sixties of 20th century. Early isolates of mastitis milk samples yielded streptococcus agalactiae, streptodisgalactiae and streptouberis infections. However, in late sixties, staph aureus and staph albus as well as less important staph citrus were isolated. This shift was probably due to development of resistance to intramammary penicillin (Ambistrin) treatment to streptococcal infection. Occasionally corynobact pyogenes was also found.

Author (Dr. S.V. Pandit) became in-charge of diagnostic centre for mastitis at D.I.S. M.S. Poona during 1970-71 periods. He developed facilities for better diagnosis of mastitis by starting various tests including Hottis test, catalase test, sodium/chloride estimation, bacterial counts, somatic cell counts, and also undertook survey work for mastitis incidence using California mastitis test (imported kits). He could demonstrate that use of penicillin streptomycin containing intramammary infusions were time barred and invalid for curing mastitis due to development of resistance against staph infection. Use of cloxicillin Terramycin/Auriomycin adjuncted with infusion of cobalt chloride, trypain and anti-inflammatory corticosteroids was advocated.

During Early Eighties Author (S.V. Pandit) while working at BAIF'S Diagnostic centres at some sugar factories which were working for giving health cover of BAIF'S crossbreeding programme, developed facilities for detection of mastitis incidence in small crossbred herds of farmers by providing "CMT" test facility on bulk milk samples received at milk collection centre (s) of sugar factories milk processing plants (such as at Pravara nagar and Malegaon taluka Baramati). The author developed commercial CMT reagent and CMT test paddle for the above programmes and for commercial use during working as R& D In-charge at BAIF, Wagholi.

Suggested Reading

Bartlett, P.C., Miller, G.Y., Lance, S.E. and L.E. Heider. (1992). Environmental and managerial determinants of somatic cell counts and clinical mastitis incidence in Ohio dairy herds. Prev. Vet. Med. 14: 195–207.

Cooray, R. (1994). Use of bovine myeloperoxidase as an indicator of mastitis in dairy cattle. Vet. Microbiol. 42(4): 317-26.

Daley, J.M., Fruda, G., Dougherty, R., Coyle, P.A., Williams, T.J., Johnston, P. (1992). Potentiation of antibiotic therapy for bovine mastitis by recombinant bovine interleukin-2. J. Dairy Sci. 75: 3330–3338.

Fox, L.K., Gay, J.M. (1993). Contagious mastitis. Vet Clin North Am Food Anim Pract. 9: 475–487.

Gröhn, Y.T., S.W. Eicker & J.A. Hertl. (1995). The association between previous 305-day milk yield and disease in New York State dairy cows. Journal of Dairy Science, 78: 1693-1702.

Miltenburg, J.D., DeLange, D., Crauwels, A.P.P. (1996). Incidence of clinical mastitis in a random sample of dairy herds in the Southern Netherlands Vet Rec 139: 204-207.

Milner, P., Page, K.L., Walton, A.W., Hillerton, J.E. (1996). Detection of clinical mastitis by changes in electrical conductivity of foremilk before visible changes in milk. J. Dairy Sci. 79: 83-86.

Morin, D.E., Constable, P.D., McCoy, G.C. (1998). Use of clinical parameters for differentiation of gram-positive and gram-negative mastitis in dairy cows vaccinated against lipopolysaccharide core antigens. J Am Vet Med Assoc. 212: 1423–1431.

Oliver, S.P. & Juneja, V.K. (1990). Growth of Corynebacterium bovis in mammary secretions during physiological transition of the bovine mammary gland. J. Dairy Sci. 73: 351-356.

□□□

Chapter 37

Strangles in Equines

Strangles is a highly contagious bacterial disease of horses, donkeys and mules which has worldwide occurence, caused by *Streptococcus equi* and is characterized by emphyema of guttural poches, caseous lymphadenopathy and mucopurulent rhinitis.

About the causative bacterial agent

Streptococcus equi, the causative agent is a gram positive coccobacillus which produces a b-haemolysin which is evident by production of a clear haemolytic zone surrounding colonies growing on blood agar at 37^0C under aerobic conditions. The organism is highly host adapted to equidae and its virulence is related to the amount of M-protein and hyaduronic capsule produced by it. A capsule deficient variant produces a milder disease (Tiamoney, 1993).

Epidemiology and disease transmission

This is a highly contagious disease affecting horses of all age groups, especially young animals. The causative agent is an obligate parasite of horses and the infection is transmitted from infected animals to other animals either directly or through fomites. The Nasal discharge from abscesses contaminate pasture, stalls, feed and water troughs, grooming instruments and the veterinarien himself or Grooms clothes and are responsible for spread of infection through contact.

Recovered animals may have persistant infection of str. equi, in their pharynx and guttural pouches for many months, which is an important source of infection (Newton *et al.,* 1997). About 25% recovered animals are susceptible for re-infection (Hamlen *et al.* 1994; Newton *et al.,* 1997). Presence of antibodies to streptococcal M. Protein in the nasopharynx is important in conferring immunity to the disease (Timoney, 1993).

Pathogenesis

Following exposure of naso pharynx to the pathogens, organisms lodge in pharyngeal and tonsillar lymphoid tissues where they multiply and subsequent migration of the neutrophils containing organisms in their cytoplasm via lymphatics to the lymph-nodes draining the area causes swelling and abscess formation with associated disruption of lymph drainage and development of oedema in tissues drained by the affected nodes. Swelling of retropharyngeal lymph-nodes interferes with deglutition and respiration. Most of the abscesses subsequently rupture and drain and infection gets resolved due to development of effective immunity. Nasal shedding begins 4-7 days after infection to persist for variable period.

Death is usually caused by aspiration of infected abscess-discharge resulting into pneumonia. Chronic disease can follow due to metastatic infection (Bastard strangles) of heart valves, brain, eyes and joints, tendon sheaths and other vital organs resulting into eventual death.

Symptoms and Postmortem lesions

After incubation period of 1 to 3 days weeks, complee anorexia, depression, fever upto 105^{0}F, severe nasal discharge, becoming mucopurulent, severe pharyngitis and laryngitis develops along with conjunctivitis.

The affected lymph-nodes in throat region are hot swollen and painful. Dyspnoea and disphagia follows resulting into death by asphyxiation in some cases. The affected retropharyngeal lymph-nodes start exudation of serum by 10th day and repture to discharge thick creamy yellow pus. The whole course runs for about 3 weeks and severe cases may last for as long as 3 months. Exudative lymphadenopathy especially in the lower limbs occurs with oedema and abscession in other organs some time. 20% of cases may show complications including fatal suppurative necrotic Broncho-pneumonia and Empyema of guttural pouches and metastatic absceses in any organ or body site like lungs, mesenteric lymph-nodes, liver, spleen, kidneys and brain, heart valves, myocarditis, joints, bones and teudon sheaths, etc. Purpura haemorrhagica may also develop as sequelae (Sweeney *et al.*, 1987).

Diagnosis

Isolation of strepto equi from nasopharyngeal swabs and discharge from abscesses will confirm the diagnosis of strangles.

Treatment

Penicillin–G or procaine 22000 IU/kg body wt. by 1/m route every 12 hours is quite effective treatment. Tetracycline (mg/kg body wt.) intravenously every 12-24 hours and sulphonamide trimethoprim combination (15-30 mg/kg) orally or I/V route every 12 hours may be efficarious but should only be used, if Penicillin is found ineffective. The treatment should start in early stage of infection to be successful.

Control

To prevent the transmission of the disease, infected horses should be isolated and treated separately. Beddings and brooms, and feed and other materials in contact of the infected horses should be burnt.

Theraputic treatment should be used for prophylaxis in case of valuable uninfected animals in contact to avoid precipitation of disease presuming that these animals are in incubation period. Newly introduced animals should be quarantined for 3 weeks before mixing them in the other healthy animals on the form Foals should be given adequate "colostrum" feeding from the vaccinated mothers or other females recovered from disease to provide maternal immunity.

Vaccination

Inactivated bacterin containing high titred M protein (capsular) of *Strepto equi.* given 3 times at 2 weeks intervals, with further administration of the same vaccine every 6 months is used to get good protective results. Vaccination of mares during last 4-6 weeks of gestation period followed by vaccination of foal at 2-3 months age reduces the incidence of disease. There are reports of occurence of purpura haemorrhagica as side effect of protein containing Bacterins. An intra-nasal vaccine of an avirulent live strain of strequi is recently developed but efficacy of the field results is yet awaited.

Strangles in equines: Indian scenario

The disease is present in India in race horses but no much literature is available for presentation.

Suggested Reading

Hamlen, H.J., Timoney, J.F., Bell, R.J. (1994). Epidemiologic and immunologic characteristics of *Streptococcus equi* infection in foals. J Am Vet Med Assoc., 204: 768–775.

Newton, J.R., Wood, J.L., Dunn, K.A., DeBrauwere, M.N.(1997). Chanter N. Naturally occurring persistent and asymptomatic infection of the guttural pouches of horses with *Streptococcus equi*. Vet Rec.; 140: 84–90.

Newton, J.R., Wood, J.L..N, Chanter, N. (1997). Strangles: Long term carriage of *Streptococcus equi* in horses. Equine Vet Educ., 9: 98–102.

Sweeney, C., Benson, C., Whitlock, R. (1987). *Streptococcus equi* infections in horses (part 2). Compend Equine., 9: 845–851.

Timoney, J.F. (1993). Strangles. Veterinary Clinics of North America, Equine Practice, 9: 365–374.

❏❏❏

Chapter 38

Swine Erysepelas

Swine erysepelas is an acute or chronic infectious bacterial disease of swine characterized by septicaemia in acute form of the disease with typical diamond shaped skin lesions and chronic form characterized by local arthritic lesions or endocarditis, caused by bacterial organism named as *Erysipelothrix rhusiopathiae*.

About the causative organism

The causative organism *Erysipelothrix rhusiopathiae* is a gram positive filamentous organism with haemolytic character, when grown on blood agar medium. There are 22 serotypes of the organism, out of which only serotype 1 and 2 are commonly found associated with clinical acute form of the disease in swines. Serotypes 1a, 3,5,6,8, 11 and 21 and type N has been isolated from chronic arthritic and lymphadenitic form of the disease. Serotype 7 is resident of tonsil of swine.

Epidemiology and transmission of the disease

Swine erysipelas occurs worldwide and produces economic loss due to mortality and carcass rejection in slaugher house due to arthritis and endocarditis.

The prevalence of infection in carrier pigs ranges from 3 to 98% (20 to 40% pigs are carries on an average), both vaccinated and unvaccinated animals can be carrying the virus in their tonsils (Takahashi *et al.*, 1987) young pigs in contact with "Carrier" sows rapidly acquire the status of "Carrier" and "Shedders" organisms from tonsils pass through stomach and intestines unaffected and thus, become continuous source of soil contamination. The organisms remain alive for several months in faeces and thus, suvage effluent from the piggery remains constant source of infection. Under natural conditions, skin abrasions and the alimentary tract mucosa are the portals of entry for these pathogens through ingestion of the contaminated feed or soil contamination of abrased skin. Pigs of all age groups are susceptible but low virulent strains can only affect adult pigs, especially recently farrowed sows are more susceptible. Piglets from an immune sow may get sufficient antibodies in colostrums to resist infection. Serotypes 1,1a and 2 are more virulent strains which produce septicaemic disease while serotypes 3,5,6,8,11, and N produce local arthritic disease.

Pathogenesis

Invasion of blood stream occurs via. skin abrasion or via alimentary mucosa in all cases of infection. Further septicaemia in organs or localization in Joints depends on characteristics of strain of pathogen. "Coagulase activity" of strain is responsible for septicaemia. Concurrant Hog Cholera virus infection increases the susceptibility of the animal.

In chronic form localisation occurs in skin, joints or on heart valves with subsequent bacteremic episodes. Selective adherence factor of some strains of the pathogen is responsible for "heart valve" affection of endocarditis form". Arthritic lesions develop probably due to "hypersensitivity" to the causative organism or other antigen. There are increased level of immunoglobulins Ig G and Ig M in the synovial fluid of pigs with polyarthritis due to this causative agent and are considered to be due to serum and increased permeability (Timoney and Groschup, 1993).

Zoonotic implications

Veterinarians are exposed to infection, when vaccinating with virulent strains cultures and they thus, become potentially susceptible to Erycepelas infection.

Symptoms and postmortem lesions

Acute form of the disease is characterized by 1-7 days of incubation period after which development of high fever upto 108^{0}F, followed by severe prostration, complete anorexia, thirst and vomiting, development of marked red to purple discolouration of skin of jaw and ventral surface, inco-ordination in walking, conjnctivities, skin lesions are almost pathogomic with diamond shaped red urticarial plaques or more diffuse oedematous eruptions with the same appearance. Pigs die after 2-3 days of illness with almost upto 75% mortality. In skin form, the above mentioned skin lesions are more marked but other lesions may be absent. In chronic form, alopecia, sloughing of tail and tips of ears, hyperkeratosis and dermatitis with lesions of joints of elbow, hips, shoulder, stitle, hock and knee showing enlargement & pain. Endocarditis (with or without arthritis) with sudden death can occur.

Postmortem lesions include skin lesions as above, wide spread ecchymotic haemorhages on kidney surface, venous infarction of stomach non-suppurative proliferative Arthritis, vegetative endocarditis are characteristic.

Diagnosis

In acute disease, blood smear examination may reveal typical gram netative filamentous organisms especially in leukocytes but blood culture will be more successful method for detection of organisms. In chronic form, repeated exam of blood smear is needed for chance detection of organisms. Final identification of organisms necessitates mouse or pigeon inoculation and "Serum protection" test in these animals using known positive Anti-erycepelas immune serum. Haematological exam reveals leukocytosis followed by leukopenia in later stages. CFT is more accurate diagnostic test but ELISA test is much quicker.

Treatment

50,000 units/kg body wt. Procaine penicillin intramuscular for 3 days is useful in acute cases but chronic cases do not respond properly to treatment. Use of Anti-Erycepelas serum prepared as per British Vet. Codex standards may be useful for therapeutic effect.

Control

Eradication is not possible, as organisms are eubiqutous.Serum simultaneous method of vaccination using preparations of bacterins containing lysates and absorbates may be useful. Vaccination at 6-10 weeks of age followed by booster vaccination at 10-14 weeks age may be used.

Swine Erycepelas: Indian scenario

Sporadic incidence of swine erycepelas came to light, when outbreaks of swine fever were recorded for the first time in India during early 1960's-62. However, no much information on incidence is available.

Suggested Reading

Takahashi, T., Sawada, T., Muramatsu, M., Tamura, Y., Fujisawa, T., Benno, Y., Mitsuoka, T. (1987). Serotype, antimicrobial susceptibility, and pathogenicity of *Erysipelothrix rhusiopathiae* isolates from tonsils of apparently healthy slaughter pigs. J. Clin. Microbiol. 25: 536–539.

Timoney, J.F., and Groschup, M.M. (1993). Properties of a protective protein antigen of Erysipelothrix rhusiopathiae. Vet Microbiol 37: 381-387.

❑❑❑

Chapter 39

Campylobacter Infections (Vibriosis) in Cattle and Sheep

Campilobacter infections (previously called vibriosis) in cattle and sheep are bacterial infections caused by campylobacter species and are characterized by abortions stillbirths and enteritis.

About the causative agent

Compylobacter foetus var venerealis is the causative agent of infertility and abortions in cattle. *Vibrio foetus* is a gram positive comma shaped organism found in singles and is aerobic and faculatative anaerobic in nature and requires 5% carbon dioxide tension for cultivation (Microaerophilic) as well as serum for its growth.

Other species of campylobacter, namely *C. Jejuni* and *C. coli* are inhabitants of intestinal tract of cattle, sheep and goats and play a role in producing afebrile infection with enteritis in farm animals.

Mode of transmission and epidemiology

The organisms present in foetal membranes and placentae and in faeces of infected animals contaminate water supplies and pasture and contaminated pastures/water is responsible for oral infection and subsequent disease.

Pathogenesis

Necrotizing and suppurative placentis results in still birth suppurative vescibulitis and endometritis of the aborted cow. The C. jejuni/coli strains produce severe gastro enteritis.

Symptoms and postmortem lesions

Vibrio foetus (*C. foetus*) causes abortions in period of late jestation (last trimester of pregnancy) with retaintion of placental and endometritis in cow resulting into further problems of infertility. Abortion and severe gastroenteritis can be even caused by strains of campylobacter jajuni/coli haemorrhagic erosive enteritis and gastritis may be present in abomasum and Jejunum.

Diagnosis

Demonstration of common shaped gram positive organisms in impression organ-smears from aborted foetus or from placental material from aborted cow confirms the diagnosis of vibrosis after biological test of the material in guinea pigs.

An adaptation of the ELISA test is available for detection of antibodies to campylobacter species for use in sero-epidemiological studies in herds of cattle and sheep (Altekruse *et al.*, 1994).

Treatment and control

Carbadox, Gentamycin and Dimetridazole are most active drugs. Clavurlanate potential amoxicillin is also effective. A vaccine containing *C. foectus* and *C. jejuni* and *S.dublin* has been used to control abortios in sheep (Hansen *et al.*, 1990).

Campylobacter (Vibrio) foetus abortions in cattle : Indian Scenario

Prof. Sane C.R. (Prof. of Gynaecology, Bombay Vet. College) recorded the 1st incidence of *Vibrio foetus* abortion in cattle in 1954. However, no much work of incidences of abortions/enteritis due to *C. foetus/C. jejuni* is found in the Indian Vet. Literature after that incidence.

Suggested Reading

Altekruse, S.F, Hunt, J.M., Tollefson, L.K., Madden, J.M. (1994). Food and animal sources of human Campylobacter jejuni infection. J Am Vet Med Assoc. 204: 57–61.

Hansen, D.E., Hedstrom, O.R., Sonn, R.J., Snyder, S.P. (1990). Efficacy of a vaccine to prevent *Chlamydia* or *Campylobacter*-induced abortions in ewes. J Am Vet Med Assoc. 196: 731–734.

□□□

Chapter 40

Bovine Theileriosis

Bovine theileriosis is an arthropod born protozon disease of bovines caused by *Theilera annulata* in India, parts of Asia and Mediterenean countries and is characterized by lymphadenopathy, Panlaukemia on one hand and haemolytic anaemia with icterous on the other hand. Similar protozoon disease is caused by theilera parva in East coast of Africa, wherein anaemia with icterus is lacking but lymphadopathy is predominant.

About the causative agent of the disease

Theileria annulata is an apicomplex protozoon parasite of class sporozoa and is belonging to the order "Piroplasmida". *Theileria annulata* is transmitted by a tick vector, namely *Hyalomma anatolicum* and *Hyalomm a dendriticum*, former is 3 host thick and later is a 2 host tick.

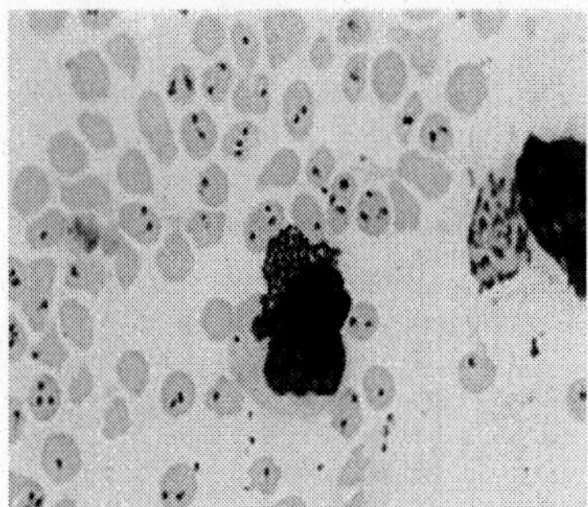

Fig. 1: Bovine *Theileria* spp.

Lifecycle

The lifecycle of theilerial parasite occurs partly in tick vector and partly in host animal. Developmental stages in tick vector are transmitted transistadially through the stages of the vector, namely larva, nymph and adult but transovarian transmission is absent. Thus, when tick larva, nymph or adult suck blood of "infected" host animal transformed merozoites (piroplasm stage) present in animals red blood cells are ingested by ticks. They undergo several developmental stages and eventually form "sporozoites" in salivary glands of ticks. This part of lifecycle of the parasite in ticks developmental stages in "sexual" part of lifecycle of the parasite. Ticks must feed for 2-4 days before sporozoites in their salivary gland will mature to become "infective" to cattle. Even one tick is sufficient for infecting cattle with sufficient no. of "sporozoites" to cause fatal infection in susceptible animal.

The infective matured sporozoites then enter lymphocytes of cattle and develop "schizonts of 1st generation" in the lymph-node draining the area of attachment of the tick. "Infected lymphocytes" are then transformed to "lymphoblasts" which continue to divide almost synchronously along with "schizonts" contained in them, so that the daughter lymphocytes are also infected with 2nd generatio schizonts. Merozoites produced by 1st generation schizonts infected lymphocytes are disseminated through out the lymphoid system of the body of cattle schizonts of 2nd generation produce, 2nd generation meroziote which invade erythrocytes (RBCS). These merozoites in RBCS get transformed into "piroplasms" which are "infective" to ticks.

When ticks (larvae, nymphs or adult ticks) get attached on animal body and suck blood of infected host cattle, infected RBCS containing piroplasms (transformed infective merozoites) are also injected by them, which undergo several developmental stages in the body of ticks, including "Gametogony" and eventually form sporozoites in the salivary glands of ticks, as mentioned previously. This completes the "lifecycle" of theilerial parasite (See Fig. 1).

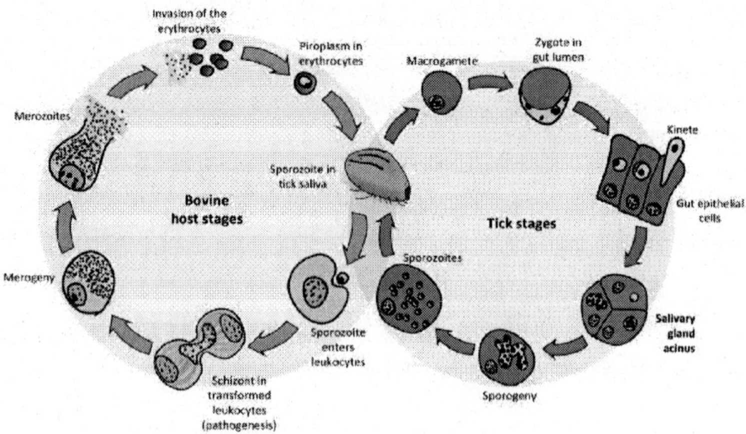

Fig. 2: Lifecycle of Theileria

Epidemiology and transmission of Theileria annulata

Theilera annulata is transmitted by 2 host tick (Hyaloma anatolicum or 3 host tick (Hyaloma dendriticum), as mentioned previously and "sexual lifecycle" is completed by the protozoon parasite in ticks while the asexual part of lifecycle is completed by the theilerial protozoon in the host animals. These developmental stages of the protozoon parasite occur in the tick and they pass trans-steadially the stages of larvae, nymph and adult but there is no trans-ovarian transmission. Consequently, larvae or nymphs become infected and transmit the infection as nymphs or adults. Mechanical transmission is of no significance. The epidemiology of the disease is, thus largely dependent on the distribution and habit of the tick and its ability to complete cyclical development. Ticks may live longer for 1 to 2 years but they loose their infection within 11 months.

In endemic areas, virtually all adult animals are infected but mortality rate is very low. In India, majority of the indigenous cattle is in this category and they almost never show any clinical disease unless otherwise they get immune suppressed due to the concurrent disease like BVD or Rinderpest. But the European cattle breeds like jersy or Holstein frezian and their indigenous crossbreeds recently introduced, may have 20 to 90% mortality due to theileriosis. The disease occurs mainly in summer, when tick activity is increased. Buffaloes may act as carriers of the disease parasite. The immunity is cell mediated but is poor in calves.

Pathogenesis

In case of *Theileria parava* infection (East coast fever) in African continent, the diamage is caused by schizonts in lymphocytes and the disease is characterized by lymphadenopathy only while in Asia and especially in India, Theileria annulata infection is characterized by both lymphedenopathy caused by schizonts in lymphocytes as well as haemolytic anaemia and icterus (Jaundice) caused by haemolysis effected by piroplasms (matured merozoites) in RBCS as over 90% RBCS are parasitized. In case of *Theileria parva* infection, there is very high level of immune suppression caused by lymphadenopathy.

In *Theileria annulata* infection in India, immune-suppression occurs in acute phase but is less marked than in case of East Coast Fever (ECF) probably due to the fact that leukocyte numbers return to normal soon after the acute phase. (Sharpe and Langley, 1983).

Symptoms and postmortem lesions

In a stable endemic situation, there may be no clinical disease in local Zebu (indigenous cattle). Clinical signs in exotic animals may last for weeks before death (Jacquiet, 1994).

The clinical signs include enlaragement of lymph-nodes draining the area of site of tick attachment 18 to 16 days after the tick attachment. One or two days later, there is high fever, depression, anorexia and drop in milk production. In later part, nasal and ocular discharges, dyspnea generalized lymph-node enlargement and splenomegaly may occur. Anaemia develops within few days and mucous membranes will become icteric. Diarrhoea and weight loss may develop later on.

Masssive pulmonary oedema, hyperemia and lung emphysema alongwith hydrothorax and hydropericardium may be revealed during postmortem examination. Copious froth is present in bronchii and trachaea haemorrhages, icherus and anaemia is evident in many tissues and organs. Enlargement of liver, lymph-nodes and spleen is marked.

Lymph-node impression smears will reveal typical schizonts in cytoplasm of lymphocytes, when stained with giema stain and examined microscopically.

Diagnosis

Examination of blood and lymph-node smears will reveal presence of typical schizonts in lymphocytes and presence of "piroplasms" either centrally or periferally located in RBCS, when stained with giemsa stain.

Schizonts of *T. annulata* are more commonly observed predominantly in liver impressions/sections as compared to lymph-nodes "Piroplasms" of *T. annulata* are more "rounded" or "oval" and centrally placed as compared to those of T. parva which are comma or rod shaped and placed at periphery of RBCS.

Reduction of W.B.C. count is less severe in East Coast Fever (ECF) compared with disease caused by *T. annulata* but lymphopenia (mainly T. lymphtocytophenia) is more severe in ECF compared to T. annulata infection (Preston *et al.*, 1992).

Treatment

"Byparvaquone" is the most effective chemotherapeutic agent which is recommended in the dose of 2.5 mg per k.g. body wt. (Sharma and Mishra, 1990). Tetracyclins were recommended as treatment for many years but they were only moderately effective. Halofuginone lactate has a much higher success rate in 2 doses 1.2 mg/kg body wt in curing clinical cases but the animals remain as "Carriers" (Morrison, 1986).

Control

Indigenous cattle do not need any intensive tick control programme as they live with the infection. For exotic animals, vaccination and strategic tick control are recommended. Vaccine can be produced from either sporozoites or schizonts. The sporozoite vaccination is based on "infection and treatment" method, using pre-fed ticks and simultaneous tetracycline treatment. In India, this methods was in use in immunization of calves and "buparvaquone" was reserved for treating the clinical cases (Singh *et al.*, 1993).

The "Schizont" vaccine was blood containing a mild strain of the parasite. "NDDB burrows welcome" produced live vaccine containing schizonts grown on lymphoid cell culture and attenuated by prolonged cell culture passaging. This vaccine has no adverse effect and immunity lasts for 3.5 years as per their claim.

Indian scenario

Indian zebu cattle and buffaloes were known to harbor *T.annulata* infection since past centuries but were not known to produce any clinical disease.

However, after introduction of exotic H.F. and Jersy cattle in India for crossbreeding programme the disease "theileriosis" started producing severe clinical disease and Nineteen sixties and seventies experienced severe theileriosis problem with high mortality in affected exotic animals.

BAIF scientists tried to produce vaccine by establishment of lymphoblastoid cell culture technique without any success. They even tried to study similar established technology from Razi Institute, Tehran, but the attempts could not be successful.

NDDB (National Dairy Development Board), Anand Scientists got technology from Burrows welcome laboratory, wey bridge, U.K. and successfully launched "schizent" based vaccine produced on lymphoblastoid cell culture. This vaccine is found very effective in protecting valuable exotic and crossbred animals.

Suggested Reading

Jacquiet, P. (1994) rev. elev. Med. Vet. Pays. Trop, 47: 147.

Morrison, W.I. (1986). The Ruminant Immuno system in health and disease ed. Cambridge University Press pp. 555.

Preston, P.M., Brown, C.G., Bell-Sakyi L., Richardson, W., Sanderson, A. (1992). Tropical theileriosis in Bos taurus and *Bos taurus* cross *Bos indicus* calves: response to infection with graded doses of sporozoites of *Theileria annulata*. Res Vet Sci. 53: 230–243.

Sharpe, R.T. & Langley, A.M. (1983). The effect of Theileria annulata infection on the immune response of cattle to foot-and-mouth disease. Br. Vet. J., 139: 378-385.

Sharma, N.N. and Mishra, A.K. (1990). Treatment of bovine tropical theileriosis with buparvaquone. Trop. Anim. Health Prod., 22: 63-65.

Singh, J., Gill, J. S.; Kwatra, M. S. and Sharma, K.K. (1993).Treatment of theileriosis in crossbred calves in Punjab, India. Tropical Animal Health and Production, 25: 75-78.

□□□

Chapter 41

Babesiosis of Cattle, Sheep and Horses (Cattle Tick Fever / Red Water Fever)

Babesiosis is an arthrapod borne protozoal disease of cattle, sheep and horses characterized by haemolytic anaemia, haemoglobinuria and Jaundice and is transmissible through tick vector in domesticated and wild animals.

About the causative agent

Babesia bigemina / babesia bovis is an apicomptex protozoon parasite belonging to the class sporozoa and order piroplasmida.

Both *Babesia bigemina* and *Babesia bovis* are infections of tropics and subtropics. *B. bigemina* occurs in South America, West Indies, Australia, Africa and India while *B. bovis* occurs in Europe, South America and Africa. Both *B. bigemina* and *B. bovis* cause cattle tick fever and red water disease in cattle while *B. equi* and *B. cabali* cause disease in equines in Southern Europe, Asia and America. *B. motasi* and *B. ovis* cause disease in ovines.

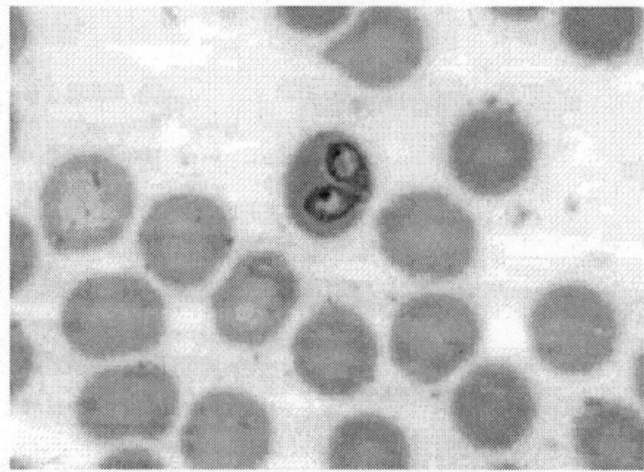

Fig. 1: *Babesia bigemina*

The infective stages of *B.bigemina* and *B. bovis* are found in pairs in red blood cells of cattle in peripheral/visceral blood vessels and are piryform in shape. Sexual cycle of the parasite probably occurs in vector ticks body and salivary glands as in case of thialerial protozoon parasites. While asexual cycle occurs in spleen and Red blood cells of the vertibrate host.

About the vectors

Ticks are the natural vectors of babesia. They persist and pass through part of their lifecycle in the invertebrate tick hosts. *B. bovis* and *B. bigemia* pass part of their lifecycle in the tick *Boophilus microplus* and *Boophilus annulatus* B. Ovis is transmitted through Rhipicephalus and *Haemophysalis punctata* species feeding on sheep and Dermacentre, *Rhipicephalus* and *Hyaloma* species on horses transmit B.caballi and B. equi.

Epidemiology and Transmission of Babesiasis

Viable protozoa (*B. bigerima* and other Babesia species) are present only in the blood stream of animals in the active stages of infection and they pass through part of their lifecycle in invertebrate host ticks. When adult animals become infected through tick bite, they act as carriers for variable periods upto 2 years. If they are constantly re-infected, as in case of endemic areas, they remain carriers throughout their life. One host ticks cause less spread of the disease and are easier to eradicate than two host/three host ticks. Control of ticks which feed both on domestic as well as wild animals are difficult to eradicate.

B. bovis persists in engorged tick Boophilus microplus "adult" after infection from cattle. Through "transovarial" passage their larvae get infected and remain infective during their active stage but the infective parasitic stage is not passed or transmitted further to "nymphal" phase of the vector. Babesia bigemina and *B. caballi* do persist through several generations of ticks in *Boophilus microplus* and *Dermacentre* species. *Babesia bigemina* and *Babesia bovis* are transmitted transovarially in *Boophilus annulatus*.

Immunity and susceptibility to infection

Immune mechanism in this infection is of complex nature. Natural infection of Babesia species imparts strong immunity in the host animal and if infection recurs repeatedly, immunity is life-long. But if infection is treated immediately in earlier stage, immunity is not produced at all and if infection is not repeated, immunity lasts only for 6 months and disappears later on. A "sterile immunity" persists for 6 months further and the host is susceptible again about a year after infection occurred. These periods of latent infection and resistance to re-infections are subject to significant variations.

Pathogenesis

When animal becomes infected through infected tick bite and multiplication of the protozoon parasite in peripheral blood vessels (*B. bigemina* / *B. ovis*) or in visceral vessels (*B. bovis*) reaches a peak with the development of clinically detectable haemolysis, after an incubation period of 7-20 days, which results into profund anaemia, jaundice and haemoglobinuria. This results into fatal outcome due to anaemic anoxia. If not, surviving animal shows ischemic changes in skeletal and heart muscle. In *B.bovis* infection profound vasodilatation and hypotension, increase in vascular permeability circulatory stasis and shock follows disseminated intravascular coagulation and resultant fatal pulmonary thrombosis occurs. *B. bigemina* in uncomplicated haemolytic agent and vascular and coagulating effects do not occur in this infection. Calves upto 5-6 months age are less susceptible to *B. bigemina* / *B. bovis* infection as compared to animals of 1-2 years and of higher age. Adults suffer more severely.

Animals surviving the infection become "Carriers" in which delicate immunological balance between protozoon and antibodies is maintained. Carrier animals become resistant to reinfection, which occurs in enzootic situation. In pregnant cow, no apparent infection occurs in the calf in utero but passive immunity is transferred to calf through colostrums after parturition.

Symptoms and postmortem lesions

Incubation period is 2-3 weeks. In young cattle, subclinical infections occur. Acute disease in characterized by onset of high fever (106^{0}F) anorexia, depression, weakness, cessation of rumination, fall of milk production, increased respiration and heart rate, brick red coloured conjunctive and mucous membranes soon changing to severe palor of anaemia. International stages, severe jaundice, coffee coloured urine with stable froth, diarrhoea are common symptoms. The febrile stage lasts for one week and total course of disease is 3 weeks. Abortion often takes place in pregnant animals. Anaemia leads to emaciation. Occasional cerebral babesiosis occurs leading to paresis, convulsions and mania. Typical lesions of acute death due to babesiosis include thin watery blood, extensive jaundice and paleness of tissues, spleenomegali, brown liver with gross enlargement, distanded gall bladder, enlarged kidneys, dark coloured urine in urinary bladder, haemorrhagic heart, with blood stained hydropericardium, severe intravascular clotting are the typical lesions found in postmortem of animal died with babesiosis.

Diagnosis

Characteristics symptoms with microscopic examination of blood smear from peripheral/visceral blood vessels, stained with giemsa stain revealed typical pyriform protozoon parasites in pairs arranged at an angle of 45^0 present in infected RBCS are quite diagnostic of Babesia infection. Thick blood smcars are recommended to detect large no. of infected RBCS in smears.

DNA probe or "PCR" are also available abroad for diagnosis but blood smear diagnosis is still a test for positive diagnosis in India. ELISA and CFT are also used abroad. Erythrocytic count as low as 2 million RBCS / ml and haemglobin level down to 3 g/dl are supportive tests to know the extent of hemolytic anaemia.

Treatment

Chemotheraputic treatment is useful only if it is carried out in early stage before RBC damage is extensive. Acaprin at a dose rate of 1 ml/50 kg B.W. (maximum 6 ml) or quinuronium sulphate at the same dose rate is safe and useful in treatment of cattle.

Babesian, Stilbamidine, propamidine, pheneramidine, Diampron are also well received by cattle for treatment by 9/m or 5/c route. Imidocarb (Imizol) at rate of 1 mg/kg B.W. completely eliminates infection without remaining in carrier stage. Blood transfusion is useful as supportive treatment.

Control

Eradication of bovine babesiosis depends on eradication of vector ticks but requires high cost.

To achieve limitations of prevalence at economically sustainable levels, requires different solutions in different circumstances as below:

1. Susceptible cattle moving into an enzootic area need prior vaccination.
2. Vaccinations before outbreak commences of forecast is available plus temporary chemoprophylasis after outbreaks have commenced is recommended.
3. Chemoprophylaxis against concurrent blood born infections like anaplosmosis is recommended, if co-current infection is present.

Vaccination

Attenuated vaccines are prepared by passaging the protozoon through susceptible. Speenectomised calves by exposure to irradiation or by repeated passage through tissue culture, thus these vaccine contain less virulent babesiae which are no longer infective to tick vector. Thus, cattle are less exposed to infection and hence, area in consistently effective because of wide fluctuations in the level of immunity produced. Vaccination concept is not practically followed in babesiosis as its utility is questionable.

Indian Scenario

Indigenous cattle and buffaloes are carriers of babesiosis (*B. bigemina*) without production of clinical symptoms. However, after introduction of cross breeding programme, the exotic cattle and cross bred animals when co-exit with the indigenous animals to B. bigenaina produce typical acute babesiosis sporadically in these animals. The high milk yielding indigenous cattle when come under stress, sporadic cases of acute babesiosis with typical coffee coloured urine and Jaundice/haemolytic anaemia develop. "Babesian" is a drug of choice for treatment of these cases in India.

Suggested Reading

Bose, R, Jorgensen, W.K., Dalgliesh, R.J., Friedhoff, K.T., De Vos, A.J. (1995). Current state and future trends in the diagnosis of babesiosis. Vet Parasitol 57(1-3): 61-74.

Papino, E. (1995).Live vaccines against haemoparasitic disease in livestock Vet. Parasital 57(1-3): 213-231.

□□□

Chapter 42

Anaplasmosis of Cattle, Sheep and Goats

Anaplasmosis is an arthropod borne disease of ruminants, characterized by anaemia, Jaundice and debilitation and is caused by Anaplasma organisms.

About the Causative Agent

Anaplasma was placed in the class sporozoa of protozoon parasites in the text books written before 1960, However, now Anaplasma species are described as obligate intraerythrocytic bacterial parasites belonging to the order Rickettsiales and infecting ruminants, *Anaplasma marginale* is the causative agent in cattle and wild ruminants, *Anaplasma ovis* in sheep and goats while *Anaplasma centrals* is closely related to *A. marginale* and causes mild anaplasmosis in cattle. There are antigenic variants among isolates of *A. marginale*, the surface proteins being antigenically polymorphic (Oberle, *et al.*, 1988).

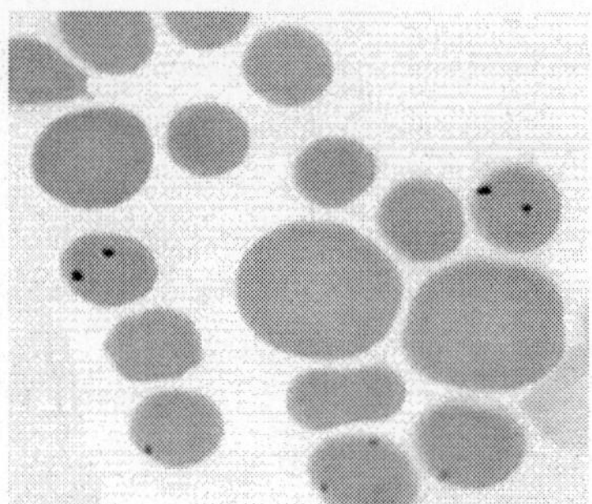

Fig. 1: *Anaplasma marginale* in blood smear

A. marginale and *A. centrale* occurs in cattle but it can get established in sheep experimentally. However, *A. ovis* cannot infect cattle many species of wild ruminants in Africa and North America get infected with A. marginale and become reservoir of disease (Jorgensen *et al.*, 1993).

Epidemiology and Transmission

Anaplasmosis occurs in all the six continents of the world, namely South Africa, Austrelia, Asia, USSR, South America and United States. Infection in cattle is endemic in tropics and subtropics. The disease is transmitted by diverse group of biological and mechanical vectors. The source of infection is always the blood of infected animals, recovery from acute infection results into persistent infection with repetitive cycles of rickettsemia. Thus, persistent carriers are the reservoirs of herd infection.

Significant natural vectors are ticks in the family Ixodidae and flies in the family Tabanidae. Boophilus species in tropical and sub-tropical regions (one host tick) and Dermacentre (3 host tick) in Western U.S. are important vectors transmitting the Anaplasma infection.

The organisms undergo a complex developmental cycle in the gut cells of ticks while final infective stage is present in the salivary glands of ticks. Transstadial transmission occurs in ticks but no trans-ovarian transmission is proved. Transmission occurs as the tick moves from one host to another while they are engorging including from cow to calf (Stiller and Coan, 1995). However, *Tabanidae* flies are mechanical transmitter of the disease. Disease can also get mechanically transmitted through blood transfusions.

Pathogenesis

After tick or Tabanid fly bite, Anaplasma infect mature erythrocytes by an endocytic process and their reproduction occurs by binary fission to produce 2-8 infective initial bodies which leave by exocytasis to infect other erythrocytes. The number of infected erythrocytes doubles every 24-48 hours and the infection becomes patent 2-4 weeks after infection.Parasitised erythrocytes are removed by Phagocytosis in the reticular endothelial system with release of acute phase inflammatory reactants and consequent development of fever phagocytic removal of parasitized erythrocytes is responsible for the development of haemolytic anaemia without development of haemoglobinuria, which is characteristics of Anaplasmosis, as opposed to Babesiosis, in which both haemolytic anaemia along with haemoglobinuria also occurs, as released haemoglobin from blood is removed out of body through urine. In Anaplasmosis, haemoglobin is removed by scavenging phagocytes of reticulo endothelial system.The appearance of antierythrocyte antibiotic late in the acute stage may exacerbate the anaemia (Richey and Palmer, 1990). The cattle surviving the acute phase of the disease become carriers and act as reservoir of the disease. Cycles of parasitemia are associated with development of new antigenic variant of the organisms to allow new cycles of invasion and perpetuation of the disease.

Symptoms and Lesions

The disease is characterized by slow rise of temperature upto 105^{0}F for one to two weeks, Anorexia, emaciation and death. Surviving animals may exhibit impaired fertility. Mucous membranes are anaemic and jaundiced but no haemoglobinuria. Animals may become hyper excitable before death. Liver is enlarged, kidneys are congested and myocardial haemorrhages may occur. Bone marrow shows increased haemopoitetic tissue. Spleen is enlarged.

Diagnosis

Blood smears show presence of typical rod shaped or comma shaped single organisms placed centrally (*A. central*) or marginally (*A.marginale*) in RBC, when stained with giemsa stain and examined microscopically.

Treatment

Clinical disease may be treated with oxytetracycline (6-10 mg/ kg b.w. daily for 3 days.Concurrently, oestradiol cypionate (14-3 mg/ kg b.w.) intramuscularly. Tetracyclines do not eliminate complete infection and carrier stage remains for rest of the life of the animal. Blood transfusion is indicated as supportive treatment.Imidocarb (3 mg/kg B.W.) is also effective for clinical cases.

Control

Eradication is difficult, as many insect vectors are responsible for its transmission weekly dipping with acaricide as helpful in control.

Vaccination

Killed vaccines of A. marginal with adjuvant base are used with 2 doses. However, problem of Neonatal isoerythrolysis can pose a risk with 2 doses. The vaccine can reduce the severity of the clinical disease but carrier stage remains, if infection occurs. Live vaccine is produced from infective blood from splenectomised animal. Single dose is used.

Indian Scenario

The problem of Anaplasmosis exists in India as "sporadic clinical incidences" in exotic animals. However, indigenous cattle are the carrier of the disease without clinical symptoms.

Suggested Reading

Oberle, S.M., Palmer, G.H., Barbet, A..F, McGuire, T.C. (1988) Molecular size variations in an immunoprotective protein complex among isolates of Anaplasma marginale. Infect Immune 56: 1567-1573.

Richey, E.J, Palmer, G.H. (1990). Bovine anaplasmosis. Compendium on Continuing Education for the Practicing Veterinarian. 12(11): 1661-1668.

Stiller, D.and Coan, M.E. (1995). Recent developments in elucidating tick vector re-lationships for anaplasmosis and equine piroplasmosis. Vet. Parasitol. 57: 97-108.

Jorgensen, W.K., Bock, R.E., de Vos A.J., Shiels, I.S.(1993). Sheep-adapted *Anaplasma marginale* maintains virulence for cattle. *Aust Vet J* 70: 192-193.

❑❑❑

Chapter 43

Coccidiosis of Calves, Lambs, Kids and Foals

Coccidiosis of young ones of domesticated animals is a universal protozoon disease of contagious nature with high morbidity and low fatality rate, showing clinical disease generally, when young ones are rared in crowded condition under unhygienic condition, and is characterized by diarrhoea and dysentery with blood and mucous in their faeces.

About the Causative Protozoon Parasite

Coccidium protozoon is a unicellular parasite with its various developmental stages occurring in epithelial cells of differet parts of the host animal's intestinal mucosa only, although schizonts have been found in mesenteric lymph-nodes of sheep and goats. In calves, different species of coccidia localize in different parts of the intestines, such as Eimeria gurundii and *E. bovis* primarily occur in caecum, colon and distant part of the ileum while *E. elipsoidales* and *E. arlongie* affect small intestine. *E. gilruthi* localises in abomasums and duodenum.

Lifecycle

The coccidial lifecycle is self-limiting. The unsporulated oocysts are passed in faeces where they develop into infective stage; the process is called as sporulation under warm temperature and moisture. Single cell of unsporulated oocyst divides into 4 sporoblasts which finally become sporocysts containing 2 sporozoites each. This occurs on the ground/soil and sporulated occcysts are protected by double wall of the oocyst. Each oocyst has specific shape as per the species of the protozoon parasite with or without terminal cap on the top of oocyst under which there is a hole known as micropile. The sporulated occyts is infective to the host animal and when feed/pasture contaminated with faeces containing sprulated oocyts is ingested by the animals or when young ones of animals lick the body haircoat contaminated with sporulated oocysts containing faeces, the sporulated oocysts are ingested in oral cavity of young ones.

The double wall of the sporulated oocysts break down in the mouth and sporocysts are released which enter the epithelial cells of intestinal mucosa. The sporocyst release sporozoites which enter the fresh epithelial cells. Once in the intestinal epithelial cells, sporozoites undergo multiple asexual fission (Schizogony) and first generation schizonts are formed. The schizents form number of "merozoites" which are released from epithelial cells, when schizonts rupture. These merozoites reinfect fresh epithelial cells and develop into second generation schizonts in large intestine and this is followed by release of another generation merozoites which invade epithelial cells and produce sexual stages, the macrogametocyte and microgametocytes. The second generation schizogony and Macro-micro gametocyte formation are the part of sexual cycle which results into fusion of gametocytes into gamete i.e. oocyst which is excreted into the faeces of host animal in unsporulated form. This completes the "lifecycle" in coccidium.

Epidemiology and transmission of coccidiosis

In young calves, lambs piglets, kids and rarely foals infection rate is high and clinical disease is much less common. High morbidity and low mortality occurs most commonly in crowded conditions both in confined pens and on pasture especially in calves and lambs moved from pasture to feed lot. The disease is transmitted by faecal oral route, oocysts shed from infected animals and immunity develops after infection. Clinical disease occurs rarely in adult animals.

Pathogenesis

After oral infection of sporulated oocysts in young ones, the sporozoites from ruptured oocyst infect the anterior part of intestinal mucosa and asexual schizogy occurs in the anterior instinal part with slight destruction of its mucosal cells. However, developmental stages of gamitogony (sexual lifecycle part) cause functional and structural lesions of the large intestine. As the second generation schizonts or gammonts mature, the cells containing them slough off from the basement membrane and cause haemorrhages and destruction of the caecum and colon. The oocysts are the result of fertilization of the gametocytes and are discharged at the time of rupture of the cells which usually coinsides with the onset of clinical signs of dysentery. "Prepatent period" varies with species of coccidium. With *E. bovis,* it is 15-20 days and with *E. zuernii* 15-17 days. These 2 species are most pathogenic to calves and their lifecycles are similar. The oocyst count is often low when the disease is at its peak, as they have not yet formed. The exfoliation of cells mucosa causes diarrhoea and haemorrhages into intestional hyman which leads to anaemia which is fatal.

Symptoms and P.M. Lesions

The first sign of clinical disease is the sudden onset of diarrhoea with foul smelling, fluid faeces containing mucous and blood, sometimes only fresh red blood is spiued in faeces. Severe straining is characteristics and rectal prolaps may occur. Haemorrhagic anaemia may develop. Inappetance is common, rarely anorexia may develop. Clinical disease in adult cattle is rare. Nervous signs are described in some cases but their relation with coceidiosis is questionable.

P.M. lesions are characterized by generalized tissue pallor and faecal staining of the hind quarters. Congestion, haemorrhages and thickening of mucosa of caecum, colon, rectum and ileum are significant necropsy findings ulceration and sloughing of the mucosa may occur in severe cases. Smears of mucosa and intestinal contents should be examined for various developmental stages of coccidia.

Diagnosis

Coccidiosis can be confirmed by faecal examination, direct microscopy showing significant number of oocysts in faeces and the developmental stages of coccidia in smears from jejunum, ileum and colon.

Treatment (Preventive and Therapeutic)

Coccidiosis is a self limiting disease and spontaneous recovery without specific treatment, occurs commonly when the multiplication stage of the coccidia has passed. Most of the coccidiostats have a depressant effect on the early first stage schizonts and are used for control. Reduction in population density of affected pens is advised. Mass medication of the feed and water supplies may be indicated in an attempt to prevent new cases and to minimize the effects of an epidemic. Calves should be brought indoors, kept well-bedded and warm and should be given fluid therapy orally and parenterally.

Following chemotherapeutics are recommended:

1.	Sulphadiamidine (or methazines)	Treatment dose 140 mg / kg daily for 3 days orally	Preventive dose 35 mg/kg B.W. daily for one week
2.	Amprolium	10 mg / kg B.W. daily for 5 days	5 mg/kg B.W. for daily for 21 days for calves / lambs
3.	Monensin	2 mg/kg B.W. daily of 220 days	16.5 to 33 g/kg continued fed for calves/lamb
4.	Lasalocid	--	25-100 mg/kg feed daily until market in lambsonly.

Coccidiosis of domestic young ones (calves, lambs, kids & foals) : Indian Scenario

This disease is prevailing universally in calves and other young one of domestic ruminants, equines and piglets but is observed seriously only when the young ones are kept in crowded conditions. Clinical disease was observed in calves of gir breed, crossbred and pure bred exotic calves, especially when they were lodged unhygienically in small crowded pens in pinjrapols. This is one of the component of calf mortality along with other enteritis conditions, namely *E. coli*, samomonellosis and rota-corna virus diarrhoeas.

Suggested Reading

Niilo, L., (1970). The effect of dexamethasone on bovine coccidiosis. Can. J. Comp. Med., 34: 325-328.

Cornelissen, A.W.C.A., Verstegen, R., van den Brand, H., Perie, N.M., Eysker, M., Lam, T.J.G.M. and Pijpers, A. (1995). An observational study of Eimeria species in housed cattle on Dutch dairy farms. Vet. Parasitol. 56: 7-16.

Gregory, M.W. & Catchpole, J. (1990). Ovine coccidiosis: the pathology of Eimeria crandalis infection. International Journal of Parasitology, 20: 849-86.

Fox, M.T., Higgins, R..J, Brown, M.E., Norten, C.C. (1991). A Case of Eimeria gilruthi infection in sheep in Northern England. Vet. Rec. 129: 141–142.

Taylor, M. (1995) Diagnosis and control of coccidiosis in sheep. In Practice. 17: 172-177.

❑❑❑

Chapter 44

Trypanosomiasis (Surra) of Cattle, Buffaloes, Horses and Camels

Surra (Trypanosomiasis) is arthropod borne disease of camels and horses mainly, but buffaloes and cattle are also affected and it is characterized by progressive anaemia, icterus, loss of body condition, terminal nervous symptoms followed by death. The disease was first identified in 1880, in India and is transmitted by Tabanid flies and other biting insects including mosquitoes. It is one of the most important diseases of camel in Africa and Asia, including India.

About the Causative Agent

The causative agent of the disease is *Trypanosoma evansi* which belongs to the family *Trypanosomidae*. It is a flagellated protozoan parasite that lives in the bood and other body fluids of vertebrate hosts. They swim in body fluids, boring their way between the cells. They generally possess a kinatoplast and undergo cyclical development in an arthropod vector, namely Tabanid fly.

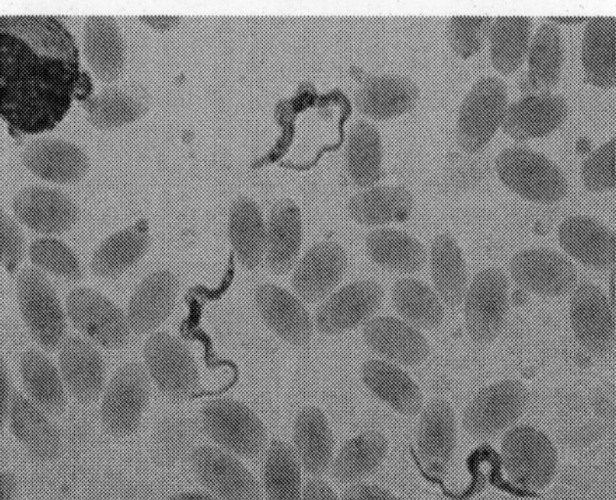

Fig. 1: *Trypanosoma evansi* in blood smear

The parasite is plemorphic and may occur as long and slender form or intermediate form or short and stumpy form. The slender and intermediate forms have a long free flagellum, pointed posterior end sub terminal kinatoplast and prominent undulating membrane. Trypanosoma evansi belongs to T. brucei group of Salvaria group of Trypanosomes but it is not having cyclical development in *Tse Tse* flies (These African flies can have "Cyclical development" of *T. virax* and T.congolensis which produce deadly disease "Nagana" in "*Tse Tse* fly (Glossina)" region of Africa. *T. evansi* produces "Surra" in South Africa beyond the "*Tse Tse* fly (Glossina)" region and in Asia, including India.

Epidemiology and Transmission

T. evansi has no cyclical development in any invertebrate arthropod host. The "*Tabanid*" flies (biting flies) and several hematophagus flies can transmit *T.evansi* "mechanically". Transmission is enhanced, when horses or camels congregate or are closely herded and when they have high numbers or parasites in their blood. Indigenous cattle and buffaloes may act as reservoirs of infection for horses and camels. During rainy season, the population of biting flies and mosquitoes are increased and they can transmit the disease from affected cattle and buffaloes to the susceptible cattle and buffaloes "mechanically".

Pathogenesis

T. evansi are inoculated into host animal from the contaminated mouth parts of biting insects or saliva of vampire bats (vampire bats are transmiters of Surra in South America).

Trypansomal parasites after entry through insect bite in animal body start multiplication in the blood and body fluids. The "metacyclic" parasites change to "trypomastigote form: and enter the blood directly and initiate characteristic intermittent parasitemias. This results into development of anaemia with complex pathogenesis involving mainly increased erythrophagocytosis, some haemolysis and dyshemopoiesis. The cerebrospinal fluid is often invaded by the parasites, with lymphoplasmacytic infiltration of the brain and spinal cord.

Symptoms and post mortem lesions

Intermittant fever, progressive anaemia, oedema of dependent parts of the body, dullness, listlessness, loss of body condition despite of good appetite, nasal and ocular discharge and terminal nervous signs including circling of the animal, paraplegia, paralysis, delirium and convulsions are the prominent symptoms shown by the animal. The disease is fatal in horses and camel. But sometimes they become chronically infected with exhibition of signs for years which include reduced milk yield and capacity reduction in working. The pregnant animals also show abortion.

Cattle and buffaloes may show milder disease which may increase if some intercurrent disease is present. Irregular oestrus, stillbirths and abortion can occur. Cattle and buffaloes can show acute disease with circling and death. P.M. findings include anaemic and icteric carcass without any gross or microscopic lesions. Trypanosomes can be demonstrated in peripheral/heart blood smears or brain smears, if stained with giemsa stain and observed microscopically.

Diagnosis

Smear examination mentioned under P.M. lesions will show diagnostic flagellated trypanosome parasites. Diagnosis during life includes injection of glucose given by route and then drawal of smears for staining or under wet smear exam microscopically under dark filed microscope facilitate appearance of parasites in blood circulation, when animal shows pyrexia. Biological test in white mice or guinea pig by inoculation of infective blood and demonstration of Trypan somes in their blood films is also used for positive diagnosis. The mercuric chloride, formal gel or stilbamidine test for demonstration of increased serum protein levels and complement fixation (CF), test, passive haemaglutination, indirect FAT and ELISA or PCR has been described recently for diagnosis of the disease in cattle (Wuyts *et al.* 1995).

Treatment and Control

Antrycide sulphate (5 mg/kg body wt.) which is Quinapyramine sulphate is given by intravenous route as "Curative treatment" for surra in camel/horse/cattle, if "Quinapyramine sulphate and chloride" which is also known as "Antrycide prosalt" is given as "prophylactic" in the dosage of 7.4 mg / kg B.W. for "protective" effect in cattle during the rainy season, when the insect population is risen to the level of precipitation of surra in endemic areas. Suramin (Naganol) at 10 mg/kg B.W. is given as both prophylactic and curative level. "Beranil" (i.e. diminazene aceturate) is used as curative in camel and cattle. No. vaccine is available for protective use.

Indian Scenario

Surra is existing in India, in camel and horses since 1880, when it was diagnosed for the first time in the world. The disease in cattle and buffaloes in the form of endemic is observed in certain parts of Maharashtra, including Dhulia, Nasik and Pune district. It is also recorded in Tonga ponies in Abibag and Panvel by the Author (S.V. Pandit), when he was working Disease Investigation Section, M.S. Pune during early sixties.

Use of "Antrycide prosalt" for prophylactic purposes was being made in Dhulia and Nasik districts during early sixties in large number of cattle by the local veterinarians. "Berenil" was being used in treatment of valuable exotic and crossbred cattle during said seventies.

Suggested Reading

Wuyts, N., Chokesajjawatee, N., Sarataphan, N. and Panyim, S. (1995): Ann. Soc. Belge Méd.Trop. 75: 229–237.

□□□

Chapter 45

Helminthic Diseases of Domesticated Animals

World of helminthic parasites is like an ocean. Unlike unicellular protozoon parasites, helminthes are multicellular living forms with more organized and with more highly evolved digestive and reproductive system which enable them to live longer pleomorphic life plemorphism outside and inside their original and intermediate hosts with extreme parasitism during their spectacular lifecycles. Probably because of their continual changing of physical and physiological forms with characteristic pleomorphism during their migratory path through the body of host animals during every stage of their lifecycle (from number of larval stages to adult stage, including egg form), host animal body and its tissues has to face a new shielding coat of antigens and has to produce protective response afresh every time which enables the helminth parasite to survive longer in the foreign territory of hosts body inspite of the parasites pathological insult during this sojurn.

The helminth parasites exist in 3 distinct classes, namely: 1) Nematodes (Roundworms), 2) Trematodes (leafy fluke-worms and 3) Cystodes (tapeworms). As mentioned in previous paragraph, they do not remain stationary in the host animals in which they spend their important part of their life as parasites but they keep on moving. The adult worms remain attached in lumen of either intestinal tract ducts like bile ducts, respiratory tract (bronchii or trachea or alveoli) or lumen of urinary tract, kidney cystern or reproductive tract or body cavities, blood vascular tract, etc. or lay eggs in those tracts which finally find their way out of the body through these tracts. These eggs under favourable conditions of temperature and moisture develop embryos and finally into the larvae which molt repeatedly and develop into the infective forms and infective forms of the immature parasite either develop in intermediate non-vertebrate hosts or develop directly on the ground or pastures and then get entry in host animal body through infestation or through skin penetration and then they develop into migrating larval or immature parasitic forms in the host animal body and finally reach their destined part of the body of animal, where they become adults and produce eggs. The lifecycle, thus continues. Every parasite undergoes its lifecycle as described above in general. However, every parasite has its own peculiarity in its life cycle which is described in the Table 1 to 4. The diseases caused by various parasites including diseases of alimentary tract produced by Nematode parasites, diseases of respiratory tract and other organs, skin and nervous system caused by Nematodes, diseases of liver and other organs caused by leaflike flukeworms (trematodes) and diseases caused by cystodes (tapeworms) are also described in consolidated table form along with the pathogenesis lesions and signs of diseases caused by them as well as diagnosed procedures, treatment and control measures are all described in Table 5.

Indian Scenario

Various climatic conditions, seasons, soils and vegetations exist in India and as India comes under tropical/subtropical region, most of these conditions are favourable for the growth and survival of helminhes as parasites in this country. Sheep and goats in India including Maharashtra are nomadic species and are migrating from place to place according to the season of availability of pasture for their grazing. Parasitic gastro-enteritis due to various genera and species of "*Trychostrongylidae*" is quite common in these animals, which include ostertagia, cooperia and Nematodirus species. In addition to these enteric parasites, Oesophagostomum species are also quite commonly occurring in ovine populations and 'nodular lesions" of intestine are quite often seen during postmortem examinations after slaughter of these animals. These "nodules' are detrimental for 'gut' industry.

The author came across serious occurrence of severe anaemia and haemorrhagic enteritis with bloody dysentery in Afghan, Bannur and exotic Russian merino as well as Ramboilet breeds of sheep at Govt. sheep breeding Farms at Pune and Thathawade which was due to the extensive infestation of those sheep with "Haemonchos contortus" during 1962 to 1965 while working at Disease Investigation Section M.S. Pune, P.M. examination revealed typical "Barbars pole" appearance of the intestines of those Haemonchus parasites. The author (Dr. S.V. Pandit) while visiting Deonar and Bandra slaughter houses during his post graduation for study of parasitism observed number of cattle carcasses with "Schistosomal" parasitic stages in mesenteric blood vessels. He also could come across number of sheep carcasses with hepatic lesions due to the presence of liver flukes belonging to Fasciola gigantic species. Occurence of hookworm infestation with Bunostemum species in sheep and cattle are quite usual slaughter house findings and presence of Ascarid worms "Toxocara viviparous in calf morlality postmortem at Pinjrapols in Maharashtra is eqully quite common. Liver fluke infestation with fasciola hepatica in sheep with typical "Bottle Jaw" symptom is the usual picture in village sheep herds.

Whipworm infestation with trichuris species in calves and lambs is also the typical occurrence with irritation in perianal region in village cattle and sheep.During late 1960's, the author (S.V. Pandit) came across the discussions with Dr. Yerawadekar well known Pathologist of Pune who was working with Govt. Chest Hospital Aundh (Sangavi) near Pune as "Consulting Pathologist". He informed that human Doctors working at Chest Hospital are suspecting few cases of "Hydatid disease" in human patients who were clinically diagnosed as "Tuberculosis like" cases and he requested to supply fluid from "Hydatid cyst" in sheep/goat for using as "antigen for allergic test". Accordingly, Dr. Pandit supplied the said "fluid" which Dr. Yerawadekar used for "skin test" and successfully diagnosed the "Hydatid Disease" in human patients.

During olden days, drenching of cattle, sheep and goats with "Phenothiazine" after opening of esophageal grove with copper sulphate administration was a common "anthalmentic" treatment followed by veterinarins. Later on "Thyabendazol came as broad spectrum antihelmintic drug. Use of beetalnut powder for treatment of tapeworms (beetalnut contain colionergic substance aerecholin which helps in paralyzing the head of tapeworms and subsequent expulsion of tapeworm). Later on other commercial anti-helmentic drugs came into markets which have broad spectrum therapeutic and preventive action against covering various class and genera of parasites. The details of dosing, etc. of those antihelmintics are given in Table 5. Vaccines were developed experimentally at IVRI, Izatnagar during early seventies (1970's) by attenuation of infective larvae of lung worms by irradiation with gamma rays (1000 infective larvae per calf as a dose) used in 8 week old calves. It is advised that exposure to lightly infected pastures will boost the immunity. Vaccine gives high levels of immunity against lung worm infestation.

Table 1: Nematode Diseases of the Alimentary Tract

Sr. No.	Disease	Etiology	Epidemiology & Life cycle	Pathogenesis	Clinical signs & lesions	Diagnostic confirmation	Treatment	Control
1	Parasitic gastro-enteritis of Ruminents (Calves, young sheep and all age groups of goats) occurs in cold as well as hot climatic conditions	Nematode genera 1) Trichostrongulus species 2) Ostertagia ostertagi & other species of ostertegia 3) Cooperia species 4) Nematodirus species	Direct life cycle without intermediate host eggs passed in faces - 2 non parasitic larval stages in eggs on groword. - 3rd stage infective larvae enter gastric glands of abomasums or crypts of small intestine and molt and return to lumen as 4th stage larvae -molt and became adult in intestine prepatent period 3 to 5 weeks as per species eggs in faeces. Hypobiosis of larvae during adverse pasture condition	Worm adult worms emerge from abomaasal/intestional glands, hyperplastic reaction in neigh boring glands, leading to reduced acid secretion, increasing pH to 6-7 with increase in incoming bacterial and protozoal flora and papsinegen is not converted to pepsin disturbing digestion. Intestinal disturbance by Trycostongyli infections and disturbed weight gain	Diarrhoea weightloss production losses. Type I disease followed recent infestation delayed due to hypobiosis of larvae in winter causing type II disease. Raised nodules on gastric mucosa and inflammation and vilus atrophy in anterior small intestine	Warm counts at Necropsy other wise largely relient on clinical signs and history. Faecal egg counts and plasma pepsin gens concentration increases	Avamectins/ milbemycins benzimidazoles prohenzimidagzols livamesole and compounds are not said able to control hypobiosis in larvae. Phenothiazine drenching was used effectively in olden days	To maintain safe grazing by reducing pasture contamination integrated management scheme with reduced dependence on drug usage due to development of drug resistance in may plces

Sr. No.	Disease	Etiology	Epidemiology & Lifecycle	Pathogenesis	Clinical signs & lesions	Diagnostic confirmation	Treatment	Control
2	Haemonchosis in ruminants (sheep, goats and cattle) occurs only in hot climatic zones (tropical and warm temperature countries)	Nematode genera 1) Haemonchus contrtus in sheep and goats 2) Haemonchus placei in cattle 3) Mecistocirus digitatus in sheep, goats and cattle & buffaloes	Direct lifecycle without intermediate host large no. of eggs produced by females and rapid development of larvae in warm wet condition and large number accumulate rapidly on pasture lifecycle in similar to trichostrongyles	Vigorous blood sucking by forth stage larvae and adults leading to severe anaemia which differs from trycostongyloid pathogenesis	Severe anaemia, wt. loss and loss in milk production in Ewes she goats and cattle and anasarca acute sudden deather. Hyperamic abomasum anaemic carcasses.	Barber's pole appearance of female worms "Reds white twists on intestine of worms.	All above mentioned broad spectrum Anthalmentics and closantel rafoxanide nitroxanile phenothiazinc drenching was used effectively in olden days.	Strategic dosing schemes using drugs mentioned under treatment

Sr. No.	Disease		Epidemiology & Life cycle	Pathogenesis	Clinical signs & lesions	Diagnostic confirmation	Treatment	Control
3	(Hook worm) disease in ruminants (Cattle & Sheep)	Nematodes of genus Bunostomum 1) Bunestomum phelbotomum in cattle. 2) Agrinostomum Asia 3) Bunsostomum trigonoceplalum found worldwide but gaigeria pachyscalis in India. 4) Globocephalus species in pigs	Transmission by skin penetration favoured by warm, humid condition,	Direct life cycle, females are prolific egg layers. Eggs hatch and 2 free living larval stages (non parasitic) follow on pasture 3rd stage infective larva in 1 week penetrates skin only in case of gaigera but by both skin penetration as well as orally in Bunostomum species. When skin penetration occurs, larvae go to heart / lung where forth stage larvae come out in air passage and pharynx and swallowed and	Stamping and licking of feet due to itching by skin penetrating larvae. Constipation mild abdominal pain followed by bouts of diarrhoea unthriptiness. Anaemia weakness Prostration death may follow.	In calves, total worm count in carcass > 100 suggests significant level of infestation >2000 suggests fatality due to this infestation, Incase of gaigeria even 24 adults can cause fatal disease.	As mentioned under haemonchosis Doramactin is specific for gaigeria infestation. Phenothiazine was used effectively by drenching.	As in case of haemonchosis

				go to intestine. They penetrate intestinal wall and returns to lumen. -11 day migration period. The prepatent period is 8-10 weeks as per species. Fourth stage larvae and adults are active blood suckers				

Sr. No.	Disease	Etiology	Epidemiology & Lifecycle	Pathogenesis	Clinical signs & lesions	Diagnostic confirmation	Treatment	Control
4	Oeso-phagestomiosis (Nodule worm disease of Ruminents and pigs)	Nematodes of genus oesophagostomum 1) Oesophagostomum columbianum, O.venulosum and O.asperum in sheep and goats. 2) O.radiabum, O.venullosum in cattle 3) O.dentatum O.equadrispinulosum in pigs	Disease confined in sheep in warm, summer, rainfall regions. In pigs, all age groups susceptible but only sows when undernourised	In cattle, O.columbianum produces massive host reaction and produce visible big size nodules. While other species do not produce so young sheep produce no	Severe diarrhoea with mucous and blood, rapid loss of condition, nodules on intestine, important	Necropsy is most reliable otherwise needs incubation of faeces and identify infective larvae in eggs.	In sheep, all modern broad spectrum dewormers listed under parasitic gastroenteritis. In pigs are compound given under stomach worms. Phenolhiazine	Strategic anthelmintic treatment adequate nutrition in sows essential.

			affected. Stout white round worms with direct lifecycle. Eggs pass in faeces 2 non-infective larval stages 3rd infective stage larvae, by ingestion go to intestine at any level and provoke nodular reaction in in the wall. Hypobiosis return to lumen as forth stage larvae prepatent period of 40-50 days before egg laying starts.	nodules or few nodules but adult sheep produces large number of nodules and no adult warms in some cases. Anorexia severe, persistant mucoid diarrhoea, loss of weight. Anaemia, Hypoprotenemia, death.	loss to gut industry and meat industry.		drenching was effectively used in olden days	

Sr. No.	Disease	Etiology	Epidemiology & Life cycle	Pathogenesis	Clinical signs & lesions	Diagnostic confirmation	Treatment	Control
5	Parasitic gastritis in pigs	Nematodes of genus Hyostrongulus 1) H. rubidus 2) Ascarops species 3) Physocephalus	H. rubidis has direct life cycle but ascarops and physocephehus has "Dung beetles" as intermediate host, where 3 stages of infective larvae are produced pigs eat beetles,	4th stage larvae from beetles or directly from eggs on ground infest pigs gastric mucosal glands and then come to lumen, gastritis occur	Asymptomatic but heavy infestation produce severe gastritis sows become thin during lactation. Nodular or ulcerative gastritis results.	Faecal sample for eggs and larval exam for H. rubidis	In sheep, all modern broad spectrum dewormers listed under parasitic gastroenteritis. In pigs are compound given under stomach worms. Phenothiazine drenching was effectively used in olden days	Strategic anthelmintic treatment adequate nutrition in sows essential.
6.	Ascariasis in pigs, horses and cattle	Nematodes worms from the Ascarid family 1) Ascaris suum in pigs 2) Paraascaris equanum in	Transmission is by injestion of highly resistance and long lived larvated eggs	Infective larvated eggs entering intestines break and larve penetrate	Heavy infestation leads to poor growth, diarrhoea sometimes obstructive	Demonstration of characteristics eggs in faeces	I-vermection Dorameetin flubenduzol febantal oxibendazole levamasole in pigs horses	Protection of young stock from sites where eggs may accumulate

		horses. 3) Toxocara vituborum in buffaloes and cattle	T. vitulorum is also transmitted via. Colostrums	intestinal wall and reach portal vein and then to liver. They cross to hepatic veins and reach lungs and then to brochii trachya and pharyn swallowed and reach intestine where they mature to adult worms prepatent perial is 6-8 week to 11-15 week as per species. Haemorrhages in liver/other migrated organs fibrosis and ahviolar injury with oedema and further pyogenesis in invaded injuries	jaundice intestinal obstruction and respiratory signs. Petechial haemorrhages in lungs and fibrotic spots on liver.		and cattle	

Sr. No.	Disease	Etiology	Epidemiology & Life cycle	Pathogenesis	Clinical signs & lesions	Diagnostic confirmation	Treatment	Control
7	Stongylosis in Horses (Red worm infestation)	Two Nematode sub families strongylina (Large strongyles) and Cyethostominae (small strongyles) Examples 1) Strongylus vulgaris (Larva migratory) 2) 40 species of cyathostomes (Larvae non-mightory)	Eggs are shed by all age groups of Horses. Lifecycle is direct. Infective larvae develop seasonally on pasture, Hypobiotic cyathostome larvae can cause severe disease in late winter. Eggs passed in faeces and develop infective 3rd stage larvae under suitable shed, moisture and moderate temperature (some eggs larvae with stand freezing temperatures). i) Non-migratory larvae enter wall of colon and caecum	Larvae of strong vulgaris are most pathogenic causing arteritis thrombosis producing complete is chemia of parts of intestine leading to colic intestional necrosis and gahgreme. Entrance mobility of intestine forximal to ischemic area leads to intussuception and ruputer of	Ill – thrift, poor performance, weight loss and anaemia verminous arteritis leading to colic and diarrhea intusception, large numbers of adult worms in intestine (colon curum) haemarrhagic inflammation of mucosa with multiple small ulcers, large and small nudules verminous	Pathognomic indicators judgement made on overall appraisal of clinical history, presenting signs and laboratory findings. Arteritis of cranial mesenteric artery sometimes palpable per rectum. Immature worms sometimes seen in faeces in larval cyathostomiasis.	Ivermection moxidection benzimidazols e.g. bebrantel fenbendazole mebendazole	Twich weekly removal of faeces from pasture mixed or alternate grazing routine doing to prevent contamination of pasture with eggs larval cyatho stomiasis 5 days treatment (preventive) fenbendazole in early winter.

			and live in small nodules sub seriously for 7-18 weeks before breaking out in lumen of intestine. ii) Migratory larvae of strongylus vulgaris molt to 4th stage larvae in sub mucosa and then pass in small arteries and reach cramical mesenteric artery and return to lumen of intestine after 3-4 months. Nodules formed in intestinal wall which rupture and adult worms go to int lumn prepatent period is 6 months.	intestine / causes cerebrospinal nematadosis due to invasion of central nervous system is also reported. Adult stonglyes cause blood sucking leading to anaemia and haemorrhages in intestional lumen the small strongyles can cause only superficial damage.	arteritis well of optimal mesenteric artery greatly thickened with thrombi and larvae on internal surface nudules in liver.			

Sr. No.	Disease	Etiology	Epidemiology & Life cycle	Pathogenesis	Clinical signs & lesions	Diagnostic confirmation	Treatment	Control
8	Miscellaneous round worm infestation i) Oxyuriasis of horses	Oxyuris equi.	Lifecycle direct worms inhabit caecum & colon worms with long taping tails. They migrate down the gut and crawl into the perianal area where they lodge eggs in yellow clusters, infective larvae develop in the egg and become infective, which are licked by fellow students or they fall on ground, adhere to dust and become airborn feed stuffs contaminated taken up by other fellow animals.	Itching due to migratory crowling in perianal area.	Itching and disturbing	Microscopic detection of operculated eggs, slightly flattened on transparent adhesive tape pressed against perianal skin or by chance observation of adult worm in faeces.	Ivermectin moxidectin or benzimidazoles for horses. Piperazine salts also effective.	Same as treatment.
	ii) Trycharis (Whip worm infestation) in ruminants and pigs	Tichurios ovis and T. globulosa in sheep and goats T. suis in pigs	Lifecycle direct eggs are very sturdy lifecycle as in case of oxyuris.	Slight inflammatory reaction in caecum and colon helps bacterial invasion and subsequent anorexia and diarrhoea (mild)	Mild diarrhoea weight loss.	Microscopic morphology of eggs specific.	Ivermectin moxidectin or benzimidazoles for horses. Piperazine salts also effective.	Same as treatment.

Table 2: Nematode Diseases of the lungs and other organs

Sr. No.	Disease	Etiology	Epidemiology& Life cycle	Pathogenesis	Clinical signs & lesions	Diagnostic confirmation	Treatment	Control
1	Lung worm infestation in cattle (bovine verminous bronchitis)	The nematode dictiocaulus viviparous (The bovine lung worm)	Disease mostly of dairy calves immunity develops relatively quickly but cattle succum is if cased to overvelming numbers of infective larvae while grazing. Adult worms in trachea and bronchi pass eggs and sare swollowed. Larve hatch from eggs in air passages or intestine. larvae passed in faeces. They develop 3rd stage infective larvae with cuticles of previous stages maintained as such moisture and temp of 65-70°F develop them fully to infective stage. They perist in pasture even for one year surrive on glycogen granules in intestine. Ingested larvae during pasture grazing penetrate intestinal wall of host and go to mesenteric lymph nodes, then migrate via venous blood to heart and then to lungs break in alveoli.	Migratory larvae do not cause damage until they reach lungs. They are blocked by mucuous of bronchii and bronchides and inflammatory cells leading to collapse of abocale coughing and dyspnea occurs pulmonary oedema as well as interstitial emphysema. Later when mature parasites are in major bronchi, eggs, fregments of worms killed by immunity and other debris are aspirated and aspiration pneumonia develops. Secondary bacterial infection occurs. Foreign body pneumonia develops and can result into death. Recovering animals develop cuboidal lining of alviclar epithelium as reaction to the foreign body. Hypersensitivity to Bronchi reaction occurs.	Characteristics larvae in faeces eosinophilia, coughing, tachypnea dyspnea larage volume of consolidation in diaphragmatic lobes of lung, emphysema worms upto 8 cm long in bronchi (only in patent phase of disease)	Clinical pathology as nriblen under clinical signs and lesions and demonstration of worms in bronchi.	Benzamidazoles and avermectins bemycines are active against all parasitic stages. The letter also have protective effects. Livamesole is also used,	Vaccination early season anthelmintic prophylactic programmes using suitable intra ruminal boluses or multiple doses of avermectin milbemycin keep susceptible animals off potentially dangerous pasture, Vaccines containing gammarays irradiated larvae is useful.

Sr. No.	Disease	Etiology	Epidemiology& Life cycle	Pathogenesis	Clinical signs & lesions	Diagnostic confirmation	Treatment	Control
2	Lung worm infestation of horses	Nematode parasite dictyocaulus arnfieldi	Infection is by ingestion of larvae on herbage, donkeys and foals shed most larvae but adult horses can perpetuate life cycle. Life cycle is direct and is similar to diction caulus viviparus described previously.	Adult worms are found in the smaller bronchi, which they completely block. In adult horses, however, few larvae reaching the lungs, develop to this stage. Pathogenesis similar as incase of Dyctiocaulus viriparus described previously.	Chronic cough in adult horses discrete areas of hyperinflation in lung tissue	Response to treatment if no eggs / larvae found in faeces.	5 days treatment with ivermectin fenbendazole (elevated dose in donkeys)	Avoid grazing donkeys and horses on the same pasture.
3	Lung worm infestation in sheep and geats	The nematode parasites dyctiocaulus filarial. Muellerius capillaris protostronyglus rufescens.	Infective D.filaria larvae are found on grass but M.Capillaris and P.rufisens are transmitted when moluscan intermediate host are accidentally injected by grazing animals.	D. fileria lives in trachea and bronchi changes similar to those described under D.Viriparus P.rufescens are found in small bronchi and hence damage smaller than P.vileria	Brochitis and loss of condition M. capilaris is asymptomatic in sheep but pathogenic in good scattered patches of consolidation	Characteristics larvae in faeces	5 days treatment with ivermectin fenbendazole (elevated dose in donkeys)	No specific measures available.
4	Lung worm infestation in pigs	Nematode parasite Metastongylus apri, M. Salmi M. pudendotectus	Epidemiology is similar to D. Viviparus but differs only in that life cycle through earthworm intermediate host	Similar to D,Viviparus these worms may provide transmission for swine influenza and swine fever from pig to pig.	Barking cough reduced growth rate. Greyish nodules nearventral border of diaphragmatic lobes of lungs	Characteristics eggs in faeces	Doramectin iIvermectin fenbendazole flerbandazole liva misole	Difficult unless pigs reared on concentrations.

Sr. No.	Disease	Etiology	Epidemiology& Life cycle	Pathogenesis	Clinical signs & lesions	Diagnostic confirmation	Treatment	Control
5	Stephanuriasis (Kidney worm disease) in pigs	Nematode parasite stephanurius dentatus	Adult worms in perirenal tissues or sometimes in other abdominal organs or spinal canal of pigs (in cysts around the renal pelvis and walls of ureters and communicate with the urinary passage. Eggs are passed out in urine of the host. The eggs hatch on the soil in favourable condition and 3rd change larvae are infective. The earthworm can act as transport host, Infective larvae are swollowed by pig through feed or penetrate skin, reach liver via lungs through systemic circulation and after moult, 4th stage larvae reach kidney and become adults.	Larval migration causes necrosis fibrosis and even abscesses along the path of migration thus producing lesions in liver kidney tissue etc.	Poor growth, emaciation, stiffness of gait in severe cases. Fibrosis and abscess formation in perirenal tissues, fibrotic scarring of liver and other abdominal organs	Eggs in urine and characteristics necropsy lesions.	Fenbendazole ivermactin doramectin livamisole for adults only	Regular Anthal mentic treatment 4 months interval. Breeding only from gilts keeping paddocks bare and dry.

Sr. No.	Disease	Etiology	Epidemiology & Life cycle	Pathogenesis	Clinical signs & lesions	Diagnostic confirmation	Treatment	Control
6	Habronemiasis (summer sores) in Horses	Nematode parasites Habronema muscae, H. majus draschia megastma	Indirect life cycle. Flies as intermediate hosts (musca domestica for H. musca and D.megastoma while stomoxis stable fly for H. majus. The thin walled larvated eggs hatch in the manure and are ingested by maggots of flies and infective larvae develop in adult fly. Horse become infested by swallowing dead flies or adult flies deposit larvae on skin or in eye,	Larvae invade gastric mucosa and produce granulmatous lesions (masses which become fibrotic, later on these tumours contain adult worms which escape in lumen of stomach. Repture of tumour result in peritonitis lavae deposited on eye and skin cause cutaneous and eye inflammation and lesions.	Extensive granulomatous tumour in stomach or skin sores and eye inflammation.	Demonstration of larvae in eye or cutaneous lesions biopsy or scrapings	Ivermection	Protect horses from flies treat all skin wounds eye wounds promptly.
7	Thaleziasis (Eye worm disease) of cattle and horses	Thalezia species	Thin worms produce indirect life cycle through faeces fly musca atonalism as intermediate host. Adult worms in conjunctiva sac of animals. Flies deposit infective larvae on eye ball.	Kerato conjunctivitis occurs due to irritation caused by the worms.	Lacrimation and purulent discharge from eyes, secondary bacterial infection occurs.	Demonstration of worms or larvae	Ivermectin in cattle effective not so much in horses	Same as treatment.

Sr. No.	Disease	Etiology	Epidemiology& Lifecycle	Pathogenesis	Clinical signs & lesions	Diagnostic confirmation	Treatment	Control
8	Cerebrospinal nematodiasis (Lumbar paralysis) or Kumari in India, Japan and Israel and Srilanka	Sataria labiatc papillosa (Or S. digitata) occurs in cattle in abodimal cavity with no pathogenesis but the infective larvae produce cerebrospinal pathology in other species like horse, sheep goats and man.	Indirect life cycle through mosquitoes as intermediate hosts. Adults are thread like filarial nematodes found in peritoneal cavity of cattle females produce motile micro filarial embryos which circulate in peripheral blood taken up by the biting mosquitoes in which infective larvae develop which are released in cattle after mosquito bite and develop into adults in cattle in 8-10 months No serious effect in cattle. But if infective larvae are released by mosquito in sheep goats or horses or man, they migrate to brain and produce serious cerebrospinal Nematodiasis.	Migrating filterial larvae produce inflammatory effects with eosinophilic infiltrations oedema in brain ad spiral cord.	Rapid onset of cerebrospinal nematodiasis with death within few days or it may occur gradually over few days. Acute or sub acute paresis with weakness and inco-ordination or paralysis involving hind legs most commonly. But sometimes all 4 legs are paralyzed. Recovery can be partial or only mild neurological disorder and subsequent full recovery. Animals affected may continue eating.	At necropsy serial sectioning of spinal cord may be required to detect the lesion, Focal Area of Malacia or micro-cavitation may be observed with adjacent site may show loss of myelin, axonal swelling, degeneration and glitter cell formation. Migratory pathways may be indicated by necrotic tracts and worm fragments may occasionally be found in section.	Ivermectin at a dose of 0.2 mg / kg B.W. given twice in sheep goats may prevent satariosis	Not described

Sr. No.	Disease	Etiology	Epidemiology & Life cycle	Pathogenesis	Clinical signs & lesions	Diagnostic confirmation	Treatment	Control
9	Stephano-fileriasis (Hump-sore) in cattle in India and (ear-sore in cattle in India.	Nematode parasites stephano-fileria assamensis. Stephanofilaria zaheeri	The adult worms are present in the skin wound on "Sores" embedded in the granulomatous tissue. The adult worms release micro filariae which later develop in flies that feed on the gores. The infective micro filariae are released in the pre existing small wound occurred due to mechanical rubbing of hump by bullock cart or plough. The microfilaria develop into adult worms after molting.	The migrating microfilariae produce extreme irritation which result into small papuls which later on coalase to produce bigger sores (3-15 cm in diameter) partial local hairloss is there due to rubbing of the sores scabs are produced on the flowing wounds.	Hump or ear sores with exudates produce thick crumbly scabs which may crack to expose blood stained fluid.	Skin scrapings may reveal broken parts of adult worms or micro filariae which can be identified under microscope.	Ointment containing insecticide may acid control oral levamisole 7.5 mg/kg BW once or have at 3-4 weeks interval is reported to be effective, Ivermactin is an effective micro filaricide and reduces the adult worms.	See treatment, simple wound prevention and treatment will reduce the risk of the disease.

Table 3 : Diseases of Liver caused by Trematodes (Liver flukes) and other flukes (like stomachflukes)

Sr. No.	Disease	Etiology	Epidemiology & Life cycle	Pathogenesis	Clinical signs & lesions	Diagnostic confirmation	Treatment	Control
1	Hepatic Fasciolasis (Liver fluke disease) in cattle sheep goats and horses.	i) Fasciola hepatica in colder regions UK/USA.Canada ii)Fasciola gigantic in warmer regions Africa/Asia	In direct life cycle through intermediate host snails (Lymnia trancatuda in UK/Europe/USA and L. Columella in Canada.. Adult Fasiolae live in bile ducts produce eggs which are excreted in faeces via. bite, Eggs hatch on wet ground to produce 1st stage larvae i.e. Miracidium at temp. 5-6⁰C which invade tissues of suitable host snail within 24-30 hours. After several cycles as a sexual multiplication circariae are formed from miracidium and they leave the snail and attach to	When warmer weather conditions prevail, metacercarial production is high with high infestation rate and they produce. Acute disease while when it is low in winter, the disease is chronic. Acute clinical disease occurs after 5-6 weeks after injestion of meta cercariae which produce substantial mechanical damage to hepatic tissue. Thus acute hepatic insufficiency and haemorrhacies results. During liver migration they also carry and activate clostr novei. Spores to produce "Black	Acute fasciolasis menifests dullness, weakness lack of appetite, pallor and oedema of mucosa and conjunctive & liver pain quick death may follow accompanied by blood stained discharge from nostrils in sheep, rarely in cattle, subacute disease in sheep with weight loss, palor of mucous membranes and "sub mandibular	Chronic ill health in sheep with debilitation condition in outbreak form should give susptition of faciodasis which can be further confirmed by misccroscopic faecal exam for typical eggs of fasciodа characteristics necropry lesions in liver with demonstration of adult flukes in hepatic parenchyma is confirmatory serological test like ELISA is promising in cattle for	Triclabendazode is a specific current treatment (10 mg/kg B.W.) for sheep and 12mg/kg B.W. for cattle higher dosase is needed for F.gigantica in buffaloes Albendazole (7.5 mg / kg B.W.) is useful in case of both nematooles and liver fluke infestations of cattle. Netobimin (20 mg/kg by S/C) route Nitroxynil (10mg / kg B.W.) oxyclozanide is also useful.	Segreatiion of stock from sources of infection eg. further tanks pounds, irrigation canals etc. by fencing. Treatment as per coloumn of treatment repeated at suitable intervals depending upon the season of metacercarial release studies. Chemical snail treatment using copper sulphate or sodium pentachlorophinate or N. tritid morpholine.

			snail and attach to herbage and become metaceracariae. After injestion of infected herbage, metacercariae release immature flukes in intestine, which penetrate intestine and migrate to peritonial cavit and then and sometimes to lungs also. Liver parasites migrate through hepatic	produce "Black disease" in cattle & sheep "Chronic hepatic faciolasis produces biliary obstruction, hypoalbuminemia and finally normochromic anaemia which results into hypochromic anaemia.	mandibular oedema" chronic disease is characterized by "bottle jaw" more prominently wool shedding, survival of sheep for longer periods for cattle milk production loss is more prominent	cattle for confirmation of disease (showing rising ELISA antibody titrus in paired sera)		

Sr. No.	Disease	Etiology	Epidemiology& Life cycle	Pathogenesis	Clinical signs & lesions	Diagnostic confirmation	Treatment	Control
2	Liver fluke disease caused by Fasciodoides magna in sheep cattle goats and deers etc.	Liver fluke parasite fascioloides magna present in north America & Europe	Life cycle similar to F.hepatica except that it grows in thin walled cysts in liver parenchyma connection between the cyst and bile ducts allow the eggs to pass in faeces. Lymnacid snails are intermediate hosts. The fluke enters the liver parenchyma after passing 3-4 week in pertionial cavity.	In sheep and goats, flukes continue to migrate and never becoming encapsulated but forming large, black tracts. Hepatic damage and haemorrhage and haemorrhage is so severe that only one or this flukes are fatal. In cattle necrotic tracts are seen in the liver parenchyma as well as dark thick walled cysts. They have no connection to bile ducts.	Clinical sign are similar to F.hepatica and infected sheep & goat can die without worming. In cattle the disease may be in apparent or can be mild with symptoms similar to Hepatic fasciolasis by F.hepatica	Eggs may be found in faeces but they are larger in size as compared to those of F.hepatica but morphologically similar to F.hepatica	Similar to that of F.hepatica	Similar to that of F.hepatica
3	Liver fluke disease caused by Dicrocoelium dendriticum	Liver fluke parasite Dicrocoelium dendriticum present in Europe and Asia & North America	Eggs passed in faeces eaten by snail Hellicella and cionella lumbrica circariae passed in slime balls used as food by ant-formica, grazing animals eat ants with grass get meta cercarial infection.	Low pathogenicity as flukes do not migrate across liver parenchyma fibrosis of parenchyma occurs are proliferation of bile ducts and thickening occurs. Infectious necrotic hepatitis develops.	Disease with mildnecrotic hepatitis.	Necropsy findings reveal lanceolate shaped small liver flukes found only in bile ducts egg in faeces are operculated asymmetrical dark brown in colour.	Treatment with Albendazole (15 mg/kg BW) Netobiminca at 20 mg/kg BW	Similar to that of F.hepatica

Sr. No.	Disease	Etiology	Epidemiology & Life cycle	Pathogenesis	Clinical signs & lesions	Diagnostic confirmation	Treatment	Control
4	Paramphistomiasis (Stomach fluke disease) in cattle sheep	Paramphistomum cervi. P.microbothrioides. P.microbothrium cotylophozon cotylophron and cotyloo phoron species occurs all over the globe but most common in Australia, Africa and India (warm region)	Infection by ingestion of metacercariae on herbage geographical distribution, seasonality and disease risk determined by occurrence of intermediate hosts (aquatic planozbid snails). Life cycle is similar to F.hepatic except that the snails are planorbid and immature flukes proximally migrate along the duodenum and through abomasums to reach their predilection site in rumen and reticulum. Maturation period is 6 weeks to 4 months	The immature flukde excyst in Jejunum or duodenum. They attach firmly to mucosa and migrate as deep as muscularis mucosa causing enteritis through patches if villus atrophy to severe descrution of mucosa. The adult worms in rumen / abomasums do not cause much damage.	Severe enteritis with number of migrating flukes in duodenum is the only manifestation of the disease fetid and persistent diarrhoea is observed along with depression dehydration and sub-maxillary oedema. Death occurs in 15-20 days, mortality rate can be high muscular atrophy, subcutaneous oedema with ascitis with gelatinous fat deposition is observed in abdominal cavity.	Demonstration of immature flukes in faeces or at necropsy in diagnostic	Oxyclozanide 18.7 mg/kg BW 2 days apart or single dose of hexachlorophene 20 mg/kg W give consistent results in cattle.	Removal of animals from infected pasture treatment is also useful for control.

Table 4 : Adult and Larval Tapeworm (Cystode) infestation

Sr. No.	Disease	Etiology	Epidemiology& Life cycle	Pathogenesis	Clinical signs & lesions	Diagnostic confirmation	Treatment	Control
1	Adult Tapewarm (Cystode) infestation in cattle and horses	Monieza species in ruminents eg. monienzia expansa M.benedeni Helictometra giardi occur globally while Avitellina specias in India and Mediterranean countries. All above species in cattle and other ruminants anaphocephela magna, A.perfoliata and Aneoplotephaloides species in Horses globally.	All have very similar life cycles. Eggs are immediately infective, pass in faeces of host singly or in clusters protected preglolid segments of tape worms which are ingested by free living pasture or botidmites and intermediate stages are formed mature tape worms develop when primary host accidentally swoolous infected mites while grazing. Most species establish in intestine, But T.actinoides invades bileducts and Pancreatic ducts S. hepatica lives in bite ducts.	Adult tapeworms compete for Nutrients in gut, excretes toxic materials or mechanically interfere with motility of gut. Moniezia expansa in lambs is associated with outbreaks of enterotoxemia, In horses A.perfoliata causes mild local infilammation around attachment area granulomatosis and occasionally pouch formation, spasmatic colic and impaction of gut as well as intussusceptions, excel tortion can occur	In ruminents, heavy burden of tapeworm infestation may result in unthriffiness, poor coat, vage digestive disturbances in colon constipation diarrhoea dysentery and sometimes anaemic	Shed segments falls of characteristic eggs can be examined by crushing under microscope for confirmation and degree of infestation. Eggs are roughly D.shaped thick shelled and contain an embryo within chitinus ring.	In ruminant praziquantal 3.75 mg/kg BW is highly effective Benzimidazole like albendazole febantal fenbendizole netobincia and oxafendazole are effective. Albendazole 7.5 mg/kg BW is effective for Horses pyranelt embonate (38 mg/kg B.W. i.e. double the standard dose for nematodes) is effective.	Ploughing of pastures helps reduction in orbatid mites and hence control of infestation of tape worms.

Sr. No.	Disease	Etiology	Epidemiology& Life cycle	Pathogenesis	Clinical signs & lesions	Diagnostic confirmation	Treatment	Control
2	Larval tapeworm infestation	Livestock my act as "Intermediate hosts" for tapeworms of man and other animals (pigs) coenurus cerebralis (cystecercoid of Tapeworm Taenia multiceps of dog.	The larval tape worms (metacystodes) develop as fluid filled cysts, each at a typical site of body. They act as space occupying lesions and cause meat condemnation during inspection but no pathogenesis.	They do not form clinical lesions. The metacystodes of taenia multicaps cause conuraisis and texian hydatigina produce multilocalor cysts but if sheep or goat swallow a whole tapeworm segment containing 190000 eggs sudden death occurs due to development of "cysticerci" larvae which migrate through the liver parenchyma. (Hepatitis cysticercosis which resembles acute hepatic faciolasis (Individual cases only). In case of multilocular conenurms cerebralis cysts developed in brain and spinal cord, of sheep goats cattle horses and wild reminents which is an intermediate stage of tapeworm taenia multicops which inhabits the intestine of dogs. The cyst causes pressure on nervous tissue and its distruction and produce irritation, wild expression salivation, frenzied running and convulsions. Development of partial or complete blindness in one eye periodic epileptic symptoms. (This disease is called as coenurosis (Gid or surely)	--	--	--	--
3	Hydatid disease of man	Taenia taenia tape worm of dog	Tenia multilocularis the meta cystoides cystic larval stage. Hydatid cyst develops in man (Intermediate host) in lung. Hydatid cyst puts pressure on lung tissue and develops "Tuber culosis" like wasting disease in human (Zoonosis)	As under pathology	Human case diagnosis can be done by "Allergic test similar to "Tuberculin" test	Surgical removal of cyst form lungs	--	--

Table 5 : Details of treatment of parasitic diseases

Sr. No.	Name of chemotherapeutic drug	Name of parasitic genera covered	Animal species for which used	Treatment dose / preventive dose
1.	Avermectins / milbemycins		Sheep and goats cattle	0.2 mg/kg BW
	i) Ivermectin	All trycostrongyle species.		0.2 mg/kg BW (injection)
	ii) Eprino mectin	Haemonchus species		Or
	iii) Moxidectin	Oesophegostomum specis		0.5 mg / kg BW (Oral)
	iv) Doramectin			
2.	Benzimidazoles / probenzigmidazoles	Bunostomum species Ascarid worms.	Horses	0.2 mg/kg BW
	i) Albendazol		Cattle	7.5 mg/kg BW
	ii) Febentol		Cattle	5.0 mg/BW (Oral)
	iii) Fenabendazole			
	iv) Oxfendazole			
	v) Mebenolozole		Horses	7.5 mg/kg BW
	vi) Triclabendazole	Fasciola worms	Cattle	12 mg/kg B.W.
	vii) Albendazole			
3.	Imidazothiazoles / LivamesoleTetrahydro pyrimidines			
	Closantel		Horses	19 mg/kg BW
	Clorozulon		Cattle	2 mg/Kg BW
	Ozyclozanide	Paramphestomum species	Cattle	18.7 mg/kg BW
	Flexaclorophene		Cattle	20 mg/kg BW
	Praziquantel	Tapeworms of various species	Cattle	1.75 mg/kg BW 1.76 to 7.5

Suggetsed Reading

Gill, H.S.and Lejambrea, I.F. (1996). Special issue novel approach to the control of helminth parasites of livestock In. J. Parasital 26 (819).

Waller, P.J. (1996). Sustainable helminth control of ruminants of developing countries Vet. Parasitol 71: 195-207.

William, J.C. *et al.* (1997). Special issue: Fourth ostertigia workshop nematode parasites of importance to reminants livestock. Vet. Parasitol 72: 3-4.

Petrov, Yu. F. & Koslov, Y.N. (1988). Veterinaria Moscow 3: 41.

Grahan, J.M. & Charleston, W.A. (1971). Vet Med. Rev. 4: 452.

Aronour, J. (1980). The epidemiology of helminth disease in farm animals. Vet. Parasitol, 6: 7-46.

Roepsdorff, A. & Nansen, P. The epidemiology diagnosis and control of helminth parasitis of swine Poone F.A.O. Hand book FAO.

Arundel, J.H. (1985). Parasitic disease of the horse, veterinary review, 28 post graduate foundation in Vety. Science, University of Sidney Australia ogoburne C.P. and Dunca J.I. (1984). Strongylus vulgaris in horse : its biology and vet important Farnhand Royal Bucks U.K. common wealth Agril. Bureca Practice 1988 20 (34) special issues.Parasitology series I & II.

Jorgensen, R.J. & Ogbourne, C.P. (1985). Bovine dictly ocautiasis a review and annotated bibliography farnham royal UK common weat Agril. Burcaux.

Urquhart, C.M. & Armous, J. (1973). Helminth disease of cattle sheep and horses in Europe. Glasgold Machose. Roepsdorff A & Nansen P. The epidemiology diagnosis and control of helminth parasites of swize FAO hand book Rome FAO.

Welsh, R.D. (1984). Equine pract 6:6 H. affman A.M. *et al.* A.M. J. Vet. Res. 54: 1615.

Batey, R.C. (1986). Pathogenesis of caseous lymphadenitis sheep and goats Aust. Vet. J. 63: 269.

Khater, A.R. *et al.* (1983). Ass. Int. Vet. Med J. 10: 88.

Dend, C.H.R. 1971. Ulcerative velvets and partitas in Australian sheep and cattle vet bull. 41: 719.

□□□

Chapter 46

Parasitic Infestations Caused by Arthropods in Domesticated Animals

Amongst the "evolution history" of animal Kingdom, Arthropod Parasites stand at higher position as compared to multicellular invertebrate helminth parasites in terms of possession of more highly developed alimentary, respiratory, vascular, reproductive, nervous and locomotary systems and therefore, they have to depend less on their hosts for their "needs" of life. Probably because of this situation, they do not need to penetrate very much deep in their hosts as compared to helminthes, the larval stages of whome require to reach even upto blood vascular, lymphatic systems and paremchyma of visceral organs, etc. for meeting their life requirements. Parasitic arthoropod adults generally live on the skin tissue either superficially or at the most in intradermal tunnels for feeding and oviposition and their larval stages have to use nasal or other sinuses or at the most lumens of alimentary canal including stomach or duodenum, etc.

The pathogenic effects of adult arthropod parasites are mainly due to the "annoyance" or "worrying" they create amongst the animal hosts while "ovipositioning" on animal body or on their external orifices or while feeding through biting/ sucking of blood which brings about "wasting" or loosening of body condition and normocytic anaemia due to reduction of their blood. The pathogenic effect of larval stages (larvae and nymphs) of some arthropod parasites bring about inflammatory reactions due to their burrowing intradermally or reaching upto nasal sinuses or even upto subdermal area or lumen of intestinal /gastric canal. All these effects are described in Table 1 to 7.

Class Arthroapoda is divided into subclass insect which includes, various flies, midges and mosquitoes and subclass Acarina which includes ticks and mites, class pediculata which includes lice and flees. Amongst the subclass insecta, larval stages of some flies like "Boat flies" warbal flies and blow flies burrow tissue after ovipositioning by adult flies and produce "Myasis" in animals. A) Disease caused by larval stages of flies while adult flies of some genera of subclass insect suck blood and produce anaemia or produce intradermal blisters and bleeding sores. They also transmit some bacterial, varial and protozoon disease agents while sucking blood miscellaneous flies midges and mosquito and Lice and Flee infestation brings about irritation of skin and damage to the fleece louse infestation.

Subclass Acarina includes ticks which spend most of their lifecycle on the body of animals hosts except during laying of eggs and they feed on blood of these animals and transmit protozoon diseases, part of whose lifecycle is completed in the body of those tickes. It can be noted that these ticks cause paralyses & warry to the animals hosting them and also they are responsible for transmission of some Bacterial, viral and ricketssial disease to the animals during blood suckings.

Subclass Acarina also includes tiny tick like creatures known as mites which burrow skin of host animals and produce allergic dermatitis (mange) reactions diseases caused by mites. The details regarding the arthropod parasites, their names, lifecycles, pathogenesis and disease signs and lesions they produce and their diagnosis as well as treatment and control measures are given in statement form.

Table 1 : Diseases caused by larval stages Arthropod Parasites

Sr. No.	Disease	Etiology	Epidemiology& Life cycle	Pathogenesis	Disease signs & lesions	Diagnostic confirmation	Treatment& Control
1	"Bot fly" infestation in horses	"Bot fly" Gastrophilus species G.nasalis G.intestinalis in Horses	Eggs are laid on hair on body or around lips. Larvae "Instars" hatch by likcing or rubbing and 1st and 2nd generations of larvae burrow through gums of molar teeth, pharynx and finally go to mucosa of stomach and Dudenum as 3rd stage larvae where they get attached to local mucosa and remain there for some months before passed out through faeces via rectum. Larvae pupate and emerge as adults on 3-5 weeks as flies.	The havering and darting of Bot flies during "Ovipostion" around lips nose with droning noise frighten the horses. Migration and burrowing of larval "Bots" produce gastritis gingivitis	Unthriftiness poor coat, occasional mild colic, lack of appetite, bad temper due to larvae bots burrowing and frightening of horses by adult flies. Gastritis and abscesses at the gastric lesion and at spleenic surface.	Eggs present on hairs and characteristics gastric lesions at autopsy	2 treatments of Ivermectin or trichlorphon or moxidection in mid and late winter, Fringes and tassels protect against fly worry.
2	Oestrus ovis (Nasal bots) in sheep and goats	Oestrus ovis in sheep & goats adult fly has sedimentary mouth parts and cannot feed	Life cycle similar to Boat files of horses fly deposits larvae at Nostrils. Larvae migrate to frontal sinses and dorsal turbinates. Where they remain for some weeks to several months. Then migrate to nasal cavity are sneezed out to ground where they pupate to produce adult flies.	Adult flies deposit larvae at external nares and annoy the host sheep spiny surface of "nasal bot" larvae irritate nasal mucosa and catarrhal rhinitis is produced.	Mucopurulent nasal discharge and sneezing production loss and occasional mortality record.	Eggs of external nares of sheep and Rhinitis lesions with Bots confirmatory.	Closantal 7.5 mg/kg B.W. and ivermection 0.2 mg/kg B.W. is effective.

Sr. No.	Disease	Etiology	Epidemiology& Life cycle	Pathogenesis	Disease signs & lesions	Diagnostic confirmation	Treatment& Control
3	"Web fly" infestation (Hypoderma) infestation In cattle	Hypoderma bovis & Hypoderma liniatum in cattle occasionally in horses	Eggs are attached to hair on body in spring to late summer. Larvae penetrate skin and migrate to oesophagus in H.liniatum and migrate to spine in H. bovis and stay for 2-3 months and then move to sub dermal tissue along the back and after 2-3 months, emerge out through breathing holes and fall on ground, pupete to emerge as adult 3-5 weeks later to "Oviposit" on hair of other bovine host.	Larvae maturing under the skin of back can produce holes on the back skin larvae produce gelaneous fluid and get sheathed to produce "Grubs" Anaphylasis can occur occasionally severe dermatitis can occur treatment during presence in oesphagus may cause inflammatory oedema and feeding my stop migration of larvae to intracranial place produces myasis and severe to moderate paraplegia	Adult fly attach for oviposition may annoy the animals. Poor growth poor production (loss of milk) 200-300 lesions on back dermis is possible with swellings. Involvement of spinal cord can cause paralytic symptoms. Larvae are found in discoloured skin tissue.	ELISA test is available for diagnosis in Great Britain for eradication programme swelling along back is characteristics.	Organo phosphates destroy migrating larvae and can be applied by spray or given by "Pour on" technique by individual oral dosing or by mixing in feed, Ivermection, moxidection or doranection as per standard dosage.
4	"Blow fly strike" cutaneous myasis	Lucilla cuprina or Blow fly (green) of sheep	Odours emanating from moist humid skin of sheep with or bacterial infection wounds attract Lucilia the blue/green flies which are gravid, to oviposit the eggs/larvae which feed on the exudates of wound and enzymes of larvae allow then to invade the wounds.	The larvae burrow into the wounds on skin with decaying fleece and tissue and spread the original round waves of "strikes" of flies come and invade and aggravate the wounds.	Sheep are restless will not feed they tend to bite and kick the "struck" area of the skin and wriggle their tails fleece rot prevails to give discoloration to fleece	Clinical signs are diagnostic	Organophosphates ivermection or cyromazine or triflubenzuron protect for 10-12 weeks

Table 2 : Diseases caused by mites

Sr. No.	Disease	Etiology	Epidemiology& Lifecycle	Pathogenesis	Disease signs & lesions	Diagnostic confirmation	Treatment& Control
1	Sarcoptic mange or scabies in all domesticated animal species	i) Sarcoptes scabiei var bovis in cattle. ii) Sarcoptes scebiei var suis in pig iii) Sarcoptes scabieivar equine in horses. iv) Sarcoptes scebiei var ovis in sheep & goats	The female mites from shallow burrny in horney layer of skin in which they lay eggs. The larval and hymphel stages live in burrow/tunnels or emerge on to skin from where any of stage of life cycle can give infestation to other animal by skin contact or through fomites lifecycle is 10-14 days duration	Development of hyper sensitivity 8-10 weeks after infestation of mites precipitates irritation, exudation of lymph and scab formation, allergic phase last for 8-9 months Ery thema, papules and intense purities occurs.	Early lesions show small red papules & general erythema of skin, loss of hair, thick brown scab formation over lying a row surface, thickening and wrinkling of skin soon follows, lesions are on face in sheep, on trunks in pigs and on inner surface of the thighs in cattle, courage in acute in sarcoptic manage.	Examination of scrapings either directly or after digestion of the same in 10% potassium hydroxide, under microscope will reveal typical scarcoptic mites and their larvae and nymphs	Ivermectin 0.3 mg / kg B.W. noxidection 0.2 mg/kg B.W. 2 doses 10 days apart work well diagnon 0.01% or prapetamphos 0.0125% or cournaphos 0.1% application.
2	Psoroptic manage or sheep scab body manage, Ear manage in all animals.	i) Psorptes ovis in sheep & goats ii) P. equi in horses iii) P.cervirus in cattle	The females abrase the surface and feed on exudates and blood from small surface haemorrhages and large scab formation under which they live eggs are laid on the skin at the edge of scab produce larvae and nymphs, after hatching and molting cycle is complete in 10-11 days. Rest of life cycle is a that of sarcoptes.	The mites profer areas covered by wool & hair. The adults pucture the epidermis to feed on lymph and cause local inflammation resulting in itchiness, resulting exudation of serum which gorm crust mites are most active at the edge of crusts and lesions spread peripherally.	In sheep, lesions are most on the sides of body. Initially papules ooze serum, wool commences to shed. Animals are emaciated and weak. In goats, external ears show crusty scabs. In horses lesions are at the base of mane and root of tail udder, prepuce and axilla. In cattle's lesions on withers, neck and tails are observed.	Examination of scrapings either directly or after digestion of the same in 10% potassium hydroxide, under microscope will reveal typical scarcoptic mites and their larvae and nymphs	Ivermectin 0.3 mg / kg B.W. noxidection 0.2 mg/kg B.W. 2 doses 10 days apart work well diagnon 0.01% or prapetamphos 0.0125% or cournaphos 0.1% application.

Sr. No.	Disease	Etiology	Epidemiology& Lifecycle	Pathogenesis	Disease signs & lesions	Diagnostic confirmation	Treatment& Control
3	Chorioptic manage (Scrotal manage) in cattle and horse in sheep Tale manage) (Leg manage)	Chorioptes bovis is one species producing manage in cattle, horse sheep and goats	Life cycle is similar to that of psoroptes and is completed in 3 weeks, In horse parasites occur in long haired parts (Tale and legs). In cattle, mostly perineum and back of udder and back of legs are affected. In sheep lesions confined to wooless area (scrotum and hind part of legs) Rams infect ewes while copulating.	Mites cause allergic excudative dermatitis, small scabby lesions are seen on the hair, severe irritation and itchiness in horses. In cattle, rapidly spreading syndrome with cornitis and marked fall in milk production, Allergic dermatitis on scrotum in sheep.	Violent stamping of feet and rubbing of back in horses with serous excudate from swollen scably cracked and gressy lesion affecting hair on legs unsightly lesions on udder thighs and escutcheon in cattle. In sheep scrotal lesions show yellowish serous exudates.	Microscopic exam of scrapings from affected area confirmatory diagnosis.	Moxidection 0.5 mg/kg B.W. applied as a pour on or 0.2 mg/kg B.W. By single injection 2 doses of flumethrin applied to the whole body (0.2 mg/kg B.W.) eliminates the infection.
4	Demodectic manage (Follicular manage)in all species of domestic animals	i) Demodex bovis in cattle. ii) D. ovis in sheep iii) D. caprein goat iv) D. equi in horse v) D. Phyloides in pigs vi) Demodex species in dog	Adult mites invade hair follicles and subaceous glands which become distended with mites and inflammatory materials eggs larval and two nymphal stages pass on the same animal transfer of mites through contact of skin directly. In horses grooming instruments and rugs transmit the infection.	Invasion of hair follicles ad sebaceous glands leads to chronic inflammation and loss of hair. Secondary staphcoccal pustules or small abscesses occur.	Initial appearance of small nodules and pustules which develop into larger abscesses. General hair loss in severe cases. Pustular contents are white cheesy. In cattle and goats lesions are on brisket, lower neck fore arm and shoulders in horses, face and around eyes. In pigs on face ad ventral surface neck.	The characteristically elongated mites in large numbers in the waxy exudates can be demonstrated under microscope.	Repeated dipping or spraying of acaricides recommended for preventing spread.

Table 3 : Diseases caused by tick infestations

Sr. No.	Disease	Etiology	Epidemiology& Lifecycle	Pathogenesis	Disease signs & lesions	Diagnostic confirmation	Treatment& Control
1		**One host ticks** Boophilus species margaropus species octobious megnini (adults not parasitic) dermacentre altripictus **Two Host Ticks** Rhipicephalus evertsi R.bursa Hyaloma species **Three Host ticks** Ixodes species Rhipicephalus species (other than R. evertric and R.bursa) Haemophysalis species Ambyloma species Hyaloma species ornithodorus species Dermacentor species	Life cycle vaies widely some species pass their entire life on one host and others may need two or three hosts as shown in column on etiology. The eggs are laid on soil and larvae attach themselves to passing hosts, on which they may develop through one or more nymphal stages before becoming adults. Adult female engorge on blood or lymph and drop to the ground to lay their eggs.	i) **Ticks causing Paralysis :** 31 species in seven genera of ixodis ticks (Hard tick) and 7 species in 3 genera of Argasid ticks (6 off ticks) are able to cause "Tick paralysis " in host animals while sucking blood. Salivary glands contain toxin which produces paralytic symptoms (see table No.1) ii) **Ticks which transmit protozoon diseases :** They are listed in table.2 attached herewith iii)**Ticks which transmit Bacterial, viral and rick attsial diseases :** They are listed in table 3 attached herewith. iv)**Ticks which cause worry :** Ticks cause damage to hides and loss of production, anaemia and death when present in large numbers.See table 4.	i) Tick paralysis Ascending flaccid paralysis with in co-ordination of hind limbs followed by paralysis of fore limbs and chest mucles. Pupils widely dialated and death may follow if ticks are not removed. ii) See account of protozoal disease to know details about tick transmission iii)See account of Bact. Viral and rickatcial diseases for details of tick transmission. iv)As ticks are blood suckers, normocytic anaemia is resulted.	Identification of adult ticks by microscopc examination of the morphological characters of ticks.	Choice of Acaricide depends on 3 factors i) Persistance of the compound on the skin and haircoat of host ii) Likelihood of residual toxic effect on man through milk or meat of host. iii) Development of resistance to particular acaricide iv) Cost of treatment of compound used as Acaricide a) Amitraz b) Combined DDT and Pyrithroid treatment c) Organo phosphates d) Ivermectin e) Moxodection f) Closantel g) Chloropyrifos

Table 4 : Summary of tick borne, protozoan and bacterial diseases transmitted through ticks

Tick	Animals affected	Protozoon	Vector tick	*Staph aureus*	*Ixodes ricing*	
Dermacentre anderrsoni D. occidentalis	Sheep, calves and goats	*Babesia bigemina* (in cattle)	*Boophilus annulatus B.microplus, B. Calcaralus, Rhipicephalus appendiculates, Haemaphysalis punctate*	*Anaplasma marginals*	*Boophilus annulatus Dermacentre alsipicus Rhy. Sanguineus Boophitus microplus*	*Octabius magini Ambyloma americanum. Ambyloam maculatum. Margarpus winthemi. Ornithodorus mobata Ornithadorus savignigic. Haemophysalis Longicormis.*
Ixodes holocyclus	Cattle lambs foals, goats	*Baberia bovis* (in calves)	*Ioxdis pursulcatus I. ricims B.annulatus B.microplus*	*Anaplasma Ovis*	*Dermacentre silvarum Ornithodorus lahorensis Rhy bursa*	
I. pilosis I. rubicundus	Sheep, goats and calves	*Babesia mortasi* (Sheep & goats)	*Dermacentre Silvarum Ixodes ricinus*	Brucellosis *B.abortus B.melitensis*	Many ticks	
Rhipicephalus ebertsi	Lambs cattle	*Babesia ovis* (Sheep)	*Rhibursa. Haemophisalis bispinosa.*	*Caudria Ruminentium* Rikettsia (Heart water)	Ambyloma spp.	
Haemophysalis punctata	Calves sheep goats	*Babesir caboli* (Horse)	*Hyaloma dromenderi H. excavates Dermacentre reticulation*	African swine fever Virus	Ornithodoras spp.	
Ornithodorus lahorensis	Sheep	*Theileria Anaulata*	*Hyaloma anaticolicum*	Nairobi sheep disease virus	Rhy. Appendiculatus	
Hyaloma Eegypticum	Sheep	*Theileria ovis*	*Rly. barsi*			
Ixodes ricinus	Sheep & goats					
Amblyoma cajanense	Calves sheep & goats					

Table 5 : Louse Infestation of livestock

Sr. No.	Disease	Etiology	Epidemiology & Lifecycle	Pathogenesis	Disease signs & lesions	Diagnostic confirmation	Treatment& Control
1		Species specific biting and sucking lice affecting all animals. **Cattle :** Linognathus vitali. (long nosed sucking loys) Haematopinus Eurysternus (Short nose sucking lice) H.quadrepertusus (tail loce) H.tuberculatus (Buffalo like) Damalinia bovis (Biting lice) **Sheep :** Linognathus avilus (sucking foot lice) Damallia ovis (biting lice) **Goat :** L. stenopsis (sucking lice) D. capre (biting lice) **Pig :** H.suis (sucking lice) Horse H. asini (sucking lice) D.equi (biting lice)	Life cycle of all lice is similar and is confined to the host. The eggs are laid, attached to body coat fibres. There are 3 nymphal stages before mature lice appear. Lifecycle varies 2 -4 weeks under optimum conditions. Hot temperatures prevent egg laying transmission occurs through direct contact.	All species cause irritation of the skin and stimulate scratching, rubbing and licking leading to rest less ness, damage to flece and hides and loss of milk production weighloss is questionable pig louce spreads swine pox pigs develop allergic dermatitis.	Hairballs may be present in infected calves due to continuous licking of hair during lice infestation. The wool looses, its brightness & become cotted andmore yellow, Heavy feetlouce infestation cause moderate to heavy stamping and biting affected parts.	Eggs and lice on hair and flece can be identified physically	Plunge or shower dipping of animals with organophosphate insecticides (diazinon, coumphos carbophenothions and synthetic pyrethroids like cypermethrine.

Table 6 : Miscellaneous flies, midges and mosquitoes

Sr. No.	Disease	Etiology	Epidemiology & Lifecycle	Pathogenesis	Disease signs & lesions	Diagnostic confirmation	Treatment& Control
1		Stable flies I. Stomoxis calcitrans II. S. nigra	It is blood sucker attacking particularly horses, cattle and less extent pigs bite is painful. The eggs are layed in rotting hey and straw when contaminated with urine andhorse manure, larvae and pupae form in rotting matter warmth and moisture favour breeding of flies.	Localised sensitivity of forelints and intradermal blister formation (bleeding sores may develop) in cattle. S.calcitrans transmits Anthrax. Infectious equine anaemia and bovine virus diarrhoea and surra, It transmits habronema major, causes allergic dermatitis is horse.	Localised sensitivity of forelints and intradermal blister formation (bleeding sores may develop) in cattle. S.calcitrans transmits Anthrax. Infectious equine anaemia and bovine virus diarrhoea and surra, It transmits habronema major, causes allergic dermatitis is horse.	Physical exam of the fly	Crotoxiphos and methoxychlor spraing.
2.		Horse flies or breeze flies (Tabanus spp.)	They are robust brown flies and worry large animals like horses and cattle. Eggs laid on leave of plants growing in or near water. Flies active in summer larval and papal stages are passed in water or mud 4-5 months lifecycle. They suck blood of animals.	They act as mechanical vectors for trypanosoma evansi,Tvivax bovine uncosis virus and anthrox. They cause anaemia as they are blood suckers.	Localised sensitivity of forelints and intradermal blister formation (bleeding sores may develop) in cattle S.calcitrans transmits Anthrax. Infectious equine anaemia and bovine virus diarrhoea and surra, It transmits habronema major causes allergic dermatitis is horse.	Physical exam of the fly	Permethrine, synthetic pyrethron used for control and treatment.

Table 7 : Biting midges, sand flies and mosquitoes

Sr. No.	Disease	Etiology	Epidemiology& Lifecycle	Pathogenesis	Disease signs & lesions	Diagnostic confirmation	Treatment& Control
1		Mosquitos belonging to genera I. *Psorophora* II. *Ades* III. *Mansonia* IV. *Culex* V. *Anophelis* feeding on various animal species	Adults suck blood of animals by biting with proboscis, they may lay eggs in shallow waters ponds, larvae and paupae mature outside animal body and adults feed on animals.	They cause annonyance and worry to animals. Kill young piglets and puppies due to blood sucking anaemia, break in productivity of animals. They act as vectorsof the disease like Japnese B. encephalitis, warbalfly disease, Ristalley fever and fileral larval disease	They cause annonyance and worry to animals. Kill young piglets and puppies due to blood sucking anaemia, break in productivity of animals. They act as vectorsof the disease like Japnese B. encophaltis, warbalfly disease, Ristalley fever and fileral larval disease	Physical exam on morphology of mosquitoes for identification	Avoid collection of water, ponds, distruction of larvae using DDT / BHC etc.
2		Biting midges i) *Culicoides* speices	Adults suck blood of animals	Cause annoyance any worrying to animals carriers of disease like blue tongue (virus) of sheep, goats and cattle, African Horse sickness virus epithmeral fever of cattle.	They cause annonyance and worry to animals. Kill young piglets and puppies due to blood sucking, anaemia, break in productivity of animals. They act as vectorsof the disease like Japnesa B. encephalitis, warbalfly disease, Rist valley fever and fileral larval disease	Physical exam on morphology of mosquitis for identification	Avoid collection of water, ponds, distruction of larvae using DDT / BHC etc.use repellent of culicoids
3		Buffalo i) Flies (Horn flies) of cattle and buffaloes horses. ii) Horse house flies	Haematobia species H. irritance H. minuta Draschia megastoma Hippobosca equina	They worry animals and interfere with their grazing, congregate on withers, shoulders,	Irritation and blood loss due to blood sucking, loss of condition and death exacerbate the ventral midline	They worry animals and interfere with their grazing congregate on withers,	Diazinon and other organo phosphates

		of horses	and H. Maculate H. ruppiens.	flanks and around eyes. Lifecycle passed on body of animal only except while oviposition they leave animal and deposit eggs in faeces of animals.	dermatitis lesions.	shoulders flanks and around eyes. Lifecycle passed on body of animal only except for while oviposition they leave animal and deposit eggs in faeces of animals.	
4	--	House fly *musca domestica*	Transmites anthrax, erycepelas and Brucellosis by mechanical means. It is intermediate host for habronema muscae eggs laid in decalying organic matter summer rise fly population	Do not produce any disease by itself.	--	Physical diagnosis	Hyginic measures and many insecticides are used. Details not given here for want to space.
5	--	Face fly *musca automanalis*	Musca automnalis in rumminents	Feeds on eye discharge, saliva of animal to nasal discharge life cycle on faces of animals.	Worrying the animals	Physical diagnosis	Repallents are used

❒❒❒

Chapter 47

Ringworm Infections in domesticated Animals (Dermatomycoses)

Ringworm is a fungal infections cused by invasion of cutaneous keratinized epithelial cells and hair fibres by dermatophytes including fungi of *Trichophyton* and *Micro-sporum* genera and is characterized by roughly circular skin lesions in domesticated animals including cattle, sheep, goats and horses.

About the causative fungi

The ringworm causing fungi are listed as below:

1. *Tricophyton equinum, Tricophyton quickeanum, Tricophyton mentagrophytes, Tricophyton Verrucosum, micro-sporum equinum* and *M. gypseum* occur in horses and donkeys.
2. *Tricophyton Verrucosum, Tricophyton mentagrophytes, Tricophyton megnini, Tricophyton Verrucosum var album* and *Var. discoides* in cattle.
3. *Tricophyton Verrucosum var ochraceum, Tricophyton quinckeanum, Tricophyton mentagrophytes, Tricophyton gypsum and M. canis* in sheep,
4. *Tricophyton verrucosum* in goats.
5. *Tricophyton mentagrophytes, Tricophyton rubrum Tricophyton verrucosum var discoides, M. canis and M. natun* in pigs.

Dermatophytic fungi show typical mycelial hypae with spores in chains in the skin lesions. Culturing of the scabs or scrapings on sabaurodls agar with acidic pH and antibiotics (Penicillin + streptomycin) produce typical cotton like growth with mycelial hyphae containing spores in chains. Hyphae are either separate or non-separate depending upon generas Tricophyton or microsporum which are differentiated on seplate/non-separate nature of mycelial growth.

Epidemiology and transmition of the infection

Ringworm (Tricophyton/micro sporum) spores are generally present on skin of about 10 to 20% normal "Carrier" animals in infected herds. Presence of humidity and crowding of animals in contaminated animal premises is condusive for the spread of infection. The infection can spread directly by animal to animal body contact between carrier and unifected animal. Spread of infection through formites, like bedding, harness, grooming kits and horse blankets also occurs.

Pathogenesis

The dermatophytic fungi mainly attack keratinizd tissues (stratum corneum and hair fibres) resulting in autolysis of the fibre structure, breaking of the hair and producing alopecia. The dry crusts are produced by exudation from invaded epithelium, its debris and fungal hyphae. The mycotic hyphae are aerobic and die out in the centre of the crust while peripheral mycelia remain active. It is this situation which is responsible for centrifugal progression of the lesion. The mycetial growth in skin tissue requires moisture and slightly alkaline pH and hence, the acidic pH of older animals (due to secretion of fatty acids in sebum) is not favourable for growth of the lesions while younger animal skin with slightly more alkaline pH is conducive for ringworm growth. Calves are more affected than the adult cattle. The severity of the infection is also dependent on the nutritional level of the animals and weaker calves show more severe infection. The spontaneous recovery can occur in wellfed calvs after short course of the disease.

Symptoms and lesions

In cattle, typical lesion is a heavy, grey-white crust raised perceptibly above the skin and is roughly circular, about 3 cm. in diameter. Earlier, the crust is moist and in older lesion, scab is detached and pityriasis and alopecia occurs. Lesions are common on neck, head and perineum in the initial stage but become generalized on entire body later on. Lesions caused by trycophyton infection are larger than those caused by microscoprum species in horses.

Diagnosis

Skin scrapings should be collected after dissolving fatty materials (defalting) by swabbing the lesion with ether or alcohol and the scrapings should be collected in 20% potassium/sodium hydroxide solution before microscopic examination of the "cover slip" preparation. Presence of highly refractile rounded or polyhedral spores in chains in fungal hyphae are diagnostic of Tricophyton species while spores in "mosaic" arrangement are diagnostic of "microsporum" species. The fungal hyphae in tissues can be identified, even down to the genus level by the use of immune fluoroscent staining for diagnosis of the specimen from necropsy or biopsy materials.

Treatment

Local or systemic treatment is carried out with the view to reduce the infection land responsible for the spread of infection rather than for "Curative" purposes as mostly there is spontaneous recovery from the infection after taking care of the infected animals by improvement in nutrition levels which is of common occurence.

Use of iodised ointment or 10% amoniated mercury ointment or ointment containing quarternary ammonium compounds, propionic or undecylenic acid and 0.25% hexadecamethylene-1, 16-bis-soquinolium chloride or antibiotics (like natamycin and nanomycin A), Povidone iodine, thia benolazole are useful topical treatments. Azole compounds like imidazole or miconazole are also effective. Rubbing of ointments with brushes is more effective. Intravenous injections of sodium iodine (1 gm/14 kg body wt.), as 10% solution repeated on several times are useful, oral administration of griseofulvin is costly but effective.

Vaccination

In Europe and Scandinavia, highly immunogenic non-virulent strains or attenuated strains of fungi or killed vaccine containing specific fraction of mycelia used effectively for prevention (Gorden P.J. et al. 1996, Vet Rec. 139:395).

Ringworm Infections: Indian Scenario

Trichophyton and microsporum infections are quite ubiquatous in India and treatments are used as above but vaccines are not available.

Suggested Reading

Gudding, R. and Lund, A. (1995).Immuno prophylasis of bovine dermatophytosis Can. Vet. J. 36: 302-306.

Pier, A.C. *et al.* (1994). Animal ringworm to etiology, public health significance & control. J. Med. Vet. Mycol 32 (Supply-1) pp. 133-150.

□□□

Chapter 48

Epizootic Lymphangitis (Equine Histoplasmosis)

Epizootic Lymphangitis (Histoplasmosis) is an infections fungal disease of equines which is caused by *Histoplasma farciminosum* and is characterized by lymphadenopaty of hind limbs in horses and donkeys.

About the fungal causative agent

The causative agent is a fungus *Histoplasma (Cryptococcus) farciminosus* which is gram positive, yeast like cell with characteristics double walled capsule and these cells are found easily in discharges. It can be cultured on special media but is a fragile organism which dies quickly in discharge, if not preserved with antibiotic, refrigerated or cultured quickly.

Epidemiology and disease transmission

The disease occurs in horses in Asia, Africa and Mediterranean areas. Outbreaks occur in autumn and winter, when horses are gathered together. Fungal spores are carried from infected animals by direct contact or on grooming instruments, horse blankets or harness and gain entry of equine body through abrasions on lower limbs. The fungus is presumed to be present in soil as saprophyte. It is also isolated from biting flies (*Stomoxys*) which also play a role in disease transmission.

Pathogenesis

After entry through skin wound, organism sets in a sub cutaneous granulome and or ulcer and spreads along the lymphatic vessels in the lower limbs.

Symptoms of disease and lesions

In cutaneous form, indulent ulcer develops at portal of entry and lymphangitis, evident as corded lymphatics with intermittent nodules develop which rupture, discharging thick creamypus. Lymphatics also enlarge and rupture, limb oedema and thickening occurs with painless lesions. Lesions are mainly near the hock but also on back, sides or neck, vulva and scrotum. Occasional nasal and occular involvement may occur, with conjunctivae sinusitis and primary pneumonia in other form of the disease. The disease can become chronic and animals may be required to be destroyed. Granulomatous lesions may be found in the lungs, liver and spleen.

Diagnosis

The demonstration of yeast like double walled capsule containing cells in discharges is diagnosic. Sterile filtrate of a culture of *H. farciminosus* can be used for "Allergic skin test" and "Mallein test' will be able to differentiate from glanders lymphangitis and confirm epizootic lymphangitis (Selim *et al.*, 1985). FAT and other serological tasts are also available (Abou Gagal,. *et al.*, 1983).

Treatment control

Parenteral iodides are found to be effective in some cases, slaughter policy was used in some countries for control. Formalin inactivated alhydrogel absorbed bacterins are widely used for prevention of disease.

Epizootic Lymphangitis in Equines: Indian Scenario

The disease occunsin military and race horses and requires development of suitable Allergic test antigen for confirmation.

Suggested Reading

Abou-Gabal, M., Hassan, F.K., Al-Siad, A.A. & Al-Karim, K.A. (1983). Study on equine histoplasmosis epizootic lymphangitis. Mykosen, 26: 145-151.

Selim, S.A., R. Soliman, K. Osman, A.A. Padhye and L. Ajello. (1985). Studies on histoplasmosis farciminosii (Epizootic lymphangitis) in Egypt. Isolation of Histoplasma farciminosum from cases of histoplasmosis farciminosii in horses and its morphological Characteristics. Eur. J. Epidemiol, 1: 84-89.

□□□

Chapter 49

Miscllaneous Fungal Infections of Domesticated Animals including Systemic Aspergillosis, Candidasis and Zygomycosis and Other Fungi

Aspergillosis, candidiasis and zygomycosis which are mainly systemic infections are widespread amongst domesticated animals but they are rarely occurring in outbreak form but mainly occur as sporadic cases. These fungal occur as sporadic cases. These fungal infections are distinctively not contagious with exception of maternal infections which cause the disease in their calves (Sarfati *et al.*, 1996).

Each infection arises from the fungal habitate as a saprophyte in organic matter commonly moudly hey or straw or moist feed like beet pulp or brewers grains which are allowed to go mouldly. Incidence of mycotic abortions is much greater in the winter months in housed cows than other groups.

The increasing incidence of mycolic placentitis leading to abortions may be related to the general use of antibiotic treated semen in A.I. programmes. In humans, increasing incidence of systemic mycoses is occurring due to frequency of human immune deficiencies infections (HIV).

Epidemiology and pathogenesis

These infections occur through inhalation of spores of mycotic agents present in dust/droplets of mouldy environments with primary focus developing in lungs and then spread through lymphatic and blood circulatory system to produce generalized microscopic nodular lesions in various other organisms including spleen, liver, kidneys and lymph-nodes. This occurs in case of aspergillosis, candidasis and zygomycotic infections.

Pneumoniac lesions of mycotic nodular type, mycotic pharyngitis, mycotic gastroenteritis can occur in this way. Fungal placentits resulting in abortions in cows usually occur at 6-8 months of their pregnancy. The fungal lesions are generally granulomatus with presence of fungal mycelia surrounded by mononuclear tissue invasion and fibrosis with presence of giant cells also. The lesions have similarity to the lesion of tuberculosis.

Aspergillus fumigatous is fungus resembling penicillium fungus while the candida abbicans is a fungus resembling yeast, both of these are involved in fungal abortion cases in animals. *Cryptococcus neophormance* is also yeast like fungus which is involved in a generalized disease or granulomatous meningo-encephalatis in various species of animals. It is also listed as a cause of bovine mastitis.

Sporotricosis is a disease of horses, cats, cattle and humans and characterized by formation of cutaneous nodules and ulcers. The spores of this fungus are gram positive and form single-walled spores.The disease is reported in Europe, India and U.S. Multiple small, cutaneous nodules develop on lower part of legs near fetlock (lymphangitis develops).

Equine phycomycosis also known as "Bursattee" occurs in tropical and semitropical climates in horses and young cattle,dogs and humans (Miller *et al.* 1985). This disease occurs in wet season of the year. The disease in characterized by ulcerative granulomas on legs and ventral abdomen. Maduromycosis is a skin disease of horses characterized by cutaneous granuloma caused by various agents including *Heliminthosporium spiciferum* and characterized by lesions on skin more frequently in coronet region in horses.

Suggested Reading

J. Sarfati, H.E. Jensen, J.P. Latgi (1996). Route of infections in bovine aspergillosis. Journal of Medical & Veterinary Mycology. 34: 379-383.

Miller, R.I. (1985). Gastrointestinal phycomycosis in 63 dogs. J. Am Vet Med Assoc 186: 473–478.

□□□